Essentials of Tests of Dyslexia™

Essentials of Psychological Assessment Series

Series Editors, Alan S. Kaufman and Nadeen L. Kaufman

Essentials of CAS2 Assessment
by Jack A. Naglieri and Tulio M. Otero

Essentials of Child and Adolescent Psychopathology, Second Edition
by Linda Wilmshurst

Essentials of Cognitive Assessment with KAIT and Other Kaufman Measures
by Elizabeth O. Lichtenberger, Debra Y. Broadbooks, and Alan S. Kaufman

Essentials of Conners Behavior Assessments™
by Elizabeth P. Sparrow

Essentials of Creativity Assessment
by James C. Kaufman, Jonathan A. Plucker, and John Baer

Essentials of Cross-Battery Assessment, Third Edition
by Dawn P. Flanagan, Samuel O. Ortiz, and Vincent C. Alfonso

Essentials of DAS-II® Assessment
by Ron Dumont, John O. Willis, and Colin D. Elliott

Essentials of Dyslexia Assessment and Intervention, Second Edition
by Nancy Mather and Barbara J. Wendling

Essentials of Evidence-Based Academic Interventions
by Barbara J. Wendling and Nancy Mather

Essentials of Executive Functions Assessment
by George McCloskey and Lisa A. Perkins

Essentials of Forensic Psychological Assessment, Second Edition
by Marc J. Ackerman

Essentials of Gifted Assessment
by Steven I. Pfeiffer

Essentials of IDEA for Assessment Professionals
by Guy McBride, Ron Dumont, and John O. Willis

Essentials of Individual Achievement Assessment
by Douglas K. Smith

Essentials of Intellectual Disability Assessment and Identification
by Alan W. Brue and Linda Wilmshurst

Essentials of KABC-II Assessment
by Alan S. Kaufman, Elizabeth O. Lichtenberger, Elaine Fletcher-Janzen, and Nadeen L. Kaufman

Essentials of KTEA™-3 and WIAT®-III Assessment
by Kristina C. Breaux and Elizabeth O. Lichtenberger

Essentials of MCMI®-IV Assessment
by Seth D. Grossman and Blaise Amendolace

Essentials of Millon™ Inventories Assessment, Third Edition
by Stephen Strack

Essentials of MMPI-A™ Assessment
by Robert P. Archer and Radhika Krishnamurthy

Essentials of MMPI-2® Assessment, Second Edition
by David S. Nichols

Essentials of Myers-Briggs Type Indicator® Assessment, Second Edition
by Naomi L. Quenk

Essentials of NEPSY®-II Assessment
by Sally L. Kemp and Marit Korkman

Essentials of Neuropsychological Assessment, Second Edition
by Nancy Hebben and William Milberg

Essentials of Nonverbal Assessment
by Steve McCallum, Bruce Bracken, and John Wasserman

Essentials of PAI® Assessment
by Leslie C. Morey

Essentials of Planning, Selecting, and Tailoring Interventions for Unique Learners
by Jennifer T. Mascolo, Vincent C. Alfonso, and Dawn P. Flanagan

Essentials of Processing Assessment, Second Edition
by Milton J. Dehn

Essentials of Psychological Assessment Supervision
by A. Jordan Wright

Essentials of Psychological Testing, Second Edition
by Susana Urbina

Essentials of Response to Intervention
by Amanda M. VanDerHeyden and Matthew K. Burns

Essentials of Rorschach® Assessment
by Tara Rose, Michael P. Maloney, and Nancy Kaser-Boyd

Essentials of Rorschach Assessment: Comprehensive System and R-PAS
by Jessica R. Gurley

Essentials of School Neuropsychological Assessment, Third Edition
by Daniel C. Miller and Denise E. Maricle

Essentials of Specific Learning Disability Identification, Second Edition
by Vincent C. Alfonso and Dawn P. Flanagan

Essentials of Stanford-Binet Intelligence Scales (SB5) Assessment
by Gale H. Roid and R. Andrew Barram

Essentials of TAT and Other Storytelling Assessments, Second Edition
by Hedwig Teglasi

Essentials of Temperament Assessment
by Diana Joyce

Essentials of Trauma-Informed Assessment and Interventions in School and Community Settings
by Kirby L. Wycoff and Bettina Franzese

Essentials of Treatment Planning, Second Edition
by Mark E. Maruish

Essentials of WAIS®-IV Assessment, Second Edition
by Elizabeth O. Lichtenberger and Alan S. Kaufman

Essentials of WISC®-IV Assessment, Second Edition
by Dawn P. Flanagan and Alan S. Kaufman

Essentials of WISC-V® Assessment
by Dawn P. Flanagan and Vincent C. Alfonso

Essentials of WISC-V Integrated Assessment
by Susan Engi Raiford

Essentials of WJ IV® Cognitive Abilities Assessment
by Fredrick A. Schrank, Scott L. Decker, and John M. Garruto

Essentials of WJ IV® Tests of Achievement
by Nancy Mather and Barbara J. Wendling

Essentials of WMS®-IV Assessment
by Lisa Whipple Drozdick, James A. Holdnack, and Robin C. Hilsabeck

Essentials of WNV™ Assessment
by Kimberly A. Brunnert, Jack A. Naglieri, and Steven T. Hardy-Braz

Essentials of Working Memory Assessment and Intervention
by Milton J. Dehn

Essentials of WPPSI™-IV Assessment
by Susan Engi Raiford and Diane L. Coalson

Essentials of WRAML2 and TOMAL-2 Assessment
by Wayne Adams and Cecil R. Reynolds

Essentials of WRAML3 and EMS Assessment
by Wayne V. Adams, David V. Sheslow, and Trevor A. Hall

Essentials of Evaluating Bias in Intelligence Testing
by Craig L. Frisby

Essentials of WJ V Assessment
by Erica M. LaForte, Nancy Mather, and W. Joel Schneider

Essentials of Tests of Dyslexia™
by Nancy Mather, R. Steve McCallum, Sherry M. Bell, and Barbara J. Wendling

Essentials

of Tests of Dyslexia™

Nancy Mather

R. Steve McCallum

Sherry M. Bell

Barbara J. Wendling

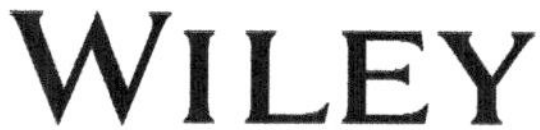

Library of Congress Cataloging-in-Publication Data
Names: Mather, Nancy author | McCallum, R. Steve author | Bell, Sherry M. author | Wendling, Barbara J. author
Title: Essentials of Tests of Dyslexia™ / Nancy Mather, R. Steve
    McCallum, Sherry M. Bell, Barbara J. Wendling
Description: Hoboken, New Jersey : Wiley, [2026] | Series: Essentials of
    psychological assessment | Includes index.
Identifiers: LCCN 2025043209 (print) | LCCN 2025043210 (ebook) | ISBN
    9781394382699 paperback | ISBN 9781394382712 adobe pdf | ISBN
    9781394382705 epub
Subjects: LCSH: Dyslexia | Dyslexia--Diagnosis
Classification: LCC RC394.W6 M385 2026 (print) | LCC RC394.W6 (ebook)
LC record available at https://lccn.loc.gov/2025043209
LC ebook record available at https://lccn.loc.gov/2025043210

Cover Design: Wiley
Cover Image: © Robert/stock.adobe.com

Set in 10/12pt Adobe Garamond Pro by Straive, Pondicherry, India

CONTENTS

In the *Essentials of Psychological Assessment Series*, we have provided the reader with books that deliver key *practical* information in the most efficient and accessible manner. Typically, books fall into one of the two categories. The first category features specific topics in a variety of domains, such as specific learning disabilities, social–emotional learning, neuropsychological assessment, cross-battery assessment, and adaptive behavior assessment. These books are intended for professionals in psychology and education—and for graduate students in these or related disciplines—who are committed to providing assessment and intervention services.

A second category of books in this series, such as *Essentials of Woodcock-Johnson V Assessment*, is devoted to a single test. These books offer a concise yet thorough review of an instrument, with special attention to the details of administration, scoring, interpretation, application, and tips for best practice use of the test. Students can rely on series books in both categories for a clear and concise overview of the important assessment tools and key topics informing skillful practice delivered efficiently, and ethically in their chosen fields. Experienced clinicians will feel equally at home with this series in their efforts to remain on the cutting edge of new research and new instruments as well as new editions of assessments in an array of diverse fields.

Wherever feasible, visual cues highlighting key points are used alongside systematic, step-by-step guidelines. Chapters are focused and succinct. Topics are organized for an easy understanding of the essential material related to a particular test or topic. Theory and research are continually woven into the fabric of each book, always to enhance the practical application of the material. With this series, we aim to challenge and assist readers interested in the psychological and educational assessment to aspire to the highest level of competency by arming them with the resources they need for knowledgeable, informed practice. We have long been advocates of "intelligent" testing—the notion that numbers are meaningless unless they are brought to life by the clinical acumen and expertise of examiners. Assessment must be used to make a difference in the child's or the adult's life, or why bother testing? All books in the series—whether devoted to specific tests or general topics—are consistent with this credo. We want this series to help our readers, novice, and veteran alike, to benefit from the intelligent assessment approaches of the authors of each book.

In *Essentials of Tests of Dyslexia*™, Mather, McCallum, Bell, and Wendling provide important insights into the administration, scoring, and interpretation of the three direct assessment components and the co-normed rating scales. In addition, they share how the TOD instructional guide facilitates linking assessment results to interventions. This book is designed for assessment professionals, reading specialists, and educators who are interested in understanding reading difficulties and evaluating and serving individuals with dyslexia. Chapters include the rationale for development of the TOD; recommendations for administering the TOD-S, TOD-E, and TOD-C; interpretation of the scores, indexes, and profiles; use of the rating scales; psychometric properties of the test; how test results can inform interventions; and illustrative case studies. An Appendix presents case reports that are designed to provide guided practice in interpreting the TOD scores and score reports. Also included is an Appendix that provides answers to commonly asked questions. This book not only focuses on administration and interpretation of the TOD but also is designed to expand understanding of the underlying linguistic abilities and related reading and spelling skills that are impacted for individuals with dyslexia.

Alan S. Kaufman, PhD, and Nadeen L. Kaufman, EdD,
Series Editors, Neag School of Education,
University of Connecticut

Note: TOD® is a registered trademark of Manson Western, LLC, dba Western Psychological Services (WPS). Used with permission.

ACKNOWLEDGMENTS

We would like to express our sincere appreciation to the numerous school and clinical psychologists, diagnosticians, reading specialists, teachers, tutors, and parents who devote their time, energy, and effort ensuring that individuals with dyslexia are accurately identified and receive appropriate assessment, accommodations, and interventions.

We are appreciative of our colleagues who contributed TOD case studies to Chapters 9 and 10: Dr. Lynne Jaffe and Dr. Janice Sammons. We also are appreciative of the individuals in our cases for allowing us to share their stories and history. We are thankful to Emily Mather for her feedback and help in editing the first draft of these chapters.

We are grateful to Mr. Nathanael Mcgavin, our managing editor, and Darren LaLonde, Christina Weyrauch, Matthew Gamerdinger, Vinoth Manoharan and the staff at Wiley for their editorial support. We are also appreciative of Drs. Alan and Nadeen Kaufman for their encouragement to write this book.

We are extremely thankful to personnel from our publishing company (WPS), including Jeff Manson, Dr. Amber Klein, and Stephanie Roberts for working with us to create and publish the TOD™. We are also thankful to Karin M. Tucker for guiding us through the permission process.

Finally, we are extremely thankful to each other for the ideas, support, and friendship.

NM, RSM, SMB, and BJW

One

OVERVIEW OF DYSLEXIA AND THE RATIONALE FOR THE TOD™

> "If these tests will give us a basis from which we can start to understand a child's difficulties, they will have justified the time spent on them. Anything which helps educators or parents to *understand* any phase of development or lack of development is of immeasurable value."
>
> (Stanger & Donohue, 1937, p. 189)

As Stanger and Donohue noted decades ago, tests are designed to help users understand an individual's difficulties. The results provide insights into an individual's developmental levels as well as educational needs. They also help diagnose the type and nature of a disability. Thompson et al. (2025) conducted interviews with teachers and parents regarding dyslexia. One central conclusion was the importance of diagnosis in increasing visibility and clarifying children's needs. Without this recognition and understanding, they found that school support was both inconsistent and ineffectual. The *Tests of Dyslexia* (TOD) (Mather et al., 2024a) was designed to help evaluators identify individuals with dyslexia so that they can receive appropriate accommodations and interventions in a timely manner.

The first section of this chapter provides a brief description of the characteristics of dyslexia. The second section includes an explanation of the rationale for the development of the major components of the TOD.

Note: TOD® is a registered trademark of Manson Western, LLC, dba Western Psychological Services (WPS). Used with permission.

WHAT IS DYSLEXIA?

Dyslexia is a neurologically based reading disorder characterized by weaknesses in word-level reading, spelling, and persistent impairments in reading fluency (Holden et al., 2025; Shaywitz & Shaywitz, 2020). It is often described as the most common specific learning disability. Although dyslexia is not primarily a problem in reading comprehension or written expression, both reading comprehension and written expression may be negatively impacted by dyslexia; difficulties in decoding affect reading comprehension, and weaknesses in spelling affect written expression. Dyslexia also affects the development of both vocabulary knowledge and general knowledge (Siegel & Hurford, 2019). Rapid

≡ *Rapid Reference 1.1 Dyslexia*

Common Symptoms and Characteristics

- Limited interest in print
- Difficulty learning to rhyme words
- Difficulty learning letter names and letter sounds
- Confusions of letters with similar sounds (e.g., /f/ and /v/)
- Reversals and transpositions of letters and words that persist past the age of 7 (e.g., b and d, on and no, was and saw)
- Trouble sequencing letters correctly when spelling
- Difficulty in learning sight words
- Difficulty reading and spelling words with irregular elements (e.g., said)
- Spelling a word in different ways on the same page (e.g., wuns, wunce, for once)
- Spelling words the way they sound rather than the way they look (e.g., sed for said)
- Slow reading rate and fluency into adulthood
- Poor spelling into adulthood
- Low motivation and self-esteem because of reading and spelling difficulties

CAUTION

Individuals with dyslexia may demonstrate any combination of the characteristics that are outlined in Rapid Reference 1.1.

Reference 1.1, adapted from Mather and Wendling (2024), lists common symptoms and characteristics of dyslexia across the age span.

REVISING THE DEFINITION OF DYSLEXIA

The most widely used definition of dyslexia in the United States was proposed over two decades ago by the International Dyslexia Association (IDA) (Lyon et al., 2003). The IDA definition specifies that the difficulties are characterized by accurate and fluent word recognition and spelling that "…typically result from a deficit in the phonological component of language" (p. 2). Recently, researchers have recommended that it is time for revisions to this definition. For example, Catts et al. (2024) offered criteria that they considered to be critical for understanding the nature of dyslexia. They proposed that a revised definition should address (a) the multifactorial causal basis acknowledging that factors beyond phonological awareness can affect reading development, (b) a prevalence rate of 5–10%, (c) a presence of severe and persistent problems in word reading accuracy and speed, (d) the cognitive precursors necessary for early intervention and treatment, (e) the early spoken language difficulties which are risk factors, (f) the comorbidity with other disorders, (g) a clarification of exclusionary factors, and (h) the secondary consequences of academic failure and the psychosocial impact of dyslexia.

In October of 2025, IDA provided the following revised definition:

Dyslexia is a specific learning disability characterized by difficulties in word reading and/or spelling that involve accuracy, speed, or both and vary depending on the orthography. These difficulties occur along a continuum of severity and persist even with instruction that is effective for the individual's peers. The causes of dyslexia are complex and involve combinations of genetic, neurobiological, and environmental influences that interact throughout development. Underlying difficulties with phonological and morphological processing are common but not universal, and early oral language weaknesses often foreshadow literacy challenges. Secondary consequences include reading comprehension problems and reduced reading and writing experience that can impede growth in language, knowledge, written expression, and overall academic achievement. Psychological well-being and employment opportunities also may be affected. Although identification and targeted instruction are important at any age, language and literacy support before and during the early years of education is particularly effective."

Adopted by the IDA Board of Directors on October 22, 2025.

Other definitions include additional characteristics and linguistic risk factors. The following definition was adapted by Nancy Mather from a Delphi study informed by opinions of over a hundred experts from across the globe (Holden et al., 2025).

Dyslexia is a neurodevelopmental language disorder characterized by difficulties in word reading, spelling, and reading rate. These difficulties exist on a continuum from mild to severe. Dyslexia is highly heritable and often unexpected given the individual's other cognitive and academic abilities. The nature and developmental trajectory of dyslexia depends upon multiple genetic and environmental influences. Dyslexia is often associated with specific linguistic risk factors that affect the development of basic reading skills, reading fluency, and spelling. Although the most commonly observed linguistic risk factor in alphabetic languages is phonological processing, additional linguistic risk factors can include working memory, processing speed, rapid automatized naming (RAN), and/or orthographic processing. Dyslexia frequently co-occurs with other neurodevelopmental disorders, including developmental language disorder (DLD), dyscalculia, and attention deficit hyperactivity disorder (ADHD). Secondary consequences can include weaknesses in reading comprehension, vocabulary, and written expression.

Various states within the United States may also have different definitions and policies regarding dyslexia. The National Center on Improving Literacy provides a source for reviewing enacted legislation and regulations for each state (stateofdyslexia.org).

INTRODUCTION TO THE TOD

The TOD consists of three direct assessments: the TOD-Screener (TOD-S, all ages), the TOD-Early (TOD-E, Grades K–2), and the TOD-Comprehensive (TOD-C, Grade 1 to Adult). The TOD-S includes three tests that are used as the first three tests in both the TOD-E and the TOD-C. The TOD typically has two main purposes: to screen for dyslexia risk with the TOD-S, in a group or individually, and to determine if further assessment is needed with the TOD-E or TOD-C (depending on age/grade). In cases where a referral question regarding dyslexia or poor reading already exists, an evaluator could administer the TOD-E or TOD-C as well as the TOD Rating Scales (parent, teacher, self). These rating

---

≡ Rapid Reference 1.2

Tests of Dyslexia

Authors: Nancy Mather, R. Steve McCallum, Sherry M. Bell, and Barbara J. Wendling
Publication date: 2024
Age range: 5–90 years
Grade range: K.0 through 12.9
Publisher: Western Psychological Services (WPS) 625 Alaska Avenue, Torrance, CA 90503
Website: https://www.wpspublish.com/ *Phone:* (844) 378-4918
Price: Contact publisher

---

scales were designed to be part of a comprehensive dyslexia evaluation. Rapid Reference 1.2 includes the authors, publication date, and publisher of the TOD.

The TOD was created to be a comprehensive assessment and was designed to include (a) the main reading and spelling skills affected by dyslexia, (b) multiple linguistic risk factors, (c) vocabulary and reasoning abilities, (d) risk and diagnostic indexes, (e) rating scales that provide information on both family history and early speech and language difficulties, and (f) an intervention guide.

READING AND SPELLING SKILLS AFFECTED BY DYSLEXIA

The TOD was designed to assess the reading and spelling skills that are often weak in individuals with dyslexia. Eleven reading and spelling tests are combined into seven composites. Measures were developed to assess both timed and untimed word reading, as well as the abilities to spell regular words and read and spell irregular words. Rapid Reference 1.3 lists the TOD reading and spelling composites.

≡ Rapid Reference 1.3

TOD Reading and Spelling Composites

- Sight Word Acquisition
- Phonics Knowledge
- Basic Reading Skills
- Decoding Efficiency
- Spelling
- Reading Fluency
- Reading Comprehension Efficiency

UNTIMED AND TIMED WORD READING

The TOD contains measures of both reading accuracy and rate. TOD-7C: Pseudoword Reading (untimed) and TOD-19C: Rapid Pseudoword Reading (timed) assess the ability to decode nonsense words. Reading of pseudowords relies on phonological processing and indicates an individual's present level of skill in applying phonics to pronounce unfamiliar words. TOD-11C: Irregular Word Reading (untimed) and TOD-20C: Rapid Irregular Word Reading (timed) assess the ability to read words that contain an irregular element. Irregular word reading relies on both phonological processing and orthographic processing (pronunciation of the irregular element of the word) and indicates the breadth of sight vocabulary. The two timed tests provide a measure of the automaticity of word reading.

Additional tests provide information about reading fluency and rate. On the TOD-3Sa: Word Reading Fluency (Grades K and 1) or TOD-3Sb: Question Reading Fluency (Grades 2 to Adult), the examinee sees a picture and selects the correct word or reads short questions and circles the correct single-word answer; both are timed (two minutes for Word Reading Fluency and three minutes for Question Reading Fluency). On the TOD-12C: Oral Reading Efficiency test, the examinee reads a grade-level passage for one minute, and on the TOD-16C: Silent Reading Efficiency test, the examinee reads passages and answers comprehension questions (Grades 1–5, five minutes; Grades 6 to Adult, eight minutes). Siegel and Hurford (2019) state: "Tests of accuracy and speed of word recognition and pseudoword reading are absolutely essential for understanding whether an individual is experiencing reading difficulties" (p. 26). Their recommended simple definition for dyslexia focuses solely on these core reading skills: "Dyslexia is a specific learning disability in reading at the word level. It involves difficulty with accurate and/or fluent word recognition and/or decoding pseudowords" (Siegel et al., 2025).

> **DON'T FORGET**
>
> Tests of word reading accuracy and speed are essential for understanding an individual's reading difficulties.

REGULAR WORD SPELLING AND IRREGULAR WORD READING AND SPELLING

TOD-15C: Regular Word Spelling measures skill in spelling words that are pronounced and spelled the way that they sound. Both blending and segmenting, two phonological awareness abilities, are required. TOD-11C: Irregular Word Reading and TOD-5C Irregular Word Spelling measure proficiency in reading and spelling words that contain one or more irregular elements. These irregular elements have to be memorized, which involves orthographic processing (i.e., primarily, the ability to recall spelling patterns). The TOD-2S: Letter and Word Choice also assesses spelling.

MULTIPLE LINGUISTIC RISK FACTORS

For years, many researchers have advocated for moving from a single-deficit model naming phonological awareness as the sole risk factor for dyslexia to a multiple-deficit

> **CAUTION**
>
> Using only phonological awareness as a criterion for dyslexia would result in missing about one-half of the cases (Pennington et al., 2012).

model that encompasses additional risk factors. In fact, as early as 1932, Monroe, in her classic book, *Children Who Cannot Read,* noted: "No one factor was present in all cases. It is probable that the reading defect is caused by a constellation of factors rather than by one isolated factor" (p. 110). Pennington et al. (2012) cautioned that if evaluators use only poor phonological awareness as a criterion for dyslexia, they would then miss about one-half of the cases.

The TOD was designed to measure multiple linguistic abilities. Although phonological awareness is the most established risk factor for dyslexia, other linguistic abilities can impede reading and spelling development. In addition to phonological awareness, the TOD also measures (a) RAN, (b) auditory working memory, (c) orthographic processing, and (d) visual-verbal paired associate learning.

PHONOLOGICAL AWARENESS

Phonological awareness is often described as the most commonly observed risk factor for dyslexia (Holden et al., 2025). Although sound blending and segmentation are the two most important phonemic awareness abilities for young children, older students may still struggle on tests involving phonological manipulation. The main reason is that measures of phonological manipulation, such as substituting or deleting sounds from words, also require working memory; the examinee must hold the information in memory while substituting or deleting phonemes to make a different word. These more complex phonological manipulation tasks are stronger predictors of reading than are the less complex tasks of blending and segmentation (Dorofeeva et al., 2020; Kilpatrick, 2012). Rapid Reference 1.4 displays the TOD tests that measure some aspect of phonological awareness.

DON'T FORGET

Phonemic manipulation tests are stronger predictors of reading skill than less complex tasks.

RAPID AUTOMATIZED NAMING

RAN requires the examinee to quickly name symbols (letters and numbers), colors, or objects. The tests are timed typically for one or two minutes. Over 25 years ago, Wolf and Bowers (1999) described what they called the "double-deficit hypothesis" suggesting that

---

≡ Rapid Reference 1.4

Phonological/Phonemic Awareness Tests

- TOD-5E: Rhyming
- TOD-8E: Early Segmenting
- TOD-4C: Phonological Manipulation: Substitution and Deletion
- TOD-13C: Blending
- TOD-14C: Segmenting

poor phonological awareness and/or slow rapid naming were the two most prominent factors that could affect reading development. Because of the complexity of the reading process, however, they also acknowledged that any single-factor, two-factor, or even three-factor explanation was inadequate for understanding reading difficulties.

Since that time, empirical research has demonstrated that slow RAN is a significant linguistic risk factor for dyslexia in all languages and should be included in assessments for reading disorders (Araújo & Faísca, 2019). The naming of pictures and colors is often used with younger children, whereas alphanumeric RAN tasks (the stronger predictors of reading achievement) are used with school-age children (McWeeny et al., 2022). In addition, RAN is not highly related to phonological awareness and phonics but is a strong predictor of future achievement in word reading and reading fluency (Araújo et al., 2015; Nelson, 2015). RAN involves several perceptual processes that are related to reading. Norton (2020) explained: "Because RAN ability depends on a large number of perceptual and cognitive factors, one can think of RAN as the "check engine light" that indicates a problem, but doesn't reveal the exact cause" (p. 26). Thus, additional testing is often needed. Sometimes, educators ask: Should I try and improve RAN? The best advice is to work on reading interventions instead.

> **DON'T FORGET**
>
> Alphanumeric RAN tasks are stronger predictors of reading achievement than colors or objects. RAN is a good predictor of slow reading, but intervention should focus on methods to build fluency.

The TOD RAN tests differ from other published RAN assessments. One notable difference with the TOD-E RAN test is that it uses the letters, A, B, C, and the numbers, 1, 2, 3. These letters and numbers were selected because they are typically the first ones that young children learn. The TOD-C RAN tests differ from other RAN tests in that confusable letters and numbers were used to make the task more sensitive to older readers with dyslexia. On letter-naming tasks, even adults with dyslexia have longer fixation times and more regressions than typical readers when the selected letters are confusing (Dahhan et al., 2020). Rapid Reference 1.5 lists the three TOD RAN tests.

> **CAUTION**
>
> Do not administer the TOD RAN tests to a child who does not recognize letters or numbers with ease. In these cases, administer a RAN test that uses colors or objects.

≋ Rapid Reference 1.5

RAN Tests

- TOD-6E: Early Rapid Number and Letter Naming
- TOD-6C: Rapid Letter Naming
- TOD-17C: Rapid Number and Letter Naming

> ## ≡ *Rapid Reference 1.6*
>
> ### Auditory Working Memory Tests
>
> - TOD 9C: Word Memory
> - TOD 18C: Letter Memory

AUDITORY WORKING MEMORY

Working memory is often measured with tests that require both simultaneous storage and processing demands (Schneider & McGrew, 2018). An individual must store information in immediate awareness while transforming that information in some way, such as rearranging a string of words in reverse order. Working memory measures can discriminate between readers with dyslexia and typically developing readers (Knoop-van Campen et al., 2018). Even many adults with dyslexia continue to show weaknesses in working memory (Fostick & Revah, 2018).

The TOD-C contains two measures of working memory, the Letter Memory and Word Memory tests, which require listening to a string of letters or words and then repeating them in reverse order. Rapid Reference 1.6 lists the two TOD Auditory Working Memory tests.

ORTHOGRAPHIC PROCESSING

Orthography refers to the writing system of a language and includes spelling patterns and the rules of capitalization and punctuation. Orthographic processing refers to the brain's ability to recall letter orientations, spelling patterns, and words with both accuracy and speed; orthographic knowledge is acquired information stored in memory regarding how spoken language is represented in written language (Mather & Jaffe, 2021). Individuals with weaknesses in orthographic processing tend to reverse letters and numbers past the age of 7, have difficulty acquiring a sight word vocabulary, and spell words the way they sound rather than the way that they look (e.g., said as *sed*). Findings from a meta-analysis indicate that individuals with dyslexia have a deficit in orthographic knowledge that is as large as that of phonological awareness and RAN (Georgiou et al., 2021).

The irregular word reading and spelling tests provide additional information regarding orthographic processing. Irregular words contain one or more elements that do not follow regular phoneme-grapheme correspondence rules and so must be memorized by sight. When spelling, individuals with weaknesses in orthographic processing tend to regularize the irregular element of a word (e.g., spelling they as *thay*). Rapid Reference 1.7 lists the TOD orthographic processing tests.

VISUAL-VERBAL PAIRED ASSOCIATE LEARNING

Paired associate learning refers to the process of pairing and recalling two pieces of information, such as symbols or words. On the TOD, this ability is measured by the TOD-21C: Symbol to Sound Learning test. One key factor in dyslexia is a letter-speech sound learning

≡ *Rapid Reference 1.7*

Orthographic Processing Tests

- TOD-2S: Letter and Word Choice
- TOD-8C: Word Pattern Choice

Supplemental

- TOD-5C: Irregular Word Spelling
- TOD-11C: Irregular Word Reading
- TOD-20C: Rapid Irregular Word Reading

deficit (Aravena et al., 2018). Individuals with dyslexia often have difficulty learning and mastering the connections between graphemes (letters) and speech sounds (phonemes). This test was designed to mimic the beginning stages of learning to read. It involves the initial stages of orthographic mapping that require forming and recalling the connections between the graphemes and phonemes and then blending the sounds together to form words.

DON'T FORGET

"Diagnostically, the multiplicity of factors means that no single cognitive deficit or combination of deficits can be used to rule in or out most neurodevelopmental disorders" (McGrath et al., 2020, p. 7).

VOCABULARY AND REASONING

The TOD also includes two tests of vocabulary and two tests of reasoning that are useful to document different types of difficulties. The Vocabulary composite can be useful to document "unexpectedness," i.e., when oral vocabulary is significantly stronger than reading. It can also be useful in cases where the Vocabulary composite is similar to reading performance, and, therefore, the difficulties can be viewed as "expected." This pattern often occurs when an individual has both dyslexia and a DLD or in individuals with low overall cognitive functioning or intelligence (Sattler, 2018; Sternberg, 2018).

The Reasoning composite can be useful with English Learners as well as to rule out intellectual impairments. Finally, the combined Vocabulary and Reasoning Composite (2 or 4 tests) can be used in both a pattern of strengths and weaknesses and an ability-achievement discrepancy model to help identify twice-exceptional students who have better than average vocabulary and/or reasoning but average or low average reading scores. Rapid Reference 1.8 lists the TOD vocabulary and reasoning tests.

RISK AND DIAGNOSTIC INDEXES

The two TOD-S tests, Letter and Word Choice and Word or Question Reading Fluency, yield the Dyslexia Risk Index (DRI); the DRI provides an estimate of the risk of dyslexia. Although the Picture Vocabulary test is not included in the DRI, if it is higher than the other two tests, additional testing is recommended. DRI scores in the "at-risk" range suggest that further testing is needed with the TOD-E or TOD-C.

The TOD-E Early Dyslexia Diagnostic Index (EDDI) and the TOD-C Dyslexia Diagnostic Index (DDI) each require administering eight tests and, as the names imply, both provide an estimate of the probability of a dyslexia diagnosis. Both the EDDI (TOD-E) and DDI (TOD-C) consist of two indexes, the Linguistic Processing Index (LPI), and the Reading and Spelling Index (RSI). Specifically, the LPI consists of tests that operationalize linguistic risk factors predictive of reading and spelling difficulties, and the RSI consists of tests that operationalize the reading and spelling skills that are most affected by dyslexia.

As noted, the vocabulary and reasoning composites are created either from one vocabulary test and one reasoning test (VR2) or two of each (VR4) and can also be compared to the LPI and RSI. Figure 1.1 shows the pattern of scores most often associated with dyslexia based on these TOD composite scores. As the graphic figure shows, there is a discrepancy between the overall cognitive composite and (a) the linguistic processing scores that are linked to and

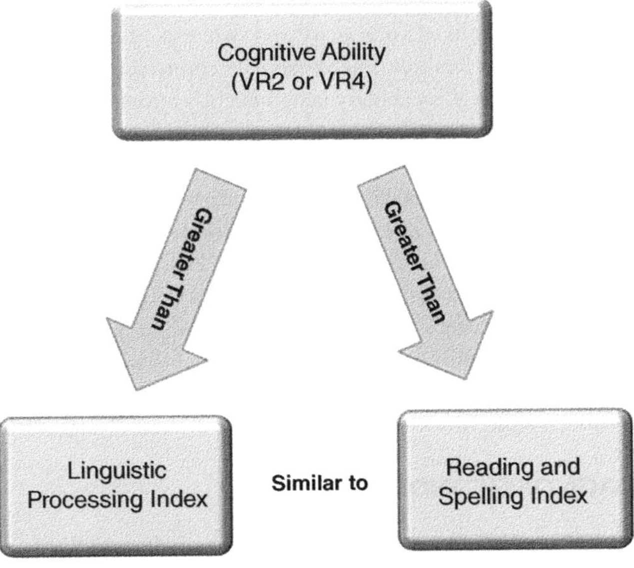

Figure 1.1   Pattern of TOD Composites Most Associated with Dyslexia

underpin the development of reading and spelling and (b) the specific reading and spelling scores most often negatively affected by dyslexia. Chapter 5 describes the content and interpretation of these indexes in detail.

CLINICAL PATTERN OF DYSLEXIA

The following table, adapted from the TOD Manual (Table 1.1. p. 3), illustrates the clinical pattern of dyslexia as measured by the TOD (Mather et al., 2024b).

CAUTION

The characteristics of dyslexia mentioned above describe a typical pattern of dyslexia, but not all of the examinee's scores will fit neatly into this pattern.

RATING SCALES

Rating scales provide a structured way to gather qualitative information. The results can provide meaningful insights that help support the scores of the direct assessments. The TOD-E includes two rating scales (parent/caregiver, teacher), and the TOD-C includes three rating scales (parent/caregiver, teacher, and self). The TOD-E and TOD-C parent/caregiver

Table 1.1 The Clinical Pattern of Dyslexia as Measured by the TOD

Significant Reading and Spelling Difficulties[1]
    Difficulty reading pseudowords
    Difficulty reading irregular words
    Slow reading rate
    Poor spelling

Low Performance on One or More Measures of Linguistic Processing Abilities[2]
    Phonological Awareness
    Rapid Automatized Naming
    Auditory Working Memory
    Orthographic Processing
    Visual-Verbal Paired Associate Learning

Average or Above Performance on Cognitive Abilities[3]
    Vocabulary
    Reasoning

Additional Risk Factors Gathered from Rating Scales and Record Review
    Family History
    Developmental Language Disorder
    Difficulties identified by parent/caregiver(s), teacher(s), and/or self

---

[1] Consider the student's age, prior reading interventions, and cognitive abilities. Twice-exceptional or high-ability students may have reading scores in the Average range but still perform well below expectations given their vocabulary and reasoning abilities.

[2] Some students with dyslexia may not have low performance on any of the linguistic processing abilities that are measured by the TOD, particularly if they have had intensive instruction in phonemic awareness.

[3] Many students with dyslexia will earn lower reading and spelling scores than they do on tests of cognitive ability (e.g., vocabulary and reasoning). Some students with dyslexia and another comorbid condition, such as a developmental language disorder, may not have such discrepancies.

rating scales are also available in Spanish. These rating scales provide important information about family history and early speech and/or language difficulties. Chapter 6 provides information on interpreting and integrating information from the rating scales into a report.

DON'T FORGET

As part of a dyslexia evaluation, always find out if a family history of reading and/or spelling problems exists.

FAMILY HISTORY

Family history of dyslexia is a key risk factor for dyslexia (Holden et al., 2025; Lasnick et al., 2022). As early as 1950, Hallgren conducted a study in Stockholm that supported the view that dyslexia is inherited. Today, we know that about 45% of children who have one parent with dyslexia will develop this reading disability (Gaab et al., 2020; Snowling & Melby-Lervåg, 2016), and if both parents have dyslexia, then the chance increases to about 75% (Gaab et al., 2020). Even though strong converging evidence indicates that dyslexia has a genetic basis, there is not one specific "reading" gene that has been identified as the sole cause of dyslexia.

EARLY SPEECH AND LANGUAGE DIFFICULTIES

Many individuals with dyslexia also have a history of early speech and language difficulties and may be identified as having a DLD. Early oral language difficulties affect the development of foundational decoding skills, including phoneme awareness and letter-sound (phoneme-grapheme) knowledge. Early weaknesses in oral language are powerful risk factors for weaknesses in both decoding and reading comprehension (Snowling & Hulme, 2024).

CATTELL–HORN–CARROLL THEORY OF COGNITIVE ABILITIES

The TOD can also play a role in different theoretical test interpretations. One well-known theory used for test interpretation is the Cattell–Horn–Carroll Theory (CHC) of Cognitive Abilities (Schneider & McGrew, 2018). CHC theory provides a taxonomy of both broad and narrow abilities. Rapid Reference 1.9 lists brief definitions of these CHC abilities. Figure 1.2 illustrates the CHC abilities that are measured by the TOD.

≡ Rapid Reference 1.9

Brief Definitions of CHC Abilities Measured by the TOD

- **Gc:** Comprehension-Knowledge: the depth and breadth of both general and specific declarative and procedural knowledge that is valued by a culture
- **Gf:** Fluid Reasoning: the ability to solve novel or unfamiliar problems
- **Ga:** Auditory Processing: the aspect of Ga that is measured is phonological processing (the ability to hear phonemes and to blend sounds into words, segment words into parts, and manipulate sounds within words)

- **Gwm:** Working Memory Capacity: the ability to maintain and manipulate information in memory
- **Gl:** Learning Efficiency or Long-term Storage: the ability to learn and store new information over time
- **Gr:** Retrieval Fluency: the rate and fluency at which known information can be accessed from memory
- **Grw:** Reading and Writing: mastery of skills and the breadth and depth of knowledge related to reading and writing

Tests of Dyslexia (TOD®)
Cattell–Horn–Carroll (CHC) Chart

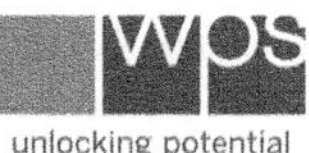

		TOD TESTS	Gc	Gf	Ga	Gwm	Gl	Gr	Grw
Section	Test #	Test Name							
TOD-Screener	1	Picture Vocabulary	X						
TOD-Screener	2	Letter and Word Choice							X
TOD-Screener	3	Word or Question Reading Fluency							X
TOD-Early	4	Sounds and Pseudowords			X				
TOD-Early	5	Rhyming			X				
TOD-Early	6	Early Rapid Number and Letter Naming						X	
TOD-Early	7	Letter and Sight Word Recognition							X
TOD-Early	8	Early Segmenting			X				
TOD-Early	9	Letter and Sound Knowledge							X
TOD-Comprehensive	4	Phonological Manipulation			X				
TOD-Comprehensive	5	Irregular Word Spelling							X
TOD-Comprehensive	6	Rapid Letter Naming						X	
TOD-Comprehensive	7	Pseudoword Reading							X
TOD-Comprehensive	8	Word Pattern Choice							X
TOD-Comprehensive	9	Word Memory				X			
TOD-Comprehensive	10	Picture Analogies		X					
TOD-Comprehensive	11	Irregular Word Reading							X
TOD-Comprehensive	12	Oral Reading Efficiency							X
TOD-Comprehensive	13	Blending			X				
TOD-Comprehensive	14	Segmenting			X				
TOD-Comprehensive	15	Regular Word Spelling							X
TOD-Comprehensive	16	Silent Reading Efficiency							X
TOD-Comprehensive	17	Rapid Number and Letter Naming						X	
TOD-Comprehensive	18	Letter Memory					X		
TOD-Comprehensive	19	Rapid Pseudoword Reading							X
TOD-Comprehensive	20	Rapid Irregular Word Reading							X
TOD-Comprehensive	21	Symbol to Sound Learning					X		
TOD-Comprehensive	22	Listening Vocabulary	X						
TOD-Comprehensive	23	Geometric Analogies		X					

Definitions of CHC abilities measured by the TOD®

Gc Comprehension-Knowledge: the depth and breadth of both general and specific declarative and procedural knowledge that is valued by a culture

Gf Fluid Reasoning: the ability to solve novel or unfamiliar problems

Ga Auditory Processing: the aspect of Ga that is measured is phonological processing (the ability to hear phonemes and to blend sounds into words, segment words into parts, and manipulate sounds within words)

Gwm Working Memory Capacity: the ability to maintain information in memory and manipulate the information

Gl Learning Efficiency or Long-Term Storage: the ability to learn and store new information over time

Gr Retrieval Fluency: the rate and fluency at which an individual can access known information in memory

Grw Reading and Writing: mastery of skills and the depth and breadth of knowledge related to reading and writing

Western Psychological Services   800.648.8857   wpspublish.com

Figure 1.2   CHC Abilities Measured by the TOD

DYSLEXIA INTERVENTIONS AND RECOMMENDATIONS GUIDE

The TOD also includes the *Dyslexia Interventions and Recommendations: A Companion Guide to the Tests of Dyslexia™* (Mather et al., 2024c). This guide provides examples of recommendations for different areas of reading and spelling intervention. It also includes examples of accommodations and an Appendix on *Teaching Students with Dyslexia.*

Results on several of the TOD tests have direct instructional implications. For example, if a child has difficulty with pseudoword reading, then an evaluator would recommend instruction to improve phonics. The evaluator would also determine if the child knows how to blend phonemes. If not, then a recommendation would be made to provide instruction in sound blending. In cases where the student has difficulty reading and spelling irregular words, a recommendation would be made to provide instruction in common spelling patterns (e.g., -ight, and -tion), as well as teaching strategies to help memorize irregular words (e.g., color code the "ai" in the word *said*).

Ideally, difficulties learning to read should be identified as early as possible so that intensive interventions can be provided. Reading difficulties have wide-reaching impacts, from activities of daily living to academic achievement to vocational prospects and beyond. The impact of dyslexia can be reduced if appropriate early intervention is provided with sufficient fidelity and intensity (Torgesen et al., 2014). In the early years of reading instruction, the main priority should be on identifying and supporting the needs of children with reading difficulties (Carroll et al., 2025). Chapter 8 of this book provides information about using the TOD results to inform the selection of interventions and accommodations. Appendix A includes commonly asked questions about the administration and interpretation of the TOD. Appendix B provides additional practice in interpreting the TOD results. Appendix C includes TOD Dyslexia Profiles that are fillable when downloaded from the WPS website.

⚔ TEST YOURSELF ⚔

1. The TOD-S is used as the first three tests in the TOD-E and TOD-C.
   True or False?

2. If the Picture Vocabulary test on the TOD-S is significantly higher than the two reading tests, an evaluator should do additional testing.
   True or False?

3. The best phonological awareness task for predicting reading achievement is

   (a) rhyming.

   (b) sound blending.

   (c) segmentation.

   (d) phoneme manipulation.

4. The TOD-C RAN tests differ from other RAN tests because they

   (a) are timed for three minutes.

   (b) use confusable letters.

   (c) use confusable letters and numbers.

   (d) both b and c.

5. **No single cognitive deficit can be used to rule in or out dyslexia.**
   True or False?

6. **Emily, a fourth-grade student, has poor spelling. She spells words the way they sound and has particular difficulty spelling irregular words, such as *was* and *said*. Most likely, she has a weakness in**

   (a) phonological awareness.

   (b) orthographic processing.

   (c) rapid automatized naming.

   (d) morphological awareness.

7. **The Vocabulary composite can be used to**

   (a) help identify a co-morbid condition, such as developmental language disorder.

   (b) demonstrate that the low reading score is unexpected compared to oral vocabulary.

   (c) help identify twice-exceptional individuals with dyslexia.

   (d) all of the above

8. **Pennington et al. (2012) indicated that adherence to a single deficit model of only poor phonological awareness would miss about what percent of cases?**

   (a) 10%

   (b) 20%

   (c) 35%

   (d) 50%

9. **The TOD EDDI and DDI consist of which two composites or indexes?**

   (a) Sight word acquisition and working memory

   (b) Phonological awareness and phonics

   (c) Linguistic processing and reading and spelling

   (d) Phonological manipulation and reading and spelling

10. **Both the TOD EDDI and DDI provide a score that indicates if an individual has dyslexia.**
    True or False?

Answers: 1. True; 2. True; 3. d; 4. d; 5. True; 6. b; 7. d; 8. d; 9. c; 10. False

REFERENCES

Araújo, S., & Faísca, L. (2019). A meta-analytic review of naming-speed deficits in developmental dyslexia. *Scientific Studies of Reading, 23*(5), 349–368. https://doi.org/10.1080/10888438.2019.1572758

Araújo, S., Reis, A., Petersson, K. M., & Faísca, L. (2015). Rapid automatized naming and reading performance: A meta-analysis. *Journal of Educational Psychology, 107*(3), 868–883. https://doi.org/10.1037/edu0000006

Aravena, S., Tijms, J., Snellings, P., & van der Molen, M. W. (2018). Predicting individual differences in reading and spelling skill with artificial script-based letter-speech sound training. *Journal of Learning Disabilities, 51*(6), 552–564. https://doi.org/10.1177/0022219417715407

Carroll, J. M., Holden, C., Kirby, P., Thompson, P. A., Snowling, M. J., & Dyslexia Delphi Panel. (2025). Toward a consensus on dyslexia: Findings from a Delphi study. *Journal of Child Psychology and Psychiatry, and Allied Disciplines, 66*(7), 1065–1076. https://doi.org/10.1111/jcpp.14123

Catts, H. W., Terry, N. P., Lonigan, C. J., Compton, D. L., Wagner, R. K., Steacy, L. M., Farquharson, K., & Petscher, Y. (2024). Revisiting the definition of dyslexia. *Annals of Dyslexia, 74*, 282–302. https://doi.org/10.1007/s11881-023-00295-3

Dahhan, N. Z. A., Kirby, J. R., Brien, D. C., Gupta, R., Harrison, A., & Munoz, D. P. (2020). Understanding the biological basis of dyslexia at a neural systems level. *Brain Communications, 2*, 1, fcaa173–16. https://doi.org/10.1093/braincomms/fcaa173

Dorofeeva, S. V., Laurinavichyute, A., Reshetnikova, V., Akhutina, T. V., Tops, W., & Dragoy, O. (2020). Complex phonological tasks predict reading in 7 to 11 years of age typically developing Russian children. *Journal of Research in Reading, 43*(4), 516–535. https://doi.org/10.1111/1467-9817.12327

Fostick, L., & Revah, H. (2018). Dyslexia as a multi-deficit disorder: Working memory and auditory temporal processing. *Acta Psychologica, 183*, 19–28. https://doi.org/10.1016/j.actpsy.2017.12.010

Gaab, N., Turesky, T. K., & Sanfilippo, J. (2020). Early identification of children at-risk for developmental dyslexia and reading impairments: Neurobiology, screening, evidence-based response to screening, and the use of educational technology. In J. A. Washington, D. L. Compton, & P. McCardle (Eds.), *Dyslexia: Revisiting etiology, diagnosis, treatment, and policy* (pp. 44–56). Brookes.

Georgiou, G. K., Martinez, D., Vieira, A. P. A., & Guo, K. (2021). Is orthographic knowledge a strength or a weakness in individuals with dyslexia? Evidence from a meta-analysis. *Annals of Dyslexia, 71*, 5–27. https://doi.org/10.1007/s11881-021-00220-6

Hallgren, B. (1950). Specific dyslexia (congenital word-blindness); A clinical and genetic study. *Acta Psychiatrica et Neurologica. Supplementum, 65*, 1–287.

Holden, C., Kirby, P., Snowling, M. J., Thompson, P. A., & Carroll, J. M. (2025). Towards a consensus for dyslexia practice: Findings of a Delphi study on assessment and identification. *Dyslexia, 31*, e1800. https://doi.org/10.1002/dys.1800

Kilpatrick, D. (2012). Phonological segmentation assessment is not enough: A comparison of three phonological awareness tests with first and second graders. *Canadian Journal of School Psychology, 27*(2), 150–165. https://doi.org/10.1177/0829573512438635

Knoop-van Campen, C. A. N., Segers, E., & & Verhoeven, L. (2018). How phonological awareness mediates the relation between working memory and word reading efficiency in children with dyslexia. *Dyslexia, 24*(2), 156–169. https://doi.org/10.1002/dys.1583

Lasnick, O., Feng, J., Quirion, A., Hart, S., & Hoeft, F. (2022). The importance of family history in dyslexia. *Reading League Journal, 3*(2), 35–40.

Lyon, G. R., Shaywitz, S. E., & Shaywitz, B. A. (2003). A definition of dyslexia. *Annals of Dyslexia, 53*, 1–14. https://doi.org/10.1007/s11881-003-0001-9

Mather, N., & Jaffe, L. (2021). Orthographic knowledge is essential for reading and spelling. *Reading League Journal, 2*(3), 15–25.

Mather, N., & Wendling, B. (2024). *Essentials of dyslexia: Assessment and intervention* (2nd ed.). Wiley.

Mather, N., McCallum, R. S., Bell, S. M., & Wendling, B. J. (2024a). *Tests of Dyslexia (TOD)*. Western Psychological Services.

Mather, N., McCallum, R. S., Bell, S. M., & Wendling, B. J. (2024b). *Tests of Dyslexia (TOD)* [Manual]. Western Psychological Services.

Mather, N., McCallum, R. S., Bell, S. M., & Wendling, B. J. (2024c). *Dyslexia Interventions and Recommendations: A Companion Guide to the Tests of Dyslexia (TOD)*. Western Psychological Services.

McGrath, L. M., Peterson, R. L., & Pennington, B. F. (2020). The Multiple Deficit Model: Progress, problems, and prospects. *Scientific Studies of Reading, 24*(1), 7–13. https://doi.org/10.1080/10888438.2019.1706180

McWeeny, S., Choi, S., Choe, J., LaTourrette, A., Roberts, M. Y., & Norton, E. S. (2022). Rapid Automatized Naming (RAN) as a kindergarten predictor of future reading in English: A systematic review and meta-analysis. *Reading Research Quarterly, 57*(4), 1187–1211. https://doi.org/10.1002/rrq.467

Monroe, M. (1932). *Children who cannot read.* University of Chicago Press.

Nelson, J. M. (2015). Examination of the double-deficit hypothesis with adolescents and young adults with dyslexia. *Annals of Dyslexia, 65*(3), 159–177. https://doi.org/10.1007/s11881-015-0105-z

Norton, E. (2020). What educators need to know about Rapid Automatized Naming (RAN). *Learning Difficulties Australia Bulletin, 52*(1), 25–28.

Pennington, B. F., Santerre-Lemmon, L., Rosenberg, J., MacDonald, B., Boada, R., Friend, A., Leopold, D. R., Samuelsson, S., Byrne, B., Willcutt, E. G., & Olson, R. K. (2012). Individual prediction of dyslexia by single versus multiple deficit models. *Journal of Abnormal Psychology, 121*(1), 212–224. https://doi.org/10.1037/a0025823

Sattler, J. M. (2018). *Assessment of children: Cognitive foundations and applications.* Sattler, Publisher.

Schneider, W. J., & McGrew, K. S. (2018). The Cattell–Horn–Carroll theory of cognitive abilities. In D. P. Flanagan & E. M. McDonough (Eds.), *Contemporary intellectual assessment: Theories, tests, and issues* (4th ed., pp. 73–163). Guilford Press. https://www.guilford.com/books/Contemporary-Intellectual-Assessment/Flanagan-McDonough/9781462552030

Shaywitz, S., & Shaywitz, J. (2020). *Overcoming dyslexia* (2nd ed.). Alfred Knopf.

Siegel, L. S., & Hurford, D. P. (2019). The case against discrepancy models in the evaluation of dyslexia. *Perspectives on Language and Literacy, 45*(1), 23–28.

Siegel, L. S., Hurford, D. P., Metsala, J. L., Ozeir, M. R., & Fender, A. C. (2025). *Thoughts on the definition of dyslexia.* Advance Online Publication. https://doi.org/10.1007/s11881-025-00337-y

Snowling, M., & Hulme, C. (2024). Do we really need a new definition of dyslexia? A commentary. *Annals of Dyslexia, 74,* 355–362. https://doi.org/10.1007/s11881-024-00305-y

Snowling, M. J., & Melby-Lervåg, M. (2016). Oral language deficits in familial dyslexia: A meta-analysis and review. *Psychological Bulletin, 142,* 498–545.

Stanger, M. A., & Donohue, E. K. (1937). *Prediction and prevention of reading difficulties.* Oxford University Press.

Sternberg, R. J. (2018). The triarchic theory of successful intelligence. In D. P. Flanagan & E. M. McDonough (Eds.), *Contemporary intellectual assessment: Theories, tests, and issues* (4th ed., pp. 174–194). Guilford Press.

Thompson, A. M., Wood, C., Thompson, I. K., & Carroll, J. M. (2025). Seeing, being seen and being able to see dyslexia in English schools: Parent and teacher perspectives. *Dyslexia: An International Journal of Research and Practice, 31*(2), Article e70003. https://doi.org/10.1002/dys.70003

Torgesen, J. K., Foorman, B. R., & Wagner, R. K. (2014). Dyslexia: A brief for educators and parents. *Asia Pacific Journal of Developmental Differences, 1*(2), 118–135. https://doi.org/10.3850/S2345734114000016

Wolf, M., & Bowers, P. (1999). The "Double-Deficit Hypothesis" for the developmental dyslexias. *Journal of Educational Psychology, 91,* 1–24. https://doi.org/10.1037/0022-0663.91.3.415

Two

GENERAL ADMINISTRATION PROCEDURES FOR THE TOD™

In general, the TOD is administered for two purposes: Screening (TOD-S) and comprehensive evaluation (TOD-C or TOD-E) (Mather et al., 2024b). While the administration of the TOD is not complicated, it is important that evaluators familiarize themselves with the test materials, as well as the administration and scoring guidelines prior to administering the TOD. Proper administration of the TOD, or any standardized test, requires training, study, and practice. Although individuals in a wide range of professions can learn the actual procedures for administering the test, a higher degree of skill is required to interpret the results or to evaluate individuals who have special problems or specific disabilities. Only properly trained individuals should interpret the results of standardized tests, especially in high-stakes situations, such as diagnosing dyslexia or making decisions for special education eligibility. Some evaluators can adequately administer a test but may lack the expertise to interpret the results. Evaluators are responsible for determining their own competence for administering and interpreting the TOD in accordance with the guidelines set forth by professional organizations and licensing boards, including the American Psychological Association *Standards for Educational and Psychological Testing* (American Educational Research Association et al., 2014). In addition, the TOD Manual includes a Principles of Use section that provides guidance on the issue of who can use the TOD. An excerpt of that section follows: "The TOD can be administered and scored by a professional who is familiar with and competent in psychological or educational testing, or by a paraprofessional with training in assessment and specific training on the TOD. Interpretation and application of the results should be performed by a professional with training and experience

DON'T FORGET

Evaluators are responsible for determining their own competence for administering and interpreting the TOD in accordance with guidelines set forth by professional organizations and licensing boards. School districts also have the responsibility of ensuring that qualified professionals are administering the tests that are used within the district.

in child development, psychology, and/or education, or a person who is supervised by such a professional, and in some cases by professionals with expertise in speech-language pathology."

GETTING READY TO TEST

Testing Environment

Prior to testing, select a testing room that is quiet, comfortable, and has adequate lighting and ventilation. Ideally, for individually administered tests, only the evaluator and the examinee should be in the room. Ensure that the room has a desk or table and two chairs, one of which is an appropriate size for the examinee. Have all the required testing materials organized and within reach. For tests that require a Test Easel, position the easel so that the stimulus page faces the examinee and the instruction page faces the evaluator. Keep the Record Form or Scoring Sheet positioned so that the examinee cannot easily see what is written. A recommended seating arrangement is to sit diagonally across from the examinee at the corner of a table. Another possible arrangement is to sit directly across the table. With this arrangement, the table must be narrow and low enough so the evaluator can see and point to the Test Easel or the examinee's Response Booklet when necessary.

Calculating Chronological Age

Before beginning an evaluation, calculate the examinee's chronological age. Verify the individual's birthdate as the calculated age is used to determine age-based standard scores. Record the test date and birth date in the designated areas on the front page of the Record Form (see Figure 2.1). When subtracting, it may be necessary to borrow a Year for the Month column (add 12) or borrow a Month for the Day column (add 30). The example shown in Figure 2.1 illustrates these steps. After obtaining the chronological age, ignore the days and do not round up when consulting the norms tables.

	Year	Month	Day
Date of testing	2025 ~~2025~~ 24	+12 20 ~~9~~ 8	+30 40 ~~10~~
Date of birth	2017	11	17
Chronological age*	7	9	23

*Days are used in age calculation but not in lookup tables. When using Appendix Tables A.3, A.9, B.1, and B.7, use Year and Month: do not round up.

Figure 2.1   Calculating Chronological Age

Testing Materials

Each of the three test batteries requires a different set of materials. The materials for each battery are described separately in this section. Some of the required materials listed are not included in the test kits, such as a stopwatch, a computer or tablet, and pencils.

TOD-SCREENER (TOD-S)

The TOD-S offers two administration formats: a print option and an online option. In either case, there are three versions of the Response Booklet: Grades K–1, Grades 2–5, and Grades 6–Adult. Make sure to have the correct Response Booklet for the individual or group being tested, or if testing online, ensure that the correct Response Booklet is cued up. The TOD-S Administration Guide provides instructions for both administration formats.

- TOD-S Print Version: Response Booklet for correct grade range, Administration Guide (use Print Administration instructions), Scoring Sheet, stopwatch, and two sharpened pencils
- TOD-S Online Version*: computer, tablet, internet connection, correct Response Booklet cued up, and Administration Guide (use Digital Administration instructions)

*NOTE: When using the online version of the TOD-S, scoring is done automatically so no Scoring Sheet is needed. Timing is done automatically so no stopwatch is needed.

TOD-COMPREHENSIVE (TOD-C) AND TOD-EARLY (TOD-E)

The TOD-C and TOD-E provide only a print administration option. Some digital materials, however, are available to purchase in an online format, including the *TOD Manual* (Mather et al. 2024b), the *Dyslexia Interventions and Recommendations: A Companion Guide to the Tests of Dyslexia™* (Mather et al., 2024c), and the *TOD Norms* book (Mather et al., 2024d). In addition, the TOD-S

CAUTION

Administering TOD-S to a Group

- Generally, a group is comprised of students in the same grade so they all use the same version of the Response Booklet..

- When a group represents multiple grades, ensure each student in the group falls within the grade range specified for the assigned Response Booklet (K–1, or Grades 2–5, or Grades 6–Adult). For example, a second grader cannot be tested with a group using the K–1 Response Booklet.

DON'T FORGET

Preparing to Administer the TOD

- Select an appropriate location for the testing session.

- Select furniture that is the appropriate size for the examinee.

- Ensure that all the necessary testing materials are organized and within reach.

- If using the TOD-S online version, make sure there is an internet connection, a computer or tablet for each individual being tested, and the correct Response Booklet is cued up.

Administration Guide, as well as the TOD-C and TOD-E easels, can be downloaded for offline use.

- TOD-E: Record Form, one Test Easel, and Stopwatch
- TOD-C: Response Booklet, two Test Easels, Record Form, stopwatch, Digital Audio Recording (for portions of Test 13C, download from WPS Online Evaluation System [OES] at the WPS website), and at least two sharpened pencils with erasers

Establishing and Maintaining Rapport

In most instances, establishing a good relationship with the examinee will not be difficult. Do not, however, begin testing until the individual seems relatively at ease. If the examinee feels sick or does not respond appropriately, do not attempt testing. Often, a testing session begins with a short period of conversation, discussing something of interest to the person, such as what sports the person plays or what they enjoy doing in leisure time. When ready to begin testing, make a brief statement such as, "I'm going to ask you to do some different things. Some will be easy and others will be hard. Please try your best."

Throughout the testing session, encourage a response when items are difficult. If the examinee appears to be struggling with an item, it is fine to say, "Would you like to take a guess on that one?" During the testing session, keep the examinee engaged by providing encouragement and praising the examinee's effort by saying "Good effort" or "You are trying really hard." Do not, however, make comments that reveal whether answers are correct or incorrect. For example, do not say "good" only when a response is correct or pause longer when a response is incorrect as if waiting for the examinee to change the response. If an examinee asks if a response was correct, say something like "That was a good answer." If you misheard or missed the examinee's response, say "I missed your answer. Say it again."

CAUTION

Examiner/Examinee Interactions

- Be careful not to reveal the correct answers to items.
- Do not indicate whether a response is correct or incorrect unless the test item's instructions allow feedback.
- Provide encouragement throughout the administration, not just when the examinee answers correctly or incorrectly.

Testing Individuals with Special Needs

Any modifications to the standardized procedures of a test may compromise the validity of the test results. Because the TOD is designed to assess an individual's level of achievement in reading, spelling, and various linguistic abilities, it is unlikely that any changes to the standardized procedures will be necessary as the goal is to determine functioning in those areas

Reading Difficulties

Accommodations are usually not provided on standardized tests for students who struggle with reading if the intent is to obtain a score that reflects their reading ability. Although an accommodation may improve performance, the resulting score will not be an accurate

> # CAUTION
>
> Modifying standardized procedures for an examinee with a particular disability is inappropriate when the purpose of a test is to diagnose the presence and degree of that disability (AERA et al., 2014). For example, if an individual is being evaluated due to limited reading fluency, then allowing that individual to have additional time to complete tasks on a timed reading test would limit the test's utility for determining the extent of the weakness.

reflection of a person's capabilities. In most instances, the purpose of the assessment is to document the nature and severity of the examinee's difficulties in reading. Clearly, the evaluator would not read the reading tests to an individual with reading difficulties, as the main purpose of the evaluation is to determine the extent and severity of the reading problem, not to measure oral language comprehension. The goal of the evaluation is to determine an individual's unique pattern of strengths and weaknesses and then use the assessment data to suggest appropriate classroom accommodations and recommend possible teaching strategies and interventions

Young Children

The TOD can be administered to children in kindergarten. Therefore, you may encounter some young children who are uncomfortable with an unfamiliar adult or an unfamiliar setting. Initially, some children may be shy and refuse to speak to a stranger. If after several rapport-building activities (e.g., talking about a favorite sport or animal; solving a puzzle), the child still refuses to speak, discontinue testing and try again at a later date. It may be helpful to visit the child in the classroom setting prior to the evaluation. This would provide an opportunity to observe the child's behavior and performance in the classroom and possibly offer a chance to interact with the child.

English Learners (ELs)

Before using the TOD (or any test that uses the English language) with an individual whose first language is not English, determine the individual's English proficiency. If the individual does not exhibit sufficient English proficiency, then it is not appropriate to base interpretation of the scores on the TOD norms. Item responses can, however, provide qualitative information.

The TOD was standardized on individuals who demonstrated fluency in English. The sample also included bilingual and multilingual individuals fluent in English, and no significant differences were noted in scores between monolingual English speakers and those who are bilingual or multilingual.

CONFIDENTIALITY OF TEST MATERIALS

Test users are responsible for carefully storing test materials and protecting test content. Do not leave the test materials (i.e., Test Easels, Response Booklets, and Record Forms) unattended where others may see them and look at the test items. During a discussion of the test results with the parent or teacher, the types of items may be described, but avoid disclosing specific test content. Use examples similar to the test items without revealing the actual test items.

Do not share test content or results with curious nonprofessionals or make materials available for public inspection. During testing, or after testing has been completed, do not inform examinees of whether answers are correct or incorrect, and do not explain the correct answers to any of the questions. Disclosing specific test content can invalidate future administrations. Occasionally, individuals will request information. Usually, it is easy to recognize whether it is appropriate or inappropriate to supply the requested information. If the requested information should not be shared, respond with a comment such as, "I'm not allowed to share that information."

Basics of Administration

The goal of standardized testing is to see how well a person can perform tasks when given instructions identical to those presented to individuals during standardization. For this reason, it is essential that each item is read exactly as it is written and that all pointing directions are followed precisely. Prior to formal administration of the TOD, administer several practice tests to develop both precise and efficient administration. Avoid unnecessary conversation during tests that may slow down the administration or distract the examinee from the test tasks. Administer the next item immediately upon completion of each item. Take short breaks, if necessary, only *between* tests; do not stop for a break *during* a test.

> **DON'T FORGET**
>
> **Precise Administration**
> - Present each item *exactly* as written.
> - Follow all instructions for pointing and providing feedback on sample items.
> - Practice administering each test several times before administering the test for an evaluation.
>
> **Efficient Administration**
> - Administer the next item *immediately* after completing each item.
> - Do not stop and visit during the testing session.
> - Use the prompts as directed in the test instructions when an examinee does not respond within the specified timeframe.

Order of Administration

In all cases, the TOD-S is administered first whether the purpose is screening or the first step of a comprehensive assessment. The TOD-S includes Tests 1S, 2S, and 3S and scores from those tests are transferred to the TOD-C or TOD-E if further testing is indicated or planned. Note that the TOD-S scores can be used in the TOD-C or TOD-E as long as the examinee is still within the same grade-based or age-based norm group. If, however, time has passed and the examinee is in a new norm group, readminister the TOD-S. To control for practice effects, allow at least three months before readministering the TOD-S. The TOD-S may be administered individually or in a group and takes approximately 10–15 minutes.

The TOD-C provides 20 additional tests. It is not required, or typical, to administer all 20 tests. Depending on the purpose for testing, select the tests to administer. For example, if the objective is to obtain the Dyslexia Diagnostic Index (DDI), administer the six tests from

DON'T FORGET

Always administer the TOD-S first. If administering the TOD-S to a group, make sure each individual is in the grade range for the same version of the Response Booklet.

the TOD-C (Tests 4C-9C) which are then combined with two of the TOD-S tests to create the DDI. These six TOD-C tests require approximately 30 minutes to administer. Chapter 4 provides detailed information about the administration and organization of the TOD-C.

The TOD-E provides six additional tests. Typically, all six tests are administered. These six tests, when combined with two of the tests from the TOD-S, create the Early Dyslexia Diagnostic Index (EDDI). The six TOD-E tests take approximately 20–25 minutes to administer. Chapter 3 provides detailed information about the organization and administration of the TOD-S and the TOD-E.

DON'T FORGET

When a test requires an oral response, do not penalize for mispronunciations that result from articulation errors, speech, or dialect differences.

CAUTION

Possible Administration Errors

- Not following standardized administration procedures
- Not using the correct Response Booklet
- Not administering the correct item set
- Not following the Start and Stop Rules for a test
- Not administering the Sample Items correctly
- On specific tests, not prompting as directed to encourage a response after a five-second pause
- On rapid naming tests, not scoring an item 0 after a three-second pause
- Providing an examinee with more assistance than is allowed by the standardization directions

General Guidelines for Item Administration and Scoring

To ensure that the information obtained from the examinee's scores on the TOD is valid and accurately reflects the examinee's abilities, adhere to the standardized administration procedures throughout the test session. Follow all instructions on each item exactly; read all bold, teal text verbatim. Do not paraphrase, translate, or change any words on the instructions. On some tests, an item may be repeated if the examinee requests it; on other tests, repeating an item is not allowed, as specified in the directions.

Learn the pronunciation of all the words in the test items prior to administering the TOD for the first time. Pronounce all words printed in bold, teal type, correctly to maintain standardized administration procedures. Study the test materials to become familiar with all of the words that may be encountered during administration. Some advanced items, in particular, include words that may be unfamiliar. Pronunciation guides for those words are included in the Record Forms and Test Easels. In addition, a chart identifying the diacritic markings for vowels is located in the TOD Manual (p. 19) as well as in each TOD Easel (p. 5).

The scoring criteria are included with each item and are shown in the Record Form and in the Easels. For the TOD-S, the correct responses are shown in the Administration Guide and the Scoring Sheet. Most of the TOD test items have only one correct response. Items in TOD-E Rhyming (5E), however, have more than one possible correct response and only the most common correct responses are listed. (See Chapter 3 for details about the administration and scoring of TOD-S and TOD-E tests.) In addition, when the examinee gives more than one response to an item or changes the response, score the last response given, even if it changes the item score from correct to incorrect or vice versa. Do not penalize the examinee for errors due to articulation or speech and dialect differences.

> ### DON'T FORGET
>
> **Competent Administration**
> - Know the correct pronunciation of all test items.
> - Be fluent in administration.
> - Have all materials organized and at hand.
> - Do not penalize for errors due to articulation or dialect and speech differences.

Tests with Start Items

Most tests on the TOD contain a range of items that are appropriate for different examinee ability levels from young children through adults. An examinee would rarely, if ever, encounter all of the items on a test. The use of different Start Items helps reduce testing time by identifying an appropriate starting item for each examinee based on their grade or ability level. If an examinee is performing above or below their grade level, a higher- or lower-grade level Start Item may be selected. For example, an individual who is low functioning may need to begin with an easier item than indicated by their present grade placement to avoid frustration; in contrast, an individual who is higher-functioning or gifted can start testing with a more difficult item to avoid spending time on items that are too easy.

> ### DON'T FORGET
>
> Select a higher- or lower-grade level Start Item when a student is performing above or below their grade level.

Tests Administered with Basal and Stop Rules

The purpose of Basal and Stop (or ceiling) Rules is to limit the number of items administered to only those that are appropriately matched to the examinee's ability, thereby avoiding items that are much too easy (i.e., lower-numbered items) or much too difficult (i.e., higher-numbered items).

Many tests in the TOD use Item 1 as the Start Point, so Item 1 serves as the basal. A number of TOD tests, however, have different Start Points for different grades. For examinees that do not start at Item 1, a basal is established after 4 consecutive correct responses.

The tests with different Start Points identify which Sample Item to administer and then the test item that begins the test. For example, for TOD-4E Sounds and Pseudowords, Grade K begins with Samples A and B, then proceeds to Item 1. In this case, Item 1 is the basal and testing continues until 4 consecutive errors are made. For Grades 1 and 2, the Start Point is Sample C, then proceeds to Item 6. If the examinee responds incorrectly to both Items 6

CAUTION

Pay close attention to the Basal Rule shown in the Test Easel and the Record Form. When there are different Start Points for grades, it may be necessary to go back to the first Start Point if a basal is not established.

and 7, the testing goes back to Samples A and B and then Items 1–5. If 4 consecutive errors have not been made, then testing continues with Item 8 until the Stop Rule has been met. Rapid Reference 2.1 lists the tests in TOD-C and TOD-E that use different Start Points which may impact establishing the basal.

≡ Rapid Reference 2.1

Tests with Different Start Points for Establishing a Basal

TOD-Comprehensive

TEST	GRADE	START POINT
4C: Phonological Manipulation	1–5	Sample A, Item 1
	6–adult	Sample C, Item 6
5C: Irregular Word Spelling	1–5	Item 1
	6–adult	Item 15*
7C: Pseudoword Reading	1–2	Sample A, Item 1
	3–adult	Sample B, Item 11
11C: Irregular Word Reading	1–2	Sample A, Item 1
	3–adult	Item 11
13C: Blending	1–5	Sample A, Item 1
	6–adult	Sample C, Item 11
14C: Segmenting	1–5	Sample A, Item 1
	6–adult	Sample C, Item 11
15C: Regular Word Spelling	1–5	Item 1
	6–adult	Item 15*
22C: Listening Vocabulary	1–5	Sample A-B, Item 1
	6–adult	Sample B, Item 10*

If a student in Grades 6 or above is functioning at a lower level, start with Item 1.

TOD-Early

TEST	GRADE	START POINT
4E: Sounds and Pseudowords	K	Sample A-B, Item 1
	1–2	Sample C, Item 6
5E: Rhyming	K	Sample A-B, Item 1
	1–2	Sample C, Item 11
7E: Letter and Sight Word Recognition	K–1	Sample A-B, Item 1
	2	Sample C, Item 11
8E: Early Segmenting	K–1	Sample A, Item 1
	2	Sample C, Item 14

Tests Administered with Item Sets

Only two tests in the TOD, both in the TOD-S, are administered using item sets: TOD-1S Picture Vocabulary and TOD-2S Letter and Word Choice. On these tests, the examinee is administered a set of items and takes *all* of the items in the assigned set, regardless of their performance.

When administering one of these two tests, consult the table in the *TOD-Screener Administration Guide* to identify the set that corresponds to the examinee's grade level. For example, in TOD-1S Picture Vocabulary, an examinee in Grades K or 1 is administered Samples A and B and then Items 1–30; an examinee in Grades 2–5 is administered Samples A and B and then Items 11–40; an examinee in Grades 6–Adult is administered Samples A and B and then Items 18–47.

> ### DON'T FORGET
>
> For the tests requiring a basal, Item 1 or 4 consecutive correct responses establish the basal. All items below the basal are considered correct and are included in the raw score. If there are two sets of 4 consecutive correct responses, always use the lowest set of four as the basal. Score items between the two sets as 1 if correct or 0 if incorrect.

> ### DON'T FORGET
>
> TOD-1S and TOD-2S require the examinee to take all of the items in the assigned set. There is no Stop Rule. Simply put, administer the complete set.

Tests Requiring a Response Booklet

Several TOD tests require a Response Booklet. Rapid Reference 2.2 lists these tests. When administering the TOD-S, there are three separate Response Booklets: Grades K–1, Grades 2–5, and Grades 6–Adult. Select the correct Response Booklet for the examinee when administering the print version of the TOD-S. When using the online version of the TOD-S, make sure to cue up the correct Response Booklet on the computer or tablet. The TOD-C has just one Response Booklet which is required for four tests. The TOD-E does not require a Response Booklet.

≡ Rapid Reference 2.2

Tests that Require a Response Booklet

TOD-Screener	TOD-Comprehensive
TOD-1S: Picture Vocabulary	TOD-5C: Irregular Word Spelling
TOD-2S: Letter and Word Choice	TOD-8C: Word Pattern Choice
TOD-3Sa: Word Reading Fluency	TOD-15C: Regular Word Spelling
TOD-3Sb: Question Reading Fluency	TOD 16C: Silent Reading Efficiency

Timed Tests

Several of the TOD tests require the examinee to complete as many items, or provide as many responses as they can, within a specific time limit. A stopwatch is required for the timed tests and conveniently most smart phones have this feature. For some tests, the examinee writes or marks responses in the Response Booklet. Other tests require the examinee to provide oral responses. Rapid Reference 2.3 lists the timed tests, response formats, and time limits.

Audio-Recorded Tests

Only one test in the TOD-C requires an audio recording, Test 13C: Blending. The recording is for Items 16–29 which are the most difficult items to present correctly. Those items range from one-syllable words with three phonemes to multisyllabic words with up to 11 phonemes. Without the recording, the evaluator would need to present each word as separate phonemes pausing one second between each phoneme. To ensure a standardized administration, use the digital recording.

Before administering this test, download the digital recording from the WPS (Online Evaluation System (OES)). Log into the OES. Select the Assessments menu option then choose My Assessments. Select

DON'T FORGET

If planning to administer Test 13-C: Blending, be sure to download the digital recording prior to beginning the evaluation.

≡ Rapid Reference 2.3

Timed Tests, Response Formats, and Time Limits

TOD-Screener-Print	Response Format	Time Limit
3Sa: Word Reading Fluency	Response Booklet	Two minutes
3Sb: Question Reading Fluency	Response Booklet	Three minutes
TOD-Screener-Online	**Response Format**	**Time Limit**
3Sa: Word Reading Fluency	Computer, Tablet	Two minutes
3Sb: Question Reading Fluency	Computer, Tablet	Three minutes
TOD-Comprehensive	**Response Format**	**Time Limit**
6C: Rapid Letter Naming	Oral	One minute
8C: Word Pattern Choice	Response Booklet	Two minutes
12C: Oral Reading Efficiency	Oral	One minute
16C: Silent Reading Efficiency	Response Booklet	Five minutes (Grade 1–5)
		Eight minutes (Grade 6–Adult)
TOD-Early	**Response Format**	**Time Limit**
6E: Early Rapid Number and Letter Naming	Oral	One minute

TOD from the drop-down list. From the TOD menu bar, select Audio and then click where indicated to download the recording. Adjust the volume to an appropriate level prior to test administration.

Sample Items

Sample items are used to ensure the examinee understands the task before the actual test items are administered. Be sure to administer the Sample Items correctly, following all pointing and corrective feedback instruction. In some cases, the first Sample Item has the evaluator demonstrate the task and then the examinee is asked to complete the second Sample Item. Acknowledge correct responses and provide feedback for incorrect responses.

Item Prompting Requirements

To help keep testing efficient, a number of TOD tests allow the evaluator to encourage a response after a specified number of seconds has elapsed and the examinee has not responded. For example, some tests prompt after a five-second delay, and if there is no response, the item is scored 0 and the next item is presented. Two of the TOD-S tests, five of the TOD-E tests, and eight of the TOD-C tests use the five-second prompting.

For the rapid naming tests or other speeded tests, if there is no response in three seconds, score the item 0 and move the examinee to the next item. Point to the next item and say "Go ahead." Tests that use the three-second prompt include one test in TOD-E and five tests in TOD-C.

Two spelling tests in the TOD-C provide a 10-second response time before moving the examinee to the next item. If an examinee requests more time, however, or is still writing, allow more time. Rapid Reference 2.4 lists the tests that use either the 3-, 5-, or 10-second prompt.

Two TOD-C tests use one other type of prompting: 9C: Word Memory and 18C: Letter Memory. Both of these tests require the examinee to repeat the stimuli backward. If the examinee repeats the stimulus as presented (forward), score the item 0 and prompt the examinee by saying, "Remember to say them backward."

≡ Rapid Reference 2.4

Tests That Use 3-, 5-, or 10-second Item Prompting

TOD-Screener	Prompt
1S: Picture Vocabulary	Five seconds
2S: Letter and Word Choice	Five seconds
TOD-Early	
4E: Sounds and Pseudowords	Five seconds
5E: Rhyming	Five seconds
6E: Early Rapid Number and Letter Naming	Three seconds
7E: Letter and Sight Word Recognition	Five seconds
8E: Early Segmenting	Five seconds
9E: Letter and Sound Knowledge	Five seconds

TOD-Comprehensive

4C: Phonological Manipulation	Five seconds
5C: Irregular Word Spelling	10 seconds
6C: Rapid Letter Naming	Three seconds
7C: Pseudoword Reading	Five seconds
9C: Word Memory	Five seconds
11C: Irregular Word Reading	Five seconds
12C: Oral Reading Efficiency	Three seconds
13C: Blending	Five seconds
14C: Segmenting	Five seconds
15C: Regular Word Spelling	10 seconds
17C: Rapid Number and Letter Naming	Three seconds
18C: Letter Memory	Five seconds
19C: Rapid Pseudoword Reading	Three seconds
20C: Rapid Irregular Word Reading	Three seconds
21C: Listening Vocabulary	Five seconds

FREE ONLINE SCORING

The WPS OES provides free scoring when the print version of the TOD-S Scoring Sheet or the Record Forms for TOD-C and TOD-E have been purchased. The item scores recorded by hand during testing or after the test administration (for tests completed in a Response Booklet) are entered into the WPS OES to obtain the appropriate score report. Intervention reports are also available at no charge. The WPS OES is located at the WPS website: wpspublish.com. Select the Assess Online (OES) tab to access the online scoring platform. Registration is required to use the scoring program.

Manual Scoring

Scoring can also be completed manually by using the Norm book that accompanies the test. Enter all item scores into the TOD-C or TOD-E Record Form or the Screener Scoring Sheet. Items scored during the test administration are already recorded in the Record Form. However, some tests that use the Response Booklet are scored after the testing is completed. Be sure to include any of those item scores in the Record Form. For each test administered, enter the total number correct in the Total Raw Score boxes in the Record Form or Scoring Sheet, with one exception. For the Oral Reading Efficiency test, 12C, the Total Raw Score is obtained by subtracting the Number of Errors from Words Read Correctly. Transfer those raw scores to the Score Summary page on the cover of the Record Form or Scoring Sheet. Consult the appropriate Appendix Tables in the Norm book to obtain the standard scores, percentiles, and age- or grade-equivalents. Fortunately, the Record Forms provide detailed directions for completing the score summary. To facilitate locating the correct tables, color-coding is used in the Norm book: Tan for TOD-S, green for TOD-C, and blue for TOD-E. There are fold-out pages on the TOD-C and TOD-E Record Forms that provide places to calculate the index and composite scores, make score comparisons, and plot profiles.

Test Observations

Qualitative information provides valuable insights into the strengths and weaknesses of the individual being assessed and can help inform instructional planning. Evaluators are encouraged to note test behaviors on the Record Form during testing and, after testing, conduct an error analysis within and across tests. To assist in collecting important examinee information, the TOD-C and TOD-E Record Forms include a Test Observation Worksheet. Figure 2.2 presents the Test Observation Worksheet.

TEST OBSERVATION WORKSHEET

Directions: *Please answer each question by circling Yes or No. Use the Observations section below if more room is needed for explanations.*

Does the examinee have prescription glasses or contact lenses?	Yes	No
If yes, were they used during testing?	Yes	No
Does the examinee have a hearing aid?	Yes	No
If yes, was the hearing aid used during testing?	Yes	No
Is English the examinee's first language? If no, what is the first language? _______	Yes	No
Did the examinee write legibly and with ease?	Yes	No
Did the examinee exhibit any unusual behaviors, such as refusing to do a task or making inappropriate comments? If yes, briefly describe: _______	Yes	No

Directions: *Please rate each statement by circling one of the options. Use the Observations section below if more room is needed for explanations.*

	Strongly Agree	Agree	Disagree	Strongly Disagree
Examinee was cooperative.	SA	A	D	SD
Examinee seemed confident.	SA	A	D	SD
Rapport was established easily.	SA	A	D	SD
Examinee's attention was age appropriate.	SA	A	D	SD
Examinee's activity level was age appropriate.	SA	A	D	SD
Examinee's oral communication was age appropriate.	SA	A	D	SD
Examinee seemed to understand the test directions.	SA	A	D	SD
Examinee persevered as items increased in difficulty. If you disagree/strongly disagree, briefly explain: _______	SA	A	D	SD
The test results represent a fair/valid estimate of the examinee's current abilities. If you disagree/strongly disagree, briefly explain: _______	SA	A	D	SD

OBSERVATIONS ____

Figure 2.2   Test Observation Worksheet

The worksheet provides additional space to add other relevant information, such as notes about the examinee's response patterns and any questions asked during the testing session. It might be helpful to think about how the examinee responds and whether the response style changes based on the skill being assessed. Was the examinee quick and accurate in responding? Slow and accurate? Quick and inaccurate? Slow and inaccurate? Noting specific types of errors and how the examinee responds when items become more difficult may help when making specific recommendations and planning an instructional program. This type of qualitative information can be useful when writing reports.

DON'T FORGET

The Importance of Qualitative Information

- Use the Test Observation Worksheet to document observational data regarding the examinee's response style, level of effort, attention, persistence, level of cooperation, and conversational proficiency.
- Analyze the errors that are made within and across tests to help inform instructional planning.
- Use the TOD Rating Scales to gather additional information from teachers, parents, and the examinee.

TEST YOURSELF

1. **The TOD-S must be administered first in all cases. True or False?**

2. **The TOD-E does not require which one of the following materials?**
   (a) Response Booklet
   (b) Record Form
   (c) Test Easel
   (d) Stopwatch

3. **Which of the following tests uses the digital audio-recording?**
   (a) 4E: Sounds and Pseudowords
   (b) 6E: Early Segmenting
   (c) 4C: Phonological Manipulation
   (d) 13C: Blending

4. **Which test is timed?**
   (a) 2S: Letter and Word Choice
   (b) 5E: Rhyming
   (c) 8C: Word Pattern Choice
   (d) 20C: Symbol to Sound Learning

5. **Which tests do not require the use of a Response Booklet? (Choose all that apply).**
   (a) 1S: Picture Vocabulary
   (b) 7E: Letter and Sight Word Recognition

(c) 12C: Oral Reading Efficiency

(d) 15C: Regular Word Spelling

6. **If an individual is performing above or below their grade level, always select the Start Point at their current grade level.**
True or False?

7. **When calculating the examinee's chronological age, ignore the days.**
True or False?

8. **On a rapid naming test, how much time is allowed for individuals to respond before scoring the item 0 and moving them to the next item?**

(a) Three seconds

(b) Two seconds

(c) One second

(d) Five seconds

9. **When may the evaluator repeat a test item?**

(a) Anytime the examinee requests it

(b) When the evaluator determines it is necessary

(c) At the request of the examinee when the directions allow

(d) Only on tests that are not timed

10. **When administering TOD-1S: Picture Vocabulary, when do you discontinue testing?**

(a) At the three-minute time limit

(b) After four consecutive errors

(c) After five consecutive errors

(d) After all items in the assigned set are administered

Answers: 1. True; 2. a; 3. d; 4. c; 5. b and c; 6. False; 7. False; 8. a; 9. c; 10. d

REFERENCES

American Educational Research Association, American Psychological Association, & National Council on Measurement in Education. (2014). *Standards for educational and psychological testing*. American Educational Research Association.

Mather, N., McCallum, R. S., Bell, S. M., & Wendling, B. J. (2024b). *Tests of Dyslexia (TOD)* [Manual]. Western Psychological Services.

Mather, N., McCallum, R. S., Bell, S. M., & Wendling, B. J. (2024c). *Dyslexia interventions and recommendations: A companion guide to the Tests of Dyslexia (TOD)*. Western Psychological Services.

Mather, N., McCallum, R. S., Bell, S. M., & Wendling, B. J. (2024d). *Tests of Dyslexia (TOD)* [Norms Book]. Western Psychological Services.

Three

ADMINISTRATION OF THE TOD-SCREENER AND THE TOD-EARLY

This chapter provides a detailed review of the administration procedures for the TOD-Screener (TOD-S) and TOD-Early (TOD-E). After studying the test administration procedures in this chapter, it is recommended to complete a few practice administrations.

TOD-SCREENER

The TOD-S is composed of three tests: 1S: Picture Vocabulary, 2S: Letter and Word Choice, and 3Sa: Word Reading Fluency or 3Sb: Question Reading Fluency. The age range for the TOD-S is five years to adult, the grade range is K to grade 12.9. The test materials include the *Administration Guide*, a Scoring Sheet, and a Response Booklet. The Response Booklets are organized into three levels: Grades K–1, Grades 2–5, and Grades 6–Adult. Each Response Booklet includes the appropriate range of items for the intended grade ranges. The TOD-S may be administered to an individual or to a group as a paper or digital version. Using either option, the evaluator uses the *Administration Guide* for each test. The *Print* directions are used for the paper version, and the *Digital* directions are used for the digital version. All items for the three TOD-S tests are in the Response Booklets or appear on the tablet. The TOD-S is always administered first before either the TOD-E or TOD-C.

The primary purpose of the TOD-S is to provide a quick and reliable screening for dyslexia. The three tests can be completed in 10–15 minutes. After testing, standard scores, age or grade equivalents, percentile ranks, significant differences between scores, and standard score profiles can be calculated. An important feature of the TOD-S is the Dyslexia Risk Index (DRI). This index provides an indication of the risk for dyslexia and whether further assessment is needed.

The TOD-S is a standalone screening test, but also serves as the first three tests for the TOD-E and TOD-C. For this reason, the TOD-S tests contribute to indexes and composites across the entire age and grade spans of the TOD-E and TOD-C. Rapid Reference 3.1

≋ Rapid Reference 3.1

Indexes, Abbreviations, and Tests Required

TOD-S: Dyslexia Risk Index (DRI)	Tests 2 and 3
TOD-E: Early Dyslexia Diagnostic Index (EDDI)	Tests, 2, 3, and 4–9
TOD-E: Early Reading and Spelling Index (ERSI)	Tests 2, 3, 4, 7, and 9
TOD-E: Early Linguistic Processing Index (ELPI)	Tests 5, 6, and 8

provides the names of the indexes and their abbreviations, and lists the tests required for each index. The abbreviations for the indexes are used throughout this chapter.

PICTURE VOCABULARY (TOD-1S)

TOD-1S: Picture Vocabulary (Rapid Reference 3.2) is a measure of receptive vocabulary which requires knowledge of the meanings of words heard or read. A person's vocabulary knowledge is a good indicator of their general language skills. The task requires the examinee to look at four pictures and choose the one that best depicts the word that the examiner says orally. This test contributes to the Vocabulary, Vocabulary and Reasoning 2, and the Vocabulary and Reasoning 4 composites.

Administration: This test requires the *Administration Guide*, a Scoring Sheet, the correct Response Booklet, and a pencil for the examinee. For the *Digital* administration, the *Administration Guide,* a computer or tablet, and an internet connection are required. The correct Response Booklet must be cued up on the tablet. The Scoring Sheet is not needed as scoring is done automatically. All examinees begin with Samples A and B. The table in the *Administration Guide* shows the Item Set to administer

DON'T FORGET

The TOD-S is administered first whether the intent is to conduct a screening test or to complete a comprehensive evaluation using the TOD-E or TOD-C. (See Chapter 4 for TOD-C information.)

CAUTION

Ensure the correct version of the three Response Booklets is used when administering the TOD-S: Grades K–1, Grades 2–5, and Grades 6–Adult. The Response Booklet includes all of the items for the TOD-S tests.

DON'T FORGET

The TOD-S can be administered to an individual or a group. All individuals in the group must use the same level of the Response Booklet. The TOD-S is available as a print or digital version.

to the examinee. All items in the assigned set are administered, and there is no Stop Rule. For example, after completing Samples A and B, examinees in Grades 2–5 are administered Items 11–40.

Present Sample Item A orally. Follow all directions and read the bolded teal words verbatim. Sample A serves as a demonstration item, illustrating what the examinee is asked to do on Sample Item B and all test items. On Sample B, if the examinee's response is correct, then confirm the response using the teal text. If the examinee is incorrect, provide the corrective feedback indicated and then move on to the start item based on the examinee's grade.

Be sure to know the correct pronunciation of all items. Pronunciation guidance is provided in the *Administration Guide* for a few of the more difficult items. Review all words in advance to ensure correct pronunciation of each item. Repeat any item if the examinee requests it.

Item Scoring: For the *Print* administration, generally the examinee's Response Booklet is used after administering the test to score each response on the Scoring Sheet. Write the number of the examinee's response in the blank provided for each item. Compare it to the correct number shown in parentheses. If the examinee's response is correct, circle the 1; if the response is incorrect, circle the 0. For the *Digital* administration, the scoring is done automatically as the examinee taps each response on the tablet.

Potential administration errors: Administration errors may include not using (or cueing up) the correct Response Booklet, mispronouncing the words, not repeating an item if requested, not administering the correct Item Set, or not completing the assigned Item Set.

≡ Rapid Reference 3.2

Important Administration Points for 1S: Picture Vocabulary

- Have the necessary materials: Administration Guide, Response Booklet, Scoring Sheet, and pencil (Digital version does not require the Scoring Sheet, Response Booklet, or pencil).
- Use the correct Response Booklet for the examinee (K–1; 2–5; 6–Adult).
- Cue up the correct Response Booklet when using the digital option.
- Know the correct pronunciation of all words on the test.
- Administer Samples A and B to all examinees.
- Administer all items in the assigned Item Set.
- Repeat any item if the examinee requests it.
- Scoring generally occurs after the test is completed when using the paper version.
- Scoring is done automatically when using the digital version.

LETTER AND WORD CHOICE (TOD-2S)

TOD-2S: Letter and Word Choice (Rapid Reference 3.3) measures the individual's ability to recognize letters and correctly spelled words. The task requires the examinee to look at four letters or four words and select the correct letter or correctly spelled word that the evaluator says. Identifying the correctly spelled word requires both phonological and orthographic knowledge. This test contributes to the DRI, the EDDI, the ERSI, and the Early Sight Word Acquisition composite. This test is also an indicator of early spelling recognition.

Administration: This test requires the *Administration Guide*, a Scoring Sheet, the correct Response Booklet, and a pencil for the examinee. For the *Digital* administration, the *Administration Guide* is required and the correct Response Booklet must be cued up on the tablet. The Scoring Sheet is not needed as scoring is done automatically and the examinee does not need a pencil. Consult the table in the *Administration Guide* to determine the correct Item Set to administer. All items in the assigned set are administered, and there is no Stop Rule. For example, for Grades K–1, after administering Samples A and B, administer Items 1–30.

For Grades K–1 only, present Sample Item A orally. Follow all directions and read the bolded teal words verbatim. Sample A serves as a demonstration item, illustrating what the examinee is asked to do on Sample Item B and all test items. On Sample B, if the examinee's response is correct, then confirm the response using the teal text. If the examinee is incorrect, provide the corrective feedback indicated and then move on to the start item which is Item 1.

For all other grades, begin administering the test with the first item in the assigned Item Set. Grades 2–5 begin with Item 12 and Grades 6–Adult begin with Item 24.

Be sure to know the correct pronunciation of all items. Pronunciation guidance is provided in the *Administration Guide* for a few of the more difficult items. Review the words in advance to ensure correct pronunciation of each item.

Allow five seconds for the examinee to respond. If no response is given, score the item 0 and then move on to the next item. Repeat any item if an examinee requests it.

Item scoring: For a *Print* administration, generally the examinee's Response Booklet is used after administering the test to score each response and record it on the Scoring Sheet. For purposes of recording an examinee's response, assign numbers 1–4 to the item response options. Write the number of the examinee's response in the blank provided for each item. Compare it to the correct number shown in parentheses. If the examinee's response is correct, circle the 1; if the response is incorrect or skipped, circle the 0. For a *Digital* administration, the scoring is done automatically as the examinee taps each response on the tablet.

DON'T FORGET

Administer the complete Item Set for each examinee on Tests 1S: Picture Vocabulary and 2S: Letter and Word Choice.

Potential administration errors: Administration errors may include not using (or cueing up) the correct Response Booklet, mispronouncing the words, not repeating an item if requested, not scoring the item 0 and then moving an examinee to the next item if there is no response after five seconds, not administering the correct Item Set, or not completing the assigned Item Set.

WORD READING FLUENCY (TOD-3Sa)

TOD-3Sa: Word Reading Fluency (Rapid Reference 3.4) measures reading automaticity, a basic word reading skill under timed conditions. The task requires the examinee to look at a picture and then select the correct word that corresponds with the picture from a row of four words as quickly as possible. This test contributes to the DRI, EDDI, and ERSI indexes.

Administration: This test requires the *Administration Guide*, a Scoring Sheet, a stopwatch or timer, the correct Response Booklet, and a pencil for the examinee. For the *Digital* administration, an internet connection and tablet with the correct Response Booklet cued up are needed in addition to the *Administration Guide*. There is no need for a stopwatch or the Scoring Sheet as timing and scoring are done automatically. Test 3Sa is administered to individuals in Grades K–1. For *Print* administration, be sure to use the K–1 Response Booklet and provide the examinee with a pencil. Also, have a stopwatch or timer available. For *Digital* administration, cue up the correct Response Booklet in advance. The examinee taps the responses on the tablet so a pencil is not needed. The program stops the test at the time limit so no stopwatch is needed. Administer Samples A, B, C, and D. Follow all directions for pointing and feedback carefully. Read the bolded teal text verbatim for each Sample Item and for the introduction to the test items. This test has a two-minute time limit. Once the test begins, do not read any words to the examinee. The directions indicate the examinees should make their best guess or skip the item if they can't decide. If an examinee pauses or stops, prompt them to move on to the next item by saying: **Go ahead. Keep going**. When administering the *Print* version, at the end of two minutes, say: **Stop. Please put your pencil down**.

≡ *Rapid Reference 3.4*

Important Administration Points for 3Sa: Word Reading Fluency

- Have the necessary materials: Administration Guide, Response Booklet, Scoring Sheet, stopwatch, and pencil (Digital version: Administration Guide, internet connection, and tablet).
- Administer to examinees in Grades K–1.
- Use the correct Response Booklet for the examinee (K–1).
- Cue up the correct Response Booklet when using the digital option.
- Administer all Sample Items (A–D).
- Once the timed test begins, if the examinee stops or pauses, prompt to continue by saying: **Go ahead. Keep going**.
- Do not read any words to the examinee once the timed test begins.
- If unsure of a response, examinees are told to guess or skip items.
- Time the test for two minutes when using a *Print* administration, then say: **Stop. Please put your pencil down**. During a *Digital* administration, the program stops the test automatically at two minutes.
- Scoring generally occurs after the test is completed when using the paper version.
- Scoring is done automatically when using the *Digital* version.

When administering the *Digital* version, the program stops the test automatically at two minutes.

Item scoring: For a *Print* administration, generally the examinee's Response Booklet is used after administering the test to score each response on the Scoring Sheet. For purposes of recording an examinee's response, assign numbers 1–4 to the item response options. Write the number of the examinee's response in the blank provided for each item. Compare it to the correct number shown in parentheses. If the examinee's response is correct, circle the 1; if the response is incorrect or skipped, circle the 0. For a *Digital* administration, the scoring is done automatically as the examinee taps each response on the tablet.

Potential administration errors: Administration errors may include not presenting the sample items correctly, not prompting the examinee to keep going, not adhering to the two-minute time limit, reading any words to the examinee once the timed test begins, or for the Digital administration, not prompting the examinee to begin responding as soon as the first item is presented.

QUESTION READING FLUENCY (TOD-3Sb)

TOD-3Sb: Question Reading Fluency (Rapid Reference 3.5) measures reading rate and comprehension under timed conditions. The task requires the examinee to read a question silently and then select the correct response from a row of four words as quickly as possible. This test contributes to the DRI, EDDI, and ERSI indexes.

> ### ≋ Rapid Reference 3.5
>
> **Important Administration Points for 3Sb: Question Reading Fluency**
>
> - Have the necessary materials: Administration Guide, Response Booklet, Scoring Sheet, stopwatch, and pencil (Digital version: Administration Guide, internet connection, and tablet).
> - Administer to examinees in Grades 2–Adult.
> - Use the correct Response Booklet for the examinee (Grades 2–5 or 6–Adult). Cue up the correct Response Booklet when using the digital option.
> - Administer all Sample Items (A–D).
> - Once the timed test begins, if the examinee stops or pauses, prompt to continue by saying: **Go ahead. Keep going**.
> - If unsure of a response, examinees are told to skip items.
> - Do not read any questions or words to the examinee once the timed test begins.
> - For *Print* administration, time the test for three minutes then say: **Stop. Please put your pencil down.** During a *Digital* administration, the program stops the test automatically at three minutes.
> - Scoring occurs after the test is completed when using the paper version.
> - Scoring is done automatically when using the digital version.

Administration: This test requires the *Administration Guide*, a Scoring Sheet, a stopwatch or timer, the correct Response Booklet, and a pencil for the examinee. For the *Digital* administration, an internet connection, tablet with the correct Response Booklet cued up, and the *Administration Guide* are required. A stopwatch and the Scoring Sheet are not needed as timing and scoring are done automatically. Test 3Sb: Question Reading Fluency is administered to individuals in Grades 2–Adult. Select the correct Response Booklet (Grades 2–5 or Grades 6–Adult), provide the examinee with a pencil, and have a stopwatch or timer available. When using a *Digital* administration, cue up the correct Response Booklet on the tablet. No pencil or stopwatch is needed. Administer Samples A, B, C, and D to all examinees. Follow all pointing and feedback instructions carefully. Read the bolded teal text verbatim for all Samples and the introduction to the test. This test has a three-minute time limit. Once the test begins, do not read any questions or words to the examinee. The directions indicate they should skip any item if they can't decide. If an examinee pauses or stops, prompt them to move on to the next item, by saying: **Go ahead. Keep going**. At the end of three minutes say: **Stop. Please put your pencil down**. When administering the *Digital* version, the program stops the test automatically at three minutes.

Item scoring: For a *Print* administration, the examinee's Response Booklet is used after administering the test to score each response on the Scoring Sheet. For purposes of recording an examinee's response, assign numbers 1–4 to the item response options. Write the number of the examinee's response in the blank provided for each item. Compare it to the correct number shown in parentheses. If the examinee's response is correct, circle the 1; if incorrect or skipped circle the 0. For a *Digital* administration, the scoring is done automatically as the examinee taps each response on the tablet.

Potential administration errors: Administration errors may include not presenting the sample items correctly, not prompting the examinee to keep going, not adhering to the three-minute time limit, or reading any questions or words to the examinee once the timed test begins.

TOD-EARLY (TOD-E)

The TOD-E is composed of an additional six tests: 4E: Sounds and Pseudowords, 5E: Rhyming, 6E: Early Rapid Number and Letter Naming, 7E: Letter and Sight Word Recognition, 8E: Early Segmenting, and 9E: Letter and Sound Knowledge. All six tests are presented in the TOD-E Stimulus Easel. The tests are organized by tabs. The first page behind each tab provides the description of the test, the start points, Basal and Stop (ceiling) Rules, scoring guidance, and directions for the test. The six TOD-E tests are used in conjunction with the three tests in the TOD-S to create a more comprehensive nine test battery. The grade range for the TOD-E is K–2. The TOD-E, as opposed to the TOD-C, would typically be administered to students in Grades 1 and 2 who are known to have low reading skills.

The TOD-E (with the TOD-S) yields three index scores: EDDI, ERSI, and ELPI. The EDDI is composed of the ERSI and the ELPI. The EDDI can help document whether a young child is exhibiting characteristics of dyslexia. Figure 3.1 presents the TOD-S and TOD-E Test Selection Chart from Table 1.5 in the TOD Manual. Consult this chart to determine which tests need to be administered to obtain any of the indexes or composites. This chart is particularly helpful if the TOD-S results indicate a need for further assessment or when specific skill areas are of interest.

SOUNDS AND PSEUDOWORDS (TOD-4E)

TOD-4E: Sounds and Pseudowords (Rapid Reference 3.6) measures knowledge of sound-letter correspondences. This test has three sections. In the first section, the evaluator presents a sound orally and the examinee points to or says the number of the picture that begins with

			Indexes			Reading and Spelling					Linguistic Processing		Vocabulary
			EDDI	ERSI	ELPI	Composites			Tests		Composite	Test	Test
	Test number	TOD-Early	Early Dyslexia Diagnostic Index	Early Reading and Spelling Index	Early Linguistic Processing Index	Early Sight Word Acquisition	Early Phonics Knowledge	Early Basic Reading Skills	Letter and Word Choice (Early Spelling Recognition)	Word or Question Reading Fluency	Early Phonological Awareness	Early Rapid Number and Letter Naming	Picture Vocabulary[a]
TOD-S	1S	Picture Vocabulary[a]											✓
TOD-S	2S	Letter and Word Choice	✓	✓		✓			✓				
TOD-S	3S	Word or Question Reading Fluency	✓	✓						✓			
TOD-E	4E	Sounds and Pseudowords	✓	✓			✓						
TOD-E	5E	Rhyming	✓		✓						✓		
TOD-E	6E	Early Rapid Number and Letter Naming	✓		✓							✓	
TOD-E	7E	Letter and Sight Word Recognition	✓	✓		✓		✓					
TOD-E	8E	Early Segmenting	✓		✓						✓		
TOD-E	9E	Letter and Sound Knowledge	✓	✓			✓	✓					

[a]Picture Vocabulary can be used in interpreting the EDDI

Figure 3.1   TOD-S and TOD-E Test Selection Chart

≡ *Rapid Reference 3.6*

Important Administration Points for 4E: Sounds and Pseudowords

- Have the necessary materials: TOD-E Easel, Record Form.
- Begin with Sample A for examinees in Grade K.
- Begin with Sample C for examinees in Grades 1–2.
- When starting with Sample C, if the examinee misses items 6 and 7, go back and administer Samples A and B and Items 1–5.
- Basal Rule: Item 1 or 4 consecutive correct responses.
- Stop Rule: 4 consecutive errors.
- When a letter is presented between slash marks (e.g., /f/) say the sound the letter makes not the letter name. Do not add a schwa (uh) to the consonant sound.
- If the examinee adds a schwa sound to a correct consonant sound (e.g., /buh/ not /b/), score it as correct.
- If an examinee pauses for more than five seconds, encourage a response, score the item 0 if there is no response after prompting, and present the next item.
- For Items 1–5, any item may be repeated one time if requested.

---

that sound. In the second section, the examinee is shown a letter and asked to say the sound the letter makes. In the third section, the examinee reads aloud phonically regular pseudowords. This test contributes to the EDDI and ERSI indexes and the Early Phonics Knowledge composite.

Administration: This test requires the TOD-E Stimulus Easel and a Record Form. Start with Samples A and B for examinees in Grade K. Begin the test with Item 1. Item 1 serves as the basal. Continue testing until the examinee has 4 consecutive errors. On Items 1–5, if the examinee requests it, the item may be repeated one time.

CAUTION

When administering the TOD-E, be careful not to add a schwa sound when pronouncing consonant sounds.

For Samples A-C and Items 1–5, when a letter is shown between slash marks (e.g., /f/) say the sound the letter makes, not the name of letter. Also, be careful not to add a schwa sound (uh) when pronouncing the consonants (e.g., /d/ not /duh/).

Examinees in Grades 1 and 2, begin with Sample C. Testing continues with Item 6. If the examinee responds *incorrectly* to Item 6 and 7, go back to Samples A and B and administer Items 1–5. If the examinee has 4 consecutive errors, discontinue testing. If not, then return to Item 8 and continue until the Stop Rule (4 consecutive errors) has been met. For Items 6–15, if the examinee adds a schwa sound to a correct consonant sound, score the item as correct. For example, if the letter is "t" and the examinee says /tuh/ or /t/, score it as correct.

In the third section of this test, reading pseudowords aloud, guidance is provided for scoring the examinee's response. The correct key includes the pseudoword and, in parentheses, provides either a real word that rhymes with the pseudoword or provides the nonsense word written in syllables. These examples illustrate acceptable pronunciations.

On all three sections of this test, if an examinee pauses on any item for more than five seconds, encourage a response. If there is still no response, score the item 0 and present the next item.

Item scoring: Score each item during the test to determine when Basal and Stop Rules are met. Score correct items as 1 and incorrect or skipped items as 0. Count all items below the basal as correct. For the second section of this test (Items 6–15), the examinee is asked to provide the sound the letter makes. In scoring these responses, if the examinee adds a schwa sound to the correct consonant sound, score it as correct. For example, for the letter "b" if the examinee says /b/ or /buh/, the response is scored as correct.

> **CAUTION**
>
> Follow the Basal Rule information carefully for examinees in Grades 1 and 2. Some examinees may need to go back to the beginning of the test.

Potential administration errors: Administration errors include not pronouncing the sounds correctly, not encouraging a response if the examinee pauses for more than five seconds, not scoring the item 0 and presenting the next item if there is no response after prompting, or not following the Basal Rule if starting with Sample C.

RHYMING (TOD-5E)

TOD-5E: Rhyming (Rapid Reference 3.7) measures one aspect of phonological awareness, an important prereading skill and strong predictor of future reading skill. Early items on this test require the examinee to point to a picture (or say the number of the picture) that rhymes with the word the evaluator presents orally. Each item presents four pictures. The first picture represents the item word the evaluator presents. The remaining three pictures are the response options, only one of which rhymes with the item word. For later items, the evaluator says a word aloud and the examinee provides a word that rhymes. To receive credit, the word must be a real word that rhymes with the item word. This test contributes to the EDDI and ELPI indexes and is an indicator of early phonological awareness.

Administration: This test requires the TOD-E Stimulus Easel and a Record Form. Begin with Sample A for examinees in Grade K. The basal is Item 1 and testing continues until 4 consecutive errors are made. For Grades 1–2, begin with Sample C and then administer Item 11. If the examinee misses Item 11, go back to Samples A and B and Items 1–10. Continue testing until the examinee makes 4 consecutive errors. Continue to Item 12 if the Stop Rule was not met after Items 1–11 were administered.

- For Items 1–10, read each item aloud. For Items 11–30, point to the appropriate picture and read the teal item text aloud.
- For Items 1–10, if requested by the examinee, repeat any item one time.
- For all items in the test, if the examinee pauses on any item for more than five seconds, encourage a response and if no response is given, score the item 0 and present the next item.

≡ *Rapid Reference 3.7*

Important Administration Points for 5E: Rhyming

- Have the necessary materials: TOD-E Easel and Record Form.
- Begin with Sample A for examinees in Grade K.
- Begin with Sample C for examinees in Grades 1–2.
- When starting with Sample C, if the examinee misses Item 11, go back and administer Samples A and B and Items 1–10.
- Basal Rule: Item 1 or 4 consecutive correct responses.
- Stop Rule: 4 consecutive errors.
- If examinee pauses for more than five seconds, encourage a response; if no response is given, score the item 0 and present the next item.
- For Items 1–10, repeat any item one time if requested.
- For Items 11–30, point to the Item's picture in the Test Easel before administering the item.

Item scoring: Score each item as testing proceeds to determine when the Basal and Stop Rules are met. Score correct items as 1 and incorrect or skipped items as 0. Count all items below the basal as correct. On Items 11–30, score real words that rhyme with the item word as correct, even if the real word is not listed in the Correct Key. Score nonsense words, even if they rhyme, as incorrect.

DON'T FORGET

For Items 11–30 in Test 5E: Rhyming, score as correct any real word that rhymes with the item word. The Correct Key does not include all possible correct responses. Score nonsense words that rhyme as incorrect.

Potential administration errors: Administration errors include not encouraging a response if the examinee pauses for more than five seconds, not scoring the item 0 and presenting the next item if no response after prompting, not following the Basal Rule if starting with Sample C, not pointing to the picture first when administering Items 11–30, or accepting a nonsense word that rhymes as correct.

EARLY RAPID NUMBER AND LETTER NAMING (TOD-6E)

TOD-6E: Early Rapid Number and Letter Naming (see Rapid Reference 3.8) measures fluency using an alphanumeric rapid naming task. The examinee is presented with rows of letters and numbers in a random sequence and names as many as possible in one minute. Three letters (A, B, C) and three numbers (1, 2, 3) are used as these are learned early by most children. Using these very familiar letters and numbers virtually eliminates limited letter or number knowledge and focuses the task on rapid naming. This test contributes to the EDDI and ELPI indexes and is an indicator of early rapid automatized naming

≋ *Rapid Reference 3.8*

Important Administration Points for 6E: Early Rapid Number and Letter Naming

- Have all necessary materials: TOD-E Easel, Record Form, and stopwatch.
- Start all examinees with Sample A. Follow the directions to continue or discontinue testing. If continuing, follow the directions for Sample B. If continuing, administer Sample C.
- Three samples must be completed correctly (after two trials) in order to administer this test. Follow the Sample Item directions carefully.
- Use the TOD-E Stimulus Easel to present all items.
- Use a stopwatch to time the test for one minute.
- When introducing the test items, point to the A in the first row as directed.
- If the examinee pauses for three seconds on any number or letter, score the item 0, point to the next number or letter, and say: **Go ahead.**
- It is easier to mark only incorrect responses in the Record Form during testing, especially when an examinee is naming the items very quickly.
- Be ready to turn the Easel page as soon as the examinee reads the last letter or number on the page (after Items 30, 60, and 90).
- The Record Form includes a note of when to turn the page in the easel (Turn Easel Page Here).
- Turn the easel page with the non-dominant hand and use the dominant hand to record the scores in the Record Form.

Administration: This test requires the TOD-E Stimulus Easel, a Record Form, and a stopwatch or timer. Begin with Sample A for all examinees (Grades K–2) which introduces the three letters A, B, and C. Provide two trials if needed. If the examinee misses one or more letters on the second trial of Sample A, discontinue the test. If continuing, administer Sample B which introduces the three numbers 1, 2, and 3. Provide two trials if needed. If the examinee misses one or more numbers on the second trial, discontinue the test. If continuing, then administer Sample C which introduces rows of the letters and number intermingled. Provide two trials if needed. If the examinee misses one or more of the letters or numbers on the second trial, discontinue the test.

Use a stopwatch for this timed test (one minute). The Test Easel is used to present the stimulus items to the examinee. If the examinee pauses for more than three seconds, score the item 0, point to the next letter or number, and say: **Go ahead.** If the examinee skips a row, redirect them by pointing to the correct row.

Once the test begins, evaluators have to multitask by paying attention to three-second delays in naming, redirecting examinees who skip a row, turning the easel pages immediately after the last item on the page is named, scoring the items, and stopping the test in one minute. It is recommended that evaluators turn the easel pages with their non-dominant hand so that scores can be recorded with their dominant hand. It is easier to mark only incorrect responses during the test rather than trying to score every item. A stopwatch or timer that can be set for one minute can help manage the timing.

Item scoring: Score correct items as 1 and incorrect or skipped items as 0.

Potential administration errors: Administration errors include not following all directions for the Sample Items (A-C), not turning the page in the Easel immediately after the last number or letter is named, not redirecting the examinee if they skip a row, not prompting after a three-second pause, or not adhering to the one-minute time limit.

LETTER AND SIGHT WORD RECOGNITION (TOD-7E)

TOD-7E: Letter and Sight Word Recognition (see Rapid Reference 3.9) is a measure of early basic reading skills. It requires the examinee to identify a named letter (Items 1–5), then name specific letters (Items 6–10), point to a word presented orally in an array of three words (Items 11–14), and then read basic sight words (Items 15–38). This test contributes to the EDDI and ERSI indexes and the Early Sight Word Acquisition and the Early Basic Reading Skills composites.

Administration: This test requires the TOD-E Stimulus Easel and a Record Form. Begin with Sample Items A and B for examinees in Grades K–1. The basal is Item 1 and testing continues until the examinee makes 4 consecutive errors. Begin with Sample C for examinees in Grade 2 and then proceed to Item 11. If the examinee responds *incorrectly* to Items 11 and 12, go back to Samples A and B and administer Items 1–10. Return to Item 13 unless 4 consecutive errors have already been made. If not, continue testing until the Stop Rule has been met.

≡ Rapid Reference 3.9

Important Administration Points for 7E: Letter and Sight Word Recognition

- Have the necessary materials: TOD-E Easel, Record Form.
- Begin with Sample A for examinees in Grades K–1.
- Begin with Sample C for examinees in Grade 2.
- When beginning with Sample C, if the examinee misses both Items 11 and 12, go back to Samples A and B and Items 1–10.
- Basal Rule: Item 1 or 4 consecutive correct responses.
- Stop Rule: 4 consecutive errors.
- For Items 6–10, if the examinee says the sound the letter makes, say: **Tell me the name, not the sound.**
- For Items 6–10 and 15–38, after a five-second pause, encourage a response; if no response, score the item 0 and move to the next item.
- Discontinue saying: **What is this word?** on Items 15–38 once the examinee understands the task.

For Items 6–10, if the examinee says the sound the letter makes, say: **Tell me the name, not the sound.** For Items 6–10 and Items 15–38, encourage a response after five seconds. If no response is given, score the item 0 and move to the next item. For Items 15–38, say: **Go ahead. Try the next one.** On Items 15–38, once it is clear that the examinee understands the task, discontinue saying: **What is this word?**

Item scoring: Score each item as testing proceeds to determine when Basal and Stop Rules are met. Score correct items as 1 and incorrect or skipped items as 0. Count all items below the basal as correct.

Potential administration errors: Administration errors may include not administering the Sample Items correctly, not following the Basal Rule, or not adhering to the directions for no response after five seconds on specific items.

EARLY SEGMENTING (TOD-8E)

TOD-8E: Early Segmenting (see Rapid Reference 3.10) measures the ability to break apart words that are pronounced orally by the evaluator. Segmenting is an essential skill for spelling. The test has three types of tasks that progress in difficulty: Breaking apart compound words (Items 1–5), breaking apart multisyllabic words into syllables (Items 6–13), and breaking apart a word into its individual phonemes (Items 14–25). This test contributes to the EDDI and ELPI indexes and the Early Phonological Awareness composite.

≡ Rapid Reference 3.10

Important Administration Points for 8E: Early Segmenting

- Have the necessary materials: TOD-E Easel, Record Form.
- Begin with Sample A for examinees in Grades K–1.
- Begin with Sample C for examinees in Grade 2.
- When beginning with Sample C, if the examinee misses both Items 14 and 15, go back to Samples A, B, and Items 1–13.
- Follow the Sample directions carefully as testing might be discontinued after Samples A and B.
- Follow the Basal Rule carefully as testing may need to go back to an earlier Start Point.
- Provide the sound a letter makes, not the name when it appears between slash marks.
- For Items 14–25, encourage a response after a five-second pause; if no response, score the item 0 and move on to the next item.
- For Items 14–25, the first time the examinee does not say all the sounds in a word, provide the reminder: **Remember to say each of the sounds in a word.**
- For Items 14–25, if the examinee adds a schwa sound after a correct consonant sound, score it as correct.
- Present all items as whole words. Do not pause between word parts, syllables or phonemes.

Administration: This test requires the TOD-E Stimulus Easel and a Record Form. The basal is either Item 1 or the lowest set of 4 consecutive correct responses. The Stop Rule, or ceiling, is 4 consecutive errors. Begin with Sample A for examinees in Grades K–1. If the examinee responds incorrectly to both trials in Sample A, discontinue the test. If Sample A is correct, then administer Items 1–5. Continue to Sample B unless the examinee has made 4 consecutive errors. If the examinee responds incorrectly to both trials in Sample B, discontinue the test. If Sample B is correct, administer Items 6–13 or until the Stop Rule is met. If the Stop Rule has not been met, then administer Sample C. When presenting Sample C, remember that a letter shown between slash marks (e.g., /m/) indicates the sound the letter makes, not the letter name. Continue to Item 14 whether or not the response to Sample C is correct.

Begin with Sample C for examinees in Grade 2 and then proceed to Item 14. If the examinee responds incorrectly to both Items 14 and 15, go back to Sample A and Items 1–13. Return to Item 16 unless the Stop Rule has been met (4 consecutive errors). Continue testing until the examinee makes 4 consecutive errors.

On Items 14–25, if the examinee pauses for more than five seconds, encourage a response. If there is still no response, score the item 0 and move on to the next item and say: **Here's another one.** Also on Items 14–25, the first time the examinee does not provide all the sounds in a word, score the item 0, and say: **Remember to say each of the sounds in a word.** To assist in the scoring of each item, the Correct Key in the Test Easel shows the individual phonemes and the number of sounds in each word. If the examinee mispronounces a consonant phoneme by adding a schwa sound (e.g., /buh/ instead of /b/), score it as correct.

Repeat any item one time if requested by the examinee. Present all words as whole words. Do not pause between syllables or phonemes.

Item scoring: Score each item as testing proceeds to determine when the Basal and Stop Rules are met. For Items 1–5, the examinee must say the two separate parts of the compound word correctly to receive credit. For Items 6–10, the examinee must say the two separate syllables correctly. For Items 11–13, the examinee must say the three separate syllables correctly. For Items 14–25, the examinee must say the individual phonemes correctly, however, adding a schwa sound to a correct consonant sound is not penalized. Score correct items as 1 and incorrect or skipped items as 0. Count all items below the basal as correct.

Potential administration errors: Administration errors include not administering the Sample Items correctly, not following the discontinue rules in the Sample Items, not following the Basal Rule correctly, saying a letter name rather than the sound when it is presented between slash marks (e.g., /m/), not presenting the items as whole words with no hesitation between the words, syllables or phonemes, or not encouraging a response on Items 14–25 after a five-second pause and then, if no response, scoring the item 0 and presenting the next item.

CAUTION

When administering Test 8E: Early Segmenting, present all words as whole words. Do not pause between the two words in a compound word, the syllables in the two- and three-syllable words, or the phonemes in the words (ranging from two to six sounds).

LETTER AND SOUND KNOWLEDGE (TOD-9E)

TOD-9E: Letter and Sound Knowledge (see Rapid Reference 3.11) measures phoneme-grapheme knowledge, important for mastering the alphabetic principle which is critical for developing literacy skills. This test has three parts. The tasks require the examinee to point to or say the letter or letters that represent the first, then last, and finally the middle sounds in words the evaluator presents orally. This test contributes to the EDDI and ERSI indexes and the Early Phonics Knowledge and Early Basic Reading Skills composites.

Administration: This test requires the TOD-E Stimulus Easel and a Record Form. Begin with Sample A for all examinees (K–2). After Samples A and B are administered, continue to Part 1. In Part 1, repeat a word if requested. Items 1–14 require identifying the letter or letters that make the first sound in a word presented orally by the evaluator. Items 1–8 provide a picture for the word and three choices of the letter or letters for the first sound in the word. Items 9–14 provide a picture for the word but require the examinee to tell what letter makes the first sound. The Stop Rule states that if there are three consecutive errors on Part 1, discontinue Part 1 and begin Part 2. If, however, the examinee misses more than three items in Part 1, then discontinue the test without administering Parts 2 and 3.

In Part 2 (Items 15–23), the task switches to identifying the letter that represents the last sound in a word. In Part 3 (Items 24–31), the examinee is required to identify the letter or letters that make the middle sound of a word. The Stop Rule for Part 2 and Part 3 is three consecutive errors. If the Stop Rule is met on Part 2, then move on to Part 3.

On all Parts (1–3), if the examinee pauses for more than five seconds, encourage a response and if there is no response, score the item 0 and present the next item. In addition, for all parts, always point to the picture before saying the word for each item. Emphasize the words *first, last,* and *middle* when presenting the items.

≡ Rapid Reference 3.11

Important Administration Points for 9E: Letter and Sound Knowledge

- Have the necessary materials: TOD-E Easel and Record Form.
- Begin with Sample A for all examinees (Grades K–2).
- Stop Rules apply to the three separate parts in the test. The rule for each part is three consecutive errors, then move to the next part.
- If the examinee has less than 3 correct responses in Part 1, discontinue the test without administering Parts 2 and 3.
- Always point to the picture before presenting the word orally.
- Emphasize the words *first, last,* or *middle* when administering those items.
- In Part 1, repeat any word if requested.
- Encourage a response after a five-second pause. If there is no response, score the item 0 and present the next item.

Item scoring: Score each item as testing proceeds to determine when to discontinue that part of the test or when to move to the next part of the test. The Stop Rule for each part is three consecutive errors. Score correct items as 1 and incorrect or skipped items as 0.

Potential administration errors: Administration errors may include not pointing to the pictures before saying the words, not repeating a word in Part 1 if requested, not encouraging a response after a five-second pause, not scoring the item 0 if no response after prompting, not moving to the next item, not discontinuing a part or the test based on the Stop Rules, or not saying the sound a letter makes when the letter is presented between slash marks.

🪶 TEST YOURSELF 🪶

1. **On tests that use Basal and Stop Rules, Item 1 is always the Basal.**
   True or False?

2. **On TOD-1S: Picture Vocabulary, the examinee names each picture that is presented.**
   True or False?

3. **With the exception of the timed tests, all TOD-E tests have a Stop rule of 4 consecutive errors.**
   True or False?

4. **For TOD-5E: Rhyming, score responses as correct if they:**
   (a) are a real word that rhymes with the target word.
   (b) are a nonsense word that rhymes with the target word.
   (c) begin with the same first sound.
   (d) both a and b

5. **Which of the following TOD tests require a Response Booklet?**
   (a) Letter and Sound Recognition (7E)
   (b) Letter and Word Choice (2S)
   (c) Early Segmenting (8E)
   (d) Both a and b

6. **On tests that use Item Sets, when is testing discontinued?**
   (a) When the examinee makes 4 consecutive errors
   (b) When the time limit is reached
   (c) When the examinee has fewer than 10 correct
   (d) When all items in the set have been administered

7. **As a general rule on untimed tests in the TOD-E, prompt examinees to keep going**
   (a) if they pause for more than 10 seconds.
   (b) if they pause for more than five seconds.

(c) if they pause for more than three seconds.

(d) never prompt on an untimed test.

8. When a letter is presented between slash marks (e.g., /f/), this means to:

(a) say the name of the letter.

(b) say the sound the letter makes.

(c) provide a word that starts with that letter.

(d) provide a word that starts with that sound.

9. Which one of the following is true about the administration of the TOD-E?

(a) Record all item scores in the Record Form.

(b) Use two Test Easels when administering the TOD-E.

(c) Administer the TOD-E before the TOD-S.

(d) Use the appropriate TOD-E Response Booklet.

10. Which one of the following is *not* true about the digital administration of the TOD-S?

(a) A Scoring Sheet is not required.

(b) A Response Booklet is not required.

(c) Item scores need to be entered into the WPS Online Evaluation System (OES).

(d) A stopwatch is not required for the timed tests.

Answers: 1. False; 2. False; 3. False; 4. a; 5. b; 6. d; 7. b; 8. b; 9. a; 10. c

Four

ADMINISTRATION OF THE TOD-COMPREHENSIVE

The TOD-Comprehensive (TOD-C) was designed to offer a thorough evaluation of the reading, spelling, and linguistic abilities that may be impacted for individuals experiencing reading delays or dyslexia. Normed with the TOD-S (see Chapter 3), the TOD-C builds on the information obtained from the screening test by providing a more complete picture of an individual's strengths and weaknesses and generates information that can help inform a diagnosis of dyslexia and the selection of instructional strategies.

ORGANIZATION OF THE TOD-C

The TOD-C is composed of 23 tests (three from the TOD-S) and may be administered to individuals in Grades 1–12.9 or Ages 6–89 years. The TOD-C test materials include two test easels, Response Booklets, Record Forms, and a digital audio recording. A stopwatch or timer is required for the tests with time limits. Other tests specify a number of seconds to wait for a response. For example, the instructions may say: If there is no response after five seconds, score the item 0 and move on to the next item. For those tests, an evaluator may find a stopwatch helpful although the use of a stopwatch is optional. Before administering any of the TOD-C tests, first administer the three tests in the TOD-S. Not only is the TOD-S a standalone screener, but the three tests are used in combination with various TOD-C tests to form composites and indexes.

The TOD-C battery includes tests 4 through 23. It is not required, nor is it likely, that an evaluator would administer all of the TOD-C tests to an examinee. In some cases, an evaluator may only administer the TOD-S and Tests 4–9 to obtain the Dyslexia Diagnostic Index (DDI), the Reading Spelling Index (RSI) and the Linguistic Processing Index (LPI).

The DDI is an important feature of the TOD-C. This index is composed of eight tests, two from the TOD-S and six from the TOD-C. The purpose of the DDI is to provide a score that indicates the probability that the individual has dyslexia. The RSI measures several important reading and spelling skills and can indicate the severity of an individual's reading and spelling difficulties. The LPI measures several underlying processing abilities that are foundational to and predictive of reading and spelling difficulties. The LPI can be

Rapid Reference 4.1

Indexes and Abbreviations and Tests Required

TOD-S: Dyslexia Risk Index (DRI)	Tests 2 and 3
TOD-C: Dyslexia Diagnostic Index (DDI)	Tests 2, 3, 4–9
TOD-C: Reading and Spelling Index (RSI)	Tests 2, 3, 5, 7
TOD-C: Linguistic Processing Index (LPI)	Tests 4, 6, 8, 9

helpful in documenting the reasons why an individual is having difficulties with reading and spelling. As noted in Chapter 3, the TOD-S yields the Dyslexia Risk Index (DRI) which provides an estimate of risk of dyslexia. Rapid Reference 4.1 lists the indexes, abbreviations, and the tests required to obtain the indexes. Figure 4.1 presents the TOD-Screener and the TOD-Comprehensive Test Selection Chart from Table 1.4 in the TOD Manual. This chart helps determine which tests to administer based on the indexes or composites of interest.

			Indexes			Reading and Spelling							Linguistic Processing					Vocabulary and Reasoning[a]			
			DDI	RSI	LPI	Composites							Composites				Test	Composites			
	Test number	TOD-Comprehensive	Dyslexia Diagnostic Index	Reading and Spelling Index	Linguistic Processing Index	Sight Word Acquisition	Phonics Knowledge	Basic Reading Skills	Decoding Efficiency	Spelling	Reading Fluency	Reading Comprehension Efficiency	Phonological Awareness	Rapid Automatized Naming	Auditory Working Memory	Orthographic Processing	Symbol to Sound Learning (Visual–Verbal PAL)	Vocabulary	Reasoning	Vocabulary and Reasoning 2	Vocabulary and Reasoning 4
TOD-S	1S	Picture Vocabulary																✓		✓	✓
TOD-S	2S	Letter and Word Choice	✓	✓												✓					
TOD-S	3S	Word or Question Reading Fluency	✓	✓							✓	✓									
TOD-C	4C	Phonological Manipulation	✓		✓								✓								
TOD-C	5C	Irregular Word Spelling	✓	✓						✓											
TOD-C	6C	Rapid Letter Naming	✓		✓									✓							
TOD-C	7C	Pseudoword Reading	✓	✓			✓	✓													
TOD-C	8C	Word Pattern Choice	✓		✓											✓					
TOD-C	9C	Word Memory	✓		✓										✓						
TOD-C	10C	Picture Analogies																	✓	✓	✓
TOD-C	11C	Irregular Word Reading				✓		✓													
TOD-C	12C	Oral Reading Efficiency									✓										
TOD-C	13C	Blending											✓								
TOD-C	14C	Segmenting											✓								
TOD-C	15C	Regular Word Spelling								✓											
TOD-C	16C	Silent Reading Efficiency										✓									
TOD-C	17C	Rapid Number and Letter Naming												✓							
TOD-C	18C	Letter Memory													✓						
TOD-C	19C	Rapid Pseudoword Reading					✓		✓												
TOD-C	20C	Rapid Irregular Word Reading				✓			✓												
TOD-C	21C	Symbol to Sound Learning															✓				
TOD-C	22C	Listening Vocabulary																✓			✓
TOD-C	23C	Geometric Analogies																	✓		✓

[a]Vocabulary and Reasoning composites can be used in interpreting the DDI.

Figure 4.1 TOD-S and TOD-C Test Selection Chart

DON'T FORGET

The TOD-Screener is administered first even if there is a plan to conduct a comprehensive evaluation using the TOD-C. To use the TOD-S scores in conjunction with the TOD-C scores, administer both tests while the examinee is within the same age- or grade-based norm group.

ADMINISTRATION AND SCORING OF THE TOD-C TESTS

This section provides a detailed review of the administration procedures for each of the TOD-C tests. After studying the test administration procedures in this chapter, it is recommended to complete several practice administrations of each test.

PHONOLOGICAL MANIPULATION (TOD-4C)

TOD-4C Phonological Manipulation (Rapid Reference 4.2) is a measure of phonological awareness skills with two subtests: Substitution and Deletion. In the Substitution subtest, the examinee is asked to change a word, a syllable, or a phoneme to make a new word. In the Deletion subtest, the examinee is asked to leave out a word, a syllable, or a phoneme to make a new word. This test contributes to both the DDI and LPI indexes as well as the Phonological Awareness composite.

Administration: This test requires the TOD-C Stimulus Easel 1 and a Record Form. A stopwatch is optional but may be helpful for timing specific items. All test items are presented using the Easel. If the examinee requests, all items may be repeated one time. As a general rule, if the examinee pauses for more than five seconds on any item, score the item 0 and present the next item. There are specific items in both subtests that have a firmer

≡ Rapid Reference 4.2

Important Administration Points for 4C: Phonological Manipulation

- Have the necessary materials: TOD-C Easel 1, Record Form, optional stopwatch or timer.
- Basal Rule: The basal is Item 1 or the lowest set of 4 consecutive correct responses. Count all items below the basal as correct.
- Stop Rule: 4 consecutive incorrect responses.
- Administer both subtests: Substitution and Deletion.
- Begin with Sample A for examinees in Grades 1–5 and Sample C for examinees in Grade 6—Adult. If starting with Sample C, follow the Basal Rule carefully as the examinee may need to go back to Sample A.
- Pronounce the sound the letter makes if the letter appears between slash marks, e.g., /b/.
- If the examinee requests, items may be repeated one time.
- For most items, if the examinee does not respond to an item *after five seconds*, score it 0 and present the next item.
- For specific items, Substitution 11–20 and Deletion 11–25, the response must be given *within the five-second* time limit or score it 0 and present the next item. Use a stopwatch or count silently to keep track of the five-second response time.

five-second rule: Substitution Items 11–20 and Deletion Items 11–23. On those items, the examinee must respond *within* five seconds, or the item is scored 0 and the next item is presented.

For both subtests, Substitution and Deletion, examinees in Grades 1–5 begin with Sample A, and those in Grade 6–Adult begin with Sample C. Although the tasks differ, the administration directions are similar on both subtests.

For examinees beginning with Sample A (substituting or deleting a word), the basal is Item 1 and testing continues until 4 consecutive errors are made. Present Sample Item A orally. Follow all directions and read the teal words verbatim. If the examinee responds correctly, confirm that the response was correct and continue to Item 1. If the examinee pauses for more than five seconds or responds incorrectly, provide the scripted corrective feedback and then present the next practice item. Again, confirm a correct response or provide the corrective feedback if the response was incorrect and then continue to Item 1 and administer Items 1–5. If the examinee pauses for more than five seconds, score the item 0, and present the next item. Continue to Sample B unless the examinee has made 4 consecutive errors.

Administer Sample B (substituting or deleting a syllable), following all directions and reading the teal text verbatim. If the examinee's response is correct, confirm that using the teal text and continue to Item 6. If the examinee is incorrect, provide the corrective feedback indicated and administer the next practice item. Provide the scripted feedback and continue to Item 6. Administer Items 6–10 and then continue to Sample C unless the examinee has made 4 consecutive errors.

Administer Sample C (substituting or deleting phonemes) following all directions carefully and providing the corrective feedback when needed. When presenting letters shown between slash marks (e.g., /f/), say the sound the letter makes not the name of the letter. Also, take care not to add a schwa sound when presenting a letter sound (e.g., /fuh/ instead of /f/). Sample C has three trials. If an examinee is incorrect on all three trials, discontinue that portion of the test.

For Grades 6–Adult, begin with Sample C and then administer Item 11. If the examinee responds correctly to 4 consecutive items (11–14), the basal has been established and testing continues. If the examinee is incorrect on all three trials of Sample C or misses Items 11 and 12, go back to Samples A and B and then administer Items 1–10. Continue to Item 13 if the Stop Rule was not met after Items 1–12 were administered. Continue testing until the examinee makes 4 consecutive errors.

On Substitution Items 11–20 and Deletion Items 11–23, examinees are told in advance that they will have five seconds to say the answer. If there is no response in five seconds, the item is scored as 0 and the next item is presented. The evaluator may either use a stopwatch/timer or silently count to five at the pace of one number per second.

Item scoring: Score each item during the test to determine when the Basal and Stop Rules are met. Using the TOD-C Record Form, circle the 1 if the response is

CAUTION

Substitution Items 11–20 and Deletion Items 11–25 have a five-second time limit. Use of a stopwatch is optional when administering these items, but the evaluator must keep careful track of examinee response times. If there is no response *within five seconds*, score the item 0 and present the next item.

correct and circle the 0 if the response is incorrect. If the examinee pauses more than five seconds on any item, score the item 0. On Substitution Items 11–20 and Deletion Items 11–23, if the examinee does not respond *within* five seconds, score the item 0.

Potential administration errors: Errors may include incorrect administration of the sample items, not repeating an item if requested, and not adhering to the five-second time limit on specified items.

> **DON'T FORGET**
>
> When starting with Item 15, if no basal is established (4 correct consecutive responses), test backward beginning with Item 14.

IRREGULAR WORD SPELLING (TOD-5C)

TOD-5C: Irregular Word Spelling (Rapid Reference 4.3) measures the individual's ability to spell words that have an element that is not phonically regular. Spelling of irregular words requires both phonological and orthographic knowledge. This test contributes to the DDI and RSI indexes and the Spelling composite.

Administration: This test requires the TOD-C Stimulus Easel 1, a Record Form, a Response Booklet, and a pencil for the examinee. Open the Response Booklet to Test 5C and place it in front of the examinee. Provide the examinee with a pencil. Read the directions and then present each item orally as scripted. Allow about 10 seconds per item. If the examinee is still writing, allow more time. If there is no response after 10 seconds, score the item 0 and present the next item. Repeat any items if requested. Examinees may print or use cursive.

Begin with Item 1 for examinees in Grades 1–5. Item 1 serves as the basal. Continue testing until the examinee makes 4 consecutive errors. If testing continues after Item 14, do not

---

≋ Rapid Reference 4.3

Important Administration Points for 5C: Irregular Word Spelling

- Have the necessary materials: TOD-C Easel 1, Record Form, Response Booklet, pencils
- Know the correct pronunciations for all words on the test.
- Begin with Item 1 for examinees in Grades 1–5.
- Begin with Item 15 for examinees in Grades 6–Adult.
- If a basal is not established (4 consecutive correct responses), begin testing backward with Item 14.
- Allow about 10 seconds for a response but allow more time if the examinee is still writing.
- If there is no response in about 10 seconds, score the item 0 and present the next item.
- If an examinee requests, all items may be repeated.
- Examinees may print or use cursive.
- Score each item during the test to determine when the Basal and Stop Rules are met.

read the instructions that appear on the next page of the Easel; just administer Item 15 and continue testing until the Stop Rule is met.

Begin with Item 15 for examinees in Grades 6–Adult. If the examinee is functioning at a lower level, testing may begin with Item 1 instead. When beginning with Item 15, if a basal is not established (4 consecutive correct responses, Items 15–18), begin testing backward with Item 14. Point to the space for Item 14 in the Response Booklet and say: **Let's do this one.** Continue testing backward one item at a time until the examinee has 4 consecutive correct responses. Resume testing forward with Item 19 and continue testing until the Stop Rule is met.

Know the correct pronunciation of all items. Pronunciation guidance is provided in the Easel for a few of the more difficult items. Review the words in advance to ensure correct pronunciation of each item.

Item scoring: Score each item during the test to determine when the Basal and Stop Rules are met. Score correct items as 1 and incorrect or skipped items as 0. Include all items below the basal as correct.

Potential administration errors: Administration errors may include mispronouncing the words, not repeating an item if requested, not scoring the item 0 and moving an examinee to the next item if there is no response after 10 seconds, or not testing backward to establish a basal.

RAPID LETTER NAMING (TOD-6C)

TOD-6C: Rapid Letter Naming (Rapid Reference 4.4) measures rapid automatized naming (RAN), an important predictor of reading rate. The task requires the examinee to look at rows of confusable letters and name them as quickly as possible. This test contributes to the DDI and LPI indexes and the RAN composite.

≡ Rapid Reference 4.4

Important Administration Points for 6C: Rapid Letter Naming

- Have the necessary materials: TOD-C Easel 1, Record Form, stopwatch or timer
- Begin with Sample A for examinees in Grades 1–2.
- Begin with Sample B for examinees in Grades 3–Adult.
- On the Sample Items, if the examinee misses one or more items on the second trial, discontinue the test.
- Once the timed test begins, if the examinee pauses for three seconds, score the item 0, point to the next letter and say: **Go ahead.**
- Be prepared to turn each Easel page as soon the examinee says the last letter on the page.
- It may be necessary to score only the incorrect items during the test, depending on how quickly the examinee is naming the letters.
- If the examinee skips a row, redirect by pointing to the correct row.
- Time the test for one minute, then say: **Stop.**

Administration: This test requires the TOD-C Stimulus Easel 1, a Record Form, and a stopwatch or timer. Begin with Sample A for Grades 1–2 and Sample B for Grades 3–Adult. Follow all directions for pointing and providing feedback carefully. Read the bolded teal text verbatim for each Sample Item and for the introduction to the test items. For both Samples A and B, if the examinee misses one or more letters on the second trial, discontinue the test.

This test has a one-minute time limit, so a stopwatch or timer is required. The Test Easel is used to present the stimulus items. If the examinee pauses for more than three seconds, score the item 0, point to the next letter, and say: **Go ahead.** If the examinee skips a row, redirect them by pointing to the correct row. At the end of one minute, say: **Stop.**

This test requires multitasking. The tasks include paying attention to three-second delays in naming, redirecting examinees who skip a row, turning the Easel pages immediately after the last item on the page is named, scoring the items, and stopping the test at one minute. A few suggestions can help. For example, use the non-dominant hand to turn the Easel pages and record scores with the dominant hand. It is easier to mark only incorrect responses during the test rather than trying to mark every item. Setting a stopwatch or timer at one minute can help manage the timing.

Item scoring: Score correct items as 1 and incorrect or skipped items as 0.

Potential administration errors: Administration errors may include not presenting the sample items correctly, not prompting the examinee to keep going after three seconds, not adhering to the one-minute time limit, or not turning the Easel pages quickly when the last letter is named.

PSEUDOWORD READING (TOD-7C)

TOD-7C: Pseudoword Reading (Rapid Reference 4.5) measures the ability to apply both phonological and orthographic knowledge to pronounce nonsense words. The initial task requires the examinee to say the sound a letter makes (Items 1–10). The next part of the test requires the examinee to read aloud nonsense words that conform to English spelling rules and patterns (Items 11–47). This test contributes to the DDI and RSI indexes and the Phonics Knowledge and Basic Reading Skills composites.

Administration: This test requires the TOD-C Stimulus Easel 1 and a Record Form. Begin with Sample A for examinees in Grades 1–2 and then administer Item 1. Item 1 serves as the basal. Continue testing until the Stop Rule is met (4 consecutive errors). Follow all pointing and feedback instructions carefully. Read the teal text verbatim. For Sample A, when a letter is presented between slash marks (e.g., /s/), say the sound the letter makes, not the letter name. Do not add a schwa sound after the letter sound. For example, say /s/ not /suh/. If, however, the examinee adds a schwa sound to the correct consonant sound, score the response as correct. If the examinee says the letter name, say: **That is the name of the letter. What sound does the letter make?** If the examinee pauses for five seconds or the response is incorrect, provide the corrective feedback and then introduce the test items. If the examinee pauses for more than five seconds on an item during the test, score the item 0, point to the next item and say: **Go ahead.** If an examinee started with Sample A and has not made 4 consecutive errors after Item 10, then administer Sample B and continue testing.

≡ *Rapid Reference 4.5*

Important Administration Points for 7C: Pseudoword Reading

- Have the necessary materials: TOD-C Easel 1, Record Form.
- Begin with Sample A for examinees in Grades 1–2.
- Begin with Sample B for examinees in Grades 3–Adult.
- Provide all of the corrective feedback when administering the Sample Items.
- Follow the Basal Rule carefully for examinees starting with Sample B as they may have to go back to Sample A if Items 11 and 12 are incorrect.
- Basal Rule: Item 1 or 4 consecutive correct responses.
- Stop Rule: 4 consecutive incorrect responses.
- Prompt examinees to go to the next item after five seconds and score the item 0.

For examinees in Grades 3–Adult, begin with Sample B and then Item 11. Follow all pointing and feedback instructions carefully for Sample B. Whether the examinee responds correctly or incorrectly to Sample B, testing continues to Item 11. Introduce the test items as scripted. Point to the first test item and say: **Start here.** If the examinee responds correctly to Items 11–14, a basal is established. Continue until the examinee makes 4 consecutive errors. If the examinee pauses for five seconds on an item during the test, score the item 0, point to the next item and say: **Go ahead.**

If, however, an examinee starts with Sample B and misses both Items 11 and 12, turn back and administer Sample A and Items 1–10. Return to Item 13 unless the Stop Rule has already been met. If not, continue testing until 4 consecutive errors have been made.

Item scoring: Score correct items as 1 and incorrect or skipped items as 0. Beginning with Item 11, the nonsense word must be pronounced as a whole word to receive credit. If the examinee sounds out the word but does not say it as a whole word, say: **Say the whole word together.** If the examinee then says the item as a whole word, score the response as correct. The Correct key in the Easel and in the Record Form provides guidance for scoring the responses by listing a rhyming word or breaking the longer words into segments. Count all items below the basal as correct.

Potential administration errors: Administration errors may include not presenting the sample items correctly, not prompting the examinee after five seconds, not following the Basal Rule for examinees starting with Sample B, or scoring a word as correct when it is not said as a whole word.

WORD PATTERN CHOICE (TOD-8C)

TOD-8C: Word Pattern Choice (Rapid Reference 4.6) measures orthographic knowledge, in particular the permissible ways that letters can be ordered in English. The task requires the examinee to look at a row of four nonwords and to choose the one that looks most like it could be a real English word. This is a timed test, so the examinee must work quickly. This test contributes to the DDI and LPI indexes, as well as the Orthographic Processing composite.

Administration: This test requires the TOD-C Stimulus Easel 1, a Record Form, a Response Booklet, a pencil for the examinee, and a stopwatch or timer. There is a two-minute time limit. Begin with Sample A for all examinees. Open the Response Booklet to Test 8C, or have the examinee turn to page 4. Administer the Sample Items as scripted. Sample A is a demonstration item and Sample B requires the examinee to complete an item. Provide the appropriate feedback for a correct response or for an incorrect response and then continue to Samples C and D. Follow all directions and provide all feedback as scripted. Read the introduction to the test. The introduction tells examinees to skip items they are unsure of and go on to the next item. There is no other prompting during the test. Have the stopwatch ready to begin timing. Ask the examinee to turn to the next page in the Response Booklet. Once the examinee has turned the page, say: **Ready? Begin**. Start timing. At the end of two minutes, say: **Stop. Put your pencil down.**

Item scoring: It is unlikely that the items can be scored during this timed test. Typically, the items are scored using the examinee's Response Booklet after the test session is completed. Score correct items as 1 and incorrect or skipped items as 0.

Potential administration errors: Administration errors may include not presenting the Sample Items as scripted, not having the examinee's Response Booklet opened to Test 8C (page 4), not presenting the introduction to the test as scripted, not having the stopwatch ready, not waiting for the examinee to turn the Response Booklet page before starting the timer, or not adhering to the two-minute time limit.

WORD MEMORY (TOD-9C)

TOD-9C: Word Memory (Rapid Reference 4.7) measures verbal working memory. The task requires the examinee to listen to a series of words and then repeat the words in reverse order. This test contributes to the DDI and LPI indexes, as well as the Auditory Working Memory composite.

≡ *Rapid Reference 4.7*

Important Administration Points for 9C: Word Memory

- Have the necessary materials: TOD-C Easel 1 and a Record Form.
- Begin with Sample A for all examinees.
- Provide all directions and corrective feedback when administering the Sample Items.
- Present the Introduction to the test as scripted.
- Present each item clearly, pausing one second between each word.
- Score items 0 if the examinee pauses for more than five seconds, then present the next item.
- Score the item 0 if the examinee says the words as presented and provide the reminder to say the words backward.
- Do not repeat any item.

Administration: This test requires the TOD-C Stimulus Easel 1 and a Record Form. Begin with Sample A for all examinees. Present the Sample Item as scripted, following all feedback directions. Introduce the test using the teal text. Present the items pausing for one second between the words. The test items can only be presented one time, so be sure to say them clearly at one word per second. During the test, if the examinee pauses for more than five seconds, score the item 0 and say: **Here's another one.** If the examinee repeats the words as presented, score the item 0 and say: **Remember to say them backward.** Continue testing until the Stop Rule of 4 consecutive errors is met.

Item scoring: Score each item during the test so the Stop Rule can be determined. Score correct items as 1 and incorrect or skipped items as 0.

Potential administration errors: Administration errors may include failure to present the sample items correctly, not scoring an item 0 if the examinee pauses for more than five seconds, not presenting the next item after the examinee has paused for five seconds, not scoring an item 0 if the examinee repeats the words as presented, not providing the reminder to say the words backward, or saying the items more than one time.

PICTURE ANALOGIES (TOD-10C)

TOD-10C: Picture Analogies (See Rapid Reference 4.8) measures reasoning ability. The task requires the examinee to select one of four response options that completes a picture analogy. The analogies are presented in a matrix format: A is to B as C is to D. To solve these analogies, the examinee must determine the relationship between the pictures in the A and B boxes and then choose one of four choices that relates in the same way to the picture in the C box. This test contributes to the Reasoning, Vocabulary and Reasoning 2, and Vocabulary and Reasoning 4 composites.

Administration: This test requires the TOD-C Stimulus Easel 1 and a Record Form. All items are presented from the Easel. Begin with Sample A for all examinees. Sample A demonstrates the task. Follow all the directions, including pointing, and read the teal text.

≡ Rapid Reference 4.8

Important Administration Points for 10C: Picture Analogies

- Have the necessary materials: TOD-C Easel 1 and a Record Form.
- Begin with Sample A for all examinees.
- Provide all directions and corrective feedback when administering the Sample Items.
- Follow all pointing directions.
- Prompt the examinee if necessary by pointing to the four response options and say: **Which one?**
- Do not provide feedback or explanations on any of the test items.
- Examinees may either point to or say the number of the response picture.

Administer Sample B which requires the examinee to point to the picture or say the number of the picture that solves the analogy. If correct, confirm it is correct by reading the teal text and continue to Item 1. If incorrect, provide the feedback and continue to Item 1. Point to item 1 on the Easel and read the teal text. After the examinee responds, provide no feedback and continue to Item 2. Follow the pointing directions and read the teal text aloud. If necessary on any item, prompt the examinee by pointing to the four response options and saying: **Which one?** After Item 2, simply turn the Easel pages to present each item. Record the examinee's response on the Record Form. Continue testing until the examinee makes 4 consecutive errors. Do not provide feedback on any of the test items.

Item scoring: Score each item during the test to determine when the Stop Rule is met (4 consecutive errors). Score correct responses as 1 and incorrect or skipped items as 0.

Potential administration errors: Administration errors may include not presenting the Sample Items as scripted including the pointing directions, providing feedback on test items, not recording item scores during the test, not prompting as necessary, or failing to discontinue after 4 consecutive errors.

IRREGULAR WORD READING (TOD-11C)

TOD-11C: Irregular Word Reading (See Rapid Reference 4.9) measures sound and word recognition, which are important basic reading skills. The first task requires the examinee to read aloud letters. The next task requires the examinee to read aloud words with an irregular element so they cannot be pronounced by phonics alone. This test contributes to the Sight Word Acquisition and the Basic Reading Skills composites.

Administration: This test requires the TOD-C Stimulus Easel 1 and a Record Form. All items are presented from the Easel. Examinees begin at one of the two Start Points based on their grade level. If an examinee is functioning above or below grade level, select the appropriate Start Point. For example, if an individual in Grade 3 is functioning at a first-grade level,

≡ Rapid Reference 4.9

Important Administration Points for 11C: Irregular Word Reading

- Have the necessary materials: TOD-C Easel 1 and a Record Form.
- Begin at the appropriate Start Point: Sample A for Grades 1–2 and Item 11 for Grades 3–Adult.
- Provide all directions and corrective feedback when administering the Sample Items.
- Follow the Basal Rule carefully for examinees starting with Item 11 as they may need to go back to the first Start Point.
- The Basal Rule is either Item 1 or 4 consecutive correct responses.
- The Stop Rule is 4 consecutive incorrect responses.
- If there is no response, prompt the examinee to go to the next item after five seconds and score the item as 0.

begin at the Start Point for Grades 1 and 2. The Basal Rule is Item 1 or 4 consecutive correct responses. The Stop Rule is 4 consecutive errors. Throughout the test, if an examinee pauses for more than five seconds on any item, score the item 0, point to the next item, and say: **Go ahead**.

Begin with Sample A for examinees in Grades 1 or 2. Read the teal text aloud and follow all pointing directions. If the examinee says the sound of the letter rather than the letter name say: **That is the sound of the letter. What is the name of the letter?** If the examinee says the correct letter name, confirm it is a correct response by reading the teal text, and then proceed to Item 1. If the examinee does not respond after five seconds or gives an incorrect response, say: **That is the letter T.** In either case, administer Item 1 which serves as the basal. Continue testing until the Stop Rule is met (4 consecutive errors). If the Stop Rule was not met after Item 10, continue by reading aloud the introduction to the word reading task and then administer those items. Discontinue the test when the examinee makes 4 consecutive errors.

For examinees in Grades 3–Adult, begin testing with Item 11. If the examinee responds incorrectly to both Items 11 and 12, go back and administer Sample A and Items 1–10. If the examinee has not made 4 consecutive errors, return to Item 13 and continue testing until the Stop Rule is met.

Item scoring: Score each item during the test to determine when the Basal (Item 1 or 4 consecutive correct responses) and Stop (4 consecutive errors) Rules are met. Score correct responses as 1 and incorrect or skipped items as 0. Count all items below the basal as correct.

Potential administration errors: Administration errors may include not presenting the Sample Items as scripted including the pointing directions, not providing the corrective feedback, not scoring an item 0 if the examinee pauses for more than five seconds, not recording item scores during the test, or not discontinuing after 4 consecutive errors.

ORAL READING EFFICIENCY (TOD-12C)

TOD-12C: Oral Reading Efficiency (See Rapid Reference 4.10) measures oral reading accuracy and efficiency. Reading efficiency relies on both accuracy and rate. The task requires the examinee to read aloud a grade-level passage for one minute. This test contributes to the Reading Fluency composite.

Administration: This test requires the TOD-C Stimulus Easel 1, a Record Form, and a stopwatch or timer. All reading passages are presented from the Easel. Open the Easel to the passage that matches the examinee's current grade level, regardless of reading ability. Introduce the passage by reading the teal text. Answer any questions the examinee may have. Then say: **Begin.** Start the stopwatch when the examinee says the first word. All passages are printed in the Record Form. As the examinee reads the passage, follow along in the Record Form. Mark any errors with a slash (/) mark. Errors include words read incorrectly, substitutions, and omissions. Do not count hesitations, insertions, or repetitions as errors. If a word is not read after three seconds, tell the examinee the word and mark it as incorrect. If the examinee misreads a word, but then self-corrects within three seconds, do not count it as an error. Stop the test after one minute. Circle the last word that was read aloud and say: **Stop.**

Item scoring: Each passage in the Record Form shows the total number of words in the passage and provides the cumulative word count by line. Locate the line total for the last line or partial line read by the examinee. If there are any unread words in that line, subtract the unread words from the cumulative total. Make a note of the total words read (including correctly and incorrectly read words), as errors will be subtracted from that total. Next, count the

---

≣ Rapid Reference 4.10

Important Administration Points for 12C: Oral Reading Efficiency

- Have the necessary materials: TOD-C Easel 1, Record Form, stopwatch.
- Use the passage at the examinee's grade level, regardless of reading ability.
- Open the Easel to the correct passage for the examinee.
- Provide the introduction to the test and answer any questions the examinee may have.
- After saying **Begin**, wait until the examinee reads aloud the first word to start the stopwatch.
- Follow along in the Record Form, marking any errors with a slash mark (/).
- Errors include substitutions, omissions, and any word told to the examinee after a three-second pause.
- Do not mark hesitations, repetitions, and insertions as errors.
- Count a self-correction within three seconds as correct.
- Circle the last word the examinee reads at the one-minute mark and say: **Stop.**
- Calculate the WRC by determining the total number of words read and subtracting the total number of errors. Enter that number in the WRC box on the Record Form. Enter the number of errors in the Number of Errors box. Subtract the errors from the number in the WRC box and record the difference in the Total Raw Score box.

number of errors (slash marks) and subtract that total from the total of words read. Enter that difference into the WRC box on the Record Form. Enter the total number of errors in the Number of Errors box on the Record Form and subtract it from the number entered in the WRC box. Enter this result into the Total Raw Score box.

Potential administration errors: Administration errors may include starting the stopwatch before the examinee says the first word; not marking errors with a slash mark; counting hesitations, repetitions, and insertions as errors; not circling the last word the examinee reads aloud; not telling the examinee words that are not read in three seconds; not marking any word provided to the examinee as an error; not marking substitutions and omissions as errors; not adhering to the one-minute time limit; not accepting a self-correction within three seconds; or not calculating the totals correctly.

BLENDING (TOD-13C)

TOD-13C: Blending (See Rapid Reference 4.11) measures one of the two most important basic phonological awareness abilities. The task requires the examinee to blend compound words, syllables, and phonemes to make whole words. This test contributes to the Phonological Awareness composite.

Administration: This test requires the TOD-C Stimulus Easel 2, a Record Form,

---

CAUTION

The scoring procedure for TOD-12C differs from the type of scoring used on traditional oral reading fluency (ORF) tests. The TOD-12C scoring procedure subtracts errors from words read correctly (WRC), whereas ORFs typically subtract errors from the total number of words attempted. The TOD-12C scoring procedure results in a standard score that can be interpreted with all of the TOD standard scores. The TOD-12C score, however, should not be directly compared to existing ORF normative data in the literature (e.g., see Hasbrouck & Tindal, 2017 Oral Reading Fluency Norms in the TOD Dyslexia Interventions and Recommendations guide) as the methodologies differ. Because the TOD-12C standard score is affected more by error rate than typical ORF tests, it was designed to be particularly sensitive to identification of those who struggle to read words quickly and accurately.

DON'T FORGET

A stopwatch is required for tests that have a time limit. TOD-C has seven tests with time limits: Rapid Letter Naming, Word Pattern Choice, Oral Reading Efficiency, Silent Reading Efficiency, Rapid Number and Letter Naming, Rapid Pseudoword Reading, and Rapid Irregular Word Reading. For all other tests, a stopwatch is optional for monitoring response times.

---

the digital recording for Items 16–29, and a device for playing the recording. Prior to administering this test, download the audio recording from the WPS Online Evaluation System and adjust the volume (https://www.wpspublish.com/tod-tests-of-dyslexia.html). The digital audio recording begins at Item 16.

Examinees begin at one of the two Start Points based on grade or functional level. The Basal Rule is Item 1 or 4 consecutive correct responses. The Stop Rule is 4 consecutive errors. Throughout the test, if an examinee pauses for more than five seconds on any item, score the item 0, present the next item by saying: **Here's another one.** Items 1–15 may each be repeated

≡ *Rapid Reference 4.11*

Important Administration Points for 13C: Blending

- Have the necessary materials: TOD-C Easel 2, Record Form, digital recording, and a device for playing the recording.
- Basal Rule: Item 1 or 4 consecutive correct responses.
- Stop Rule: 4 consecutive errors
- To be correct, the examinee's response must be pronounced as a whole word.
- If an examinee pauses for more than five seconds on Items 1–15, score the item 0 and present the next item.
- When presenting sample items or test items, pause one second between each compound word, syllable, or phoneme.
- Pronounce the phonemes correctly; do not add a schwa sound to the consonants.
- Items 1–15: Each item may be repeated one time if requested.
- Items 16–29: Do not repeat any item.
- Download the digital recording and adjust the volume prior to administration.
- For the digitally recorded Items 16–29, if the examinee has not finished responding in the five seconds that follow each recorded item, pause the recording to allow the examinee to finish responding.

one time if requested by the examinee. The recorded items, Items 16–29, may not be repeated.

Begin with Sample A for examinees in Grades 1–5. Read the teal text aloud. This section of the test presents compound words as two separate parts, which the examinee must blend together to say the whole word. Be sure to pause for about one second between the two parts when presenting the sample items as well as the test items. Provide the scripted feedback based on the examinee's response to Sample A. Continue to Item 1. If the examinee has not made 4 consecutive errors after Items 1–5 have been administered, present Sample B. This section of the test presents words as syllables, which the examinee blends together to say the whole word. Pause for about one second between the syllables when presenting the sample items and the test items. Continue to Item 6. If the examinee has not met the Stop Rule after Items 1–10 have been administered, present Sample C and continue testing until the examinee has 4 consecutive errors.

Begin with Sample C for examinees in Grades 6–Adult. This section of the test presents words as individual phonemes, which the examinee must blend together to say the whole word. When a letter is shown between slash marks (e.g., /d/), say the sound the letter makes. Do not add a schwa sound /uh/ to the end of the consonant sounds, e.g., say /d/ not /duh/. Read the teal text in Sample C, pausing about one second between each sound when presenting the sample item. Provide the appropriate feedback based on whether the examinee's response was correct or incorrect. In either case, continue to Item 11. Provide the directions as scripted. For examinees who started at Sample C, if the responses to both Items 11 and 12 are incorrect, go back and administer Sample A and Items 1–10. If the examinee has not made 4 consecutive errors, return to Item 13 and continue testing until the Stop Rule is met. Any examinee who started at Sample A and has continued to Sample C does not go back to Sample A if Items 11 and 12 are incorrect. Just continue testing until 4 consecutive errors are made.

Present Items 11–15, pausing one second between each phoneme. For Items 16–29, use the digital recording for item presentation. Introduce these items by reading the teal text. The recording presents each item phoneme by phoneme and then beeps, which is the signal for the examinee to say the whole word. The recording provides five seconds for a response. If the examinee has begun responding but needs more time, pause the recording. Do not repeat or replay any of the recorded items.

Item scoring: Score each item during the test to determine when the Basal and Stop Rules have been met. Count all items below the basal as correct. To be correct, the examinee's response must be pronounced as a whole word. Score correct responses as 1 and incorrect or skipped items as 0.

Potential administration errors: Administration errors may include forgetting to download the digital recording in advance, not adjusting the volume prior to testing; not pausing the recording if examinee has not finished responding in five seconds; not pausing one second between compound words, syllables, and phonemes when presenting items; not pronouncing letter sounds correctly; not following the Basal Rule for examinees who start with Sample C and miss Items 11 and 12; not repeating any item upon request for Items 1–15; or repeating any item for Items 16–29.

SEGMENTING (TOD-14C)

TOD-14C: Segmenting (See Rapid Reference 4.12) measures one of the two most important basic phonological awareness abilities for early reading and spelling. The task requires the examinee to segment whole words into compound words, syllables, and phonemes. This test contributes to the Phonological Awareness composite.

Administration: This test requires the TOD-C Stimulus Easel 2 and a Record Form. Examinees begin at one of the two Start Points based on grade or functional level. The Basal Rule is Item 1 or 4 consecutive correct responses. The Stop Rule is 4 consecutive errors. Throughout the test, if an examinee pauses for more than five seconds on any item, score the item 0, present the next item by saying: **Here's another one**. Items may be repeated one time if requested by the examinee.

Begin with Sample A for examinees in Grades 1–5. Read the teal text aloud. This section of the test presents compound words, which the examinee must segment into the two separate parts. Be sure to say the item word as a whole word when presenting the sample items as well as the test items. Do not pause between the parts. Provide the scripted feedback based on the examinee's response to Sample A. Continue to Item 1. If the examinee has not reached a Stop point after Items 1–5 have been administered, present Sample B. This section of the test presents whole words, which the examinee must segment into two syllables. Do not pause between the syllables when presenting the sample items and the test items. Continue to Item 6. If the examinee has not reached a Stop point after Items 1–10 have

***

≡ *Rapid Reference 4.12*

Important Administration Points for 14C: Segmenting

- Have the necessary materials: TOD-C Easel 2 and a Record Form.
- Basal Rule: Item 1 or 4 consecutive correct responses.
- Stop Rule: 4 consecutive errors.
- To be correct, the examinee must pronounce the two words in the compound words, the two syllables in the words, and the correct number of phonemes in the word.
- If an examinee pauses for more than five seconds on any item score the item 0 and present the next item.
- When presenting sample items or test items, do not pause between each word, syllable, or phoneme.
- Pronounce the phonemes correctly on the Sample Items; do not add a schwa sound to the consonants.
- Do not penalize examinees if they add a schwa sound to consonants when segmenting phonemes. If the phoneme is /d/ and the examinee says /duh/, score it as correct.
- Each item may be repeated one time if requested.

***

been administered, present Sample C and continue testing until the examinee has 4 consecutive errors.

For examinees in Grades 6–Adult begin with Sample C. This section of the test presents words, which the examinee must segment into the individual phonemes. Read the teal text in Sample C. When a letter is shown between slash marks (e.g., /d/), say the sound the letter makes. Do not add a schwa sound /uh/ to the end of the consonant sounds, e.g., say /d/ not /duh/. However, if the examinee adds a schwa sound when pronouncing the consonant phonemes, do not count that as an error. Provide the appropriate feedback based on whether the examinee's response was correct or incorrect. In either case, continue to Item 11. Provide the directions as scripted. For examinees that started at Sample C, if the responses to both Items 11 and 12 are incorrect, go back and administer Sample A and Items 1–10. If the examinee has not made 4 consecutive errors, return to Item 13 and continue testing until a Stop Rule is met. Any examinee who started at Sample A and has continued to Sample C does not go back to Sample A if Items 11 and 12 are incorrect. Just continue testing until 4 consecutive errors are made. On Items 11–29, the first time an examinee does not provide

DON'T FORGET

Present each test item in TOD-14C: Segmenting as a whole word. Do not pause between parts of a compound word, syllables, or phonemes.

CAUTION

For Items 11–29, if the examinee mispronounces a consonant phoneme by adding the schwa sound, e.g., saying /buh/ instead of /b/, score it as correct.

all of the sounds in a word, score the item 0 and say: **Remember to say all of the sounds in a word**. Then continue to the next item.

Item scoring: Score each item during the test to determine when the Basal and Stop Rules have been met. Count all items below the basal as correct. To be correct, the examinee's response must be pronounced as two separate words for Items 1–5, as two separate syllables in Items 6–10, and the indicated number of separate phonemes for Items 11–29. To facilitate scoring of responses, the Easel and the Record Form show the items as the correct separate parts, syllables, and phonemes. For Items 11–29, the number of sounds in each word is also shown. Score correct items as 1 and incorrect items as 0. Items with no response after five seconds are scored 0.

Potential administration errors: Administration errors may include pausing between word parts, syllables, or phonemes when presenting items, not pronouncing letter sounds correctly, not following the Basal Rule for examinees who start with Sample C, not repeating any item upon request, or not scoring as correct an examinee's mispronunciation of a consonant phoneme by adding a schwa sound (e.g., /buh/ instead of /b/).

REGULAR WORD SPELLING (TOD-15C)

TOD-15C: Regular Word Spelling (See Rapid Reference 4.13) assesses spelling skills using words that are phonically regular and are mostly spelled the way they sound. Examinees write the words in the Response Booklet and may write in either print or cursive. This test contributes to the Spelling composite.

Administration: This test requires the TOD-C Stimulus Easel 2, a Record Form, a Response Booklet, and a pencil. Examinees begin at one of the two Start Points based on grade or functional level. The Basal Rule is Item 1 or 4 consecutive correct responses. The Stop Rule is 4 consecutive errors. Throughout the test, allow about 10 seconds for the examinee to start writing on each item. If the examinee is still writing, wait to administer the next

≡ *Rapid Reference 4.13*

Important Administration Points for 15C: Regular Word Spelling

- Have the necessary materials: TOD-C Easel 2, Record Form, Response Booklet, pencil.
- Basal Rule: Item 1 or 4 consecutive correct responses.
- Stop Rule: 4 consecutive errors.
- Choose the appropriate Start Point (Item 1 or Item 15) based on Grade level or functioning.
- When starting at Item 15 and a basal is not established, test backward beginning with Item 14 until the Basal Rule is met. Resume testing forward until the Stop Rule is met.
- Each spelling word may be repeated if requested.
- Allow about 10 seconds for each response, but allow more time if the examinee is still writing.
- If no response occurs within about 10 seconds, score the item 0 and present the next item.
- Score each item during the test to determine the Basal and Stop Rules.

item. If there is no response after 10 seconds, score the item 0 and present the next item. Items may be repeated if requested by the examinee. Pronunciations are provided in the Easel for some of the words in Items 37–44. Review all items prior to testing to ensure correct pronunciation.

Begin with Item 1 for examinees in Grades 1–5, or older examinees who are functioning at a lower level. Open the Response Booklet to Test 15C or have the examinee turn to page 10. Give the examinee a pencil. Introduce the test by reading the teal text. Read each item as scripted; say the item number, the word, the sentence, and then say the word again. If the Stop Rule has not been met after Item 14, skip the directions on the next page and go directly to Item 15. Continue testing until the examinee has 4 consecutive errors.

Begin with Item 15 for examinees in Grades 6–Adult, or younger examinees who are functioning at a higher level. Open the Response Booklet to Test 15C, or have the examinee turn to page 10. Give the examinee a pencil. Introduce the test by reading the teal text. Read each item as scripted. If a basal is not established on Items 15–18 (4 consecutive correct responses), begin testing backward with Item 14. Point to the space for Item 14 in the Response Booklet and say: **Let's do this one.** Continue testing backward until a basal is established. Then resume testing forward until a Stop Rule is met (4 consecutive errors).

Item scoring: Score each item during the test to determine when the Basal and Stop Rules have been met. Count all items below the basal as correct. Score correct responses as 1 and incorrect or skipped responses as 0. Examinees are asked to write neatly and they can print or use cursive. To score a response, it must be legible. Remind an examinee to write neatly if responses are difficult to score.

Potential administration errors: Administration errors may include not pronouncing items correctly, not following the Basal Rule for examinees who start with Sample C, not repeating any item upon request, not scoring an item 0 if there is no response in about 10 seconds, or not allowing more than 10 seconds if the examinee is still writing.

SILENT READING EFFICIENCY (TOD-16C)

TOD-16C: Silent Reading Efficiency (See Rapid Reference 4.14) measures reading comprehension efficiency under timed conditions. The task requires the examinee to read passages of increasing difficulty and answer comprehension questions. This test contributes to the Reading Comprehension Efficiency composite.

Administration: This test requires the TOD-C Stimulus Easel 2, a Record Form, a Response Booklet, a pencil, and a stopwatch. Examinees begin at one of the two Start points depending on grade or functional level. Grades 1–5 begin with Samples A, B, and C, and then Item 1. Grades 6–Adult begin with Samples D and E and then Item 13. The Samples are administered using the Easel and the Response Booklet. Continuation Rules follow Samples C and E that determine whether or not testing will continue. The examinee reads the passages in the TOD-C Response Booklet and answers the comprehension questions, which are multiple choice, by circling the letter of the chosen answer. Although examinees are asked to read silently, do not penalize an examinee who chooses to read orally, or subvocalizes while reading. Once the test begins, do not help the examinee with any words.

For examinees starting with Samples A–C, open the Response Booklet to Test 16C or ask the examinee to turn to page 12. Give the examinee a pencil. Read the teal text to introduce the task in Sample A. Continue reading the teal text for Sample B. Provide the appropriate

---

≡ Rapid Reference 4.14

Important Administration Points for 16C: Silent Reading Efficiency

- Have the necessary materials: TOD-C Easel 2, Record Form, Response Booklet, stopwatch or timer, pencil.
- Choose the appropriate Start Point (Sample A or Sample D) based on Grade level.
- Follow the Continuation Rules located after Sample C and Sample E.
- Be sure examinees are on the correct page in the Response Booklet before beginning the timed test.
- After one minute, promptly examinees who do not appear to be reading or answering questions. If the examinee does not respond, discontinue and do not score the test.
- Prompt examinees to turn the page and keep going if they stop after completing a story or passage.
- Do not tell the examinee any words during the test.
- Do not penalize an examinee who reads orally or subvocalizes.
- Adhere to the time limits: five minutes for Grades 1–5, eight minutes for Grades 6–Adult.
- After the test is completed, use the Response Booklet to score the items.

---

feedback for correct or incorrect responses. Continue by administering Sample C. Check the examinee's responses. If the examinee has 2 or 3 correct on Samples B and C combined (total possible is 3), then continue to the test introduction. If the examinee has only 1 or 0 correct responses on Samples B and C combined, discontinue the test. For examinees continuing to the test items, read the teal text to introduce the test. The examinees are told to read each story carefully but quickly; to try to answer each question but skip a question if they don't know the answer; to move to the next story after finishing the questions; and that they will have five minutes. Tell

> ### DON'T FORGET
>
> Do not help the examinee with any words during the test.
>
> Do not penalize an examinee who chooses to read orally or subvocalize.

> ### CAUTION
>
> Do not begin timing until the examinee is on the correct page in the Response Booklet.

the examinee to turn to page 16 and begin. Once the examinee is on page 16, begin timing. After one minute, if the examinee does not appear to be reading or answering questions, say: **Please keep reading**. If the examinee does not respond, discontinue and do not score the test. For all other examinees, at the end of five minutes, say: **Stop. Put your pencil down.**

Begin with Sample D for examinees in Grades 6–Adult. Open the Response Booklet to Test 16C or ask the examinee to turn to page 14. Give the examinee a pencil. Read the teal text to introduce the task in Sample D. Provide the scripted feedback for correct or incorrect responses to question 1. Read the teal text to complete Sample D and provide the feedback for correct or incorrect responses. Continue to Sample E and administer it as scripted and then consult the Continuation Rules to determine whether testing will continue. If the examinee has 3 or 4 correct responses on Samples D and E combined, continue to the test. If the examinee has 2 or fewer correct responses on those samples, discontinue the test. For examinees continuing to the test items, read the teal text to introduce the test. The examinees are told to try to answer all the questions, but they can skip a question if they don't know the answer; to move to the next passage when finishing questions; to work carefully but quickly; and that they will have eight minutes. Ask the examinee to turn to page 20 and begin. Once the examinee has turned to page 20, begin timing. After one minute, if the examinee does not appear to be reading or answering questions, say: **Please keep reading**. If the examinee does not respond, discontinue and do not score the test. For all other examinees, at the end of eight minutes say: **Stop. Put your pencil down.**

Item scoring: Because all answers are marked in the Response Booklet, scoring occurs after the test is finished. Score correct responses as 1 and incorrect or skipped responses as 0. The correct answers are found only in the Record Form.

Potential administration errors: Administration errors may include not administering the sample items as scripted, not following the Continuation Rules, not making sure the examinee is on the correct page in the Response Booklet before starting the time, not prompting an examinee who appears not to be reading or answering questions, telling an examinee a word during the test, penalizing an examinee who reads orally or subvocalizes, or not adhering to the time limit.

RAPID NUMBER AND LETTER NAMING (TOD-17C)

TOD-17C: Rapid Number and Letter Naming (See Rapid Reference 4.15) measures retrieval and fluency under timed conditions. The task requires the examinee to name a mix of three letters (E, F, L) and three numbers (3, 6, 9) presented in random sequence as quickly as possible within a one-minute time limit. Confusable stimuli were selected because individuals with dyslexia are slower to discriminate between similar letters (e.g., F and E). This test contributes to the Rapid Automatized Naming composite.

Administration: This test requires the TOD-C Stimulus Easel 2, a Record Form, and a stopwatch or timer. All items are presented from the Easel. Examinees begin at one of two Start points based on Grade or functional level. Begin with Sample A for examinees in Grades 1 or 2; the first sample assesses whether the examinee knows the names of the letters and numbers. Begin with Sample B for Grade 3–Adult. Sample B requires the examinee to name the letters and numbers as quickly as possible.

For Grades 1–2, administer Sample A. If the examinee reads the numbers and letters accurately on the first trial, continue to Sample B. If the examinee pauses for more than three seconds, or responds incorrectly, point to the number or letter and say its name. Repeat this procedure for any number or letter that was named incorrectly or not responded to in time. Then have the examinee read the row of numbers and letters again. If correct, continue to Sample B. If the examinee still misses one or more on the second trial, discontinue the test.

For examinees in Grades 3–Adult, or those continuing from Sample A, administer Sample B. The examinee is asked to read the row of letters and numbers as quickly as possible. If the

≡ Rapid Reference 4.15

Important Administration Points for 17C: Rapid Letter and Number Naming

- Have the necessary materials: TOD-C Easel 2, Record Form, stopwatch or timer.
- Begin with Sample A for examinees in Grades 1–2.
- Begin with Sample B for examinees in Grades 3–Adult.
- If the examinee misses one or more of the Sample items on the second trial, discontinue the test.
- Once the timed test begins, if the examinee pauses for three seconds, score the item 0, point to the next letter or number and say: **Go ahead.**
- Be prepared to turn each Easel page as soon as the examinee says the last letter or number on the page.
- It may be necessary to score only the incorrect items during the test, depending on how quickly the examinee names the letters and numbers.
- If the examinee skips a row, redirect by pointing to the correct row.
- Time the test for one minute, then say: **Stop.**

examinee says the numbers and letters correctly, continue to the test items. If the examinee is incorrect or pauses for more than three seconds on the first trial, provide the error correction. Then have the examinee say the row again quickly. If the examinee reads the row correctly, continue to the test items. If the examinee misses one or more of the numbers or letters on this second trial, discontinue the test.

Introduce the test items and follow the pointing directions. After saying **Begin**, start timing. If the examinee pauses for more than three seconds on any item, score it 0, point to the next number or letter and say: **Go ahead**. If the examinee skips a row, redirect by pointing to correct row. At the end of one minute say: **Stop.**

This test requires the evaluator to multitask. The tasks include paying attention to three-second delays in naming, redirecting examinees who skip a row, turning the Easel pages immediately after the last item on the page is named, scoring the items, and stopping the test at one minute. A few suggestions can help. For example, use the non-dominant hand to turn the Easel pages and record scores with the dominant hand. It is easier to mark only incorrect responses during the test rather than trying to score every item. Setting a stopwatch or timer at one minute can help manage the timing.

Item scoring: Score correct items as 1 and incorrect or skipped items as 0.

Potential administration errors: Administration errors may include not presenting the sample items correctly, not discontinuing the test as directed after the second trial on Sample A and B, not prompting the examinee to keep going after three seconds, not redirecting the examinee if a row is skipped, not turning the Easel pages quickly when the last letter or number is named, or not adhering to the one-minute time limit.

LETTER MEMORY (TOD-18C)

TOD-18C: Letter Memory (See Rapid Reference 4.16) measures working memory. The task requires the examinee to listen to a series of letters presented orally and then repeat them in reverse order. This test contributes to the Auditory Working Memory composite.

Administration: This test requires the TOD-C Stimulus Easel 2 and a Record Form. All examinees begin with Sample A. Read the teal text and provide the appropriate feedback for a correct or incorrect response to the sample. If there is no response in more than five seconds, treat it as an incorrect response to the sample and provide the appropriate feedback. Whether the examinee responded correctly or incorrectly to the sample item, continue to Item 1. During the test, score a pause of more than five seconds as 0 and say: **Here is another one.** When presenting the sample and all test items, pause for one second between each letter. If the examinee repeats the letters as presented, score the item 0 and say: **Remember to say them backward.** Discontinue the test when an examinee makes 4 consecutive errors. Do not repeat any items on this test.

DON'T FORGET

Pause one second between each letter when presenting the items.

Item scoring: Score each item during the test to determine when the Stop Rule has been met. Score correct responses as 1 and incorrect responses as 0. Incorrect responses include any item that is not recalled in the correct reverse order, a pause of more than five seconds, or saying the letters forward.

Potential administration errors: Administration errors may include not pausing one second between each letter when presenting the sample or test items, not scoring an item 0 if the examinee pauses for more than five seconds, not scoring an item 0 if the examinee says the letters forward, not providing the reminder to say the letters backward, or not discontinuing after the examinee makes 4 consecutive errors.

≡ Rapid Reference 4.16

Important Administration Points for 18C: Letter Memory

- Have the necessary materials: TOD-C Easel 2, Record Form.
- Begin all examinees with Sample A.
- All examinees start with Item 1.
- When presenting the sample item or test items, pause for one second between each letter.
- Do not repeat any items.
- If the examinee pauses for more than five seconds, score the item 0 and present the next item.
- If the examinee says the letters forward, score the item 0 and provide the reminder to say them backward.
- Discontinue the test when the examinee makes 4 consecutive errors.

RAPID PSEUDOWORD READING (TOD-19C)

TOD-19C: Rapid Pseudoword Reading (See Rapid Reference 4.17) measures automaticity of applying phonological and orthographic knowledge and requires the examinee to read aloud phonically regular nonsense words as quickly as possible within a one-minute time limit. This test contributes to the Phonics Knowledge and the Decoding Efficiency composites.

Administration: This test requires the TOD-C Stimulus Easel 2, a Record Form, and a stopwatch or timer. Use the Easel to present all items. Begin with Sample A for all examinees. Read the teal text and follow all pointing directions. If the examinee pauses for more than three seconds or responds incorrectly, provide the correct pronunciation and have them repeat the sample items again. Read the teal instructions to introduce the test and then turn to the next page. Read the teal text and then, after saying **Begin**, start timing for one minute. If the examinee pauses for more than three seconds, score the item 0, point to the next item and say: **Go ahead.** At the end of one minute say: **Stop.**

This test requires the evaluator to multitask. The tasks include paying attention to three-second delays in reading the nonsense word, turning the Easel pages immediately after the last item on the page is read, scoring the items, and stopping the test in one minute. The Record Form includes a reminder of when to turn the Easel page. Each Easel page has eight items, and the reminder note appears after each group of eight (e.g., after Items 8, 16, 24, 32, and so on). A few suggestions may help. For example, use the non-dominant hand to turn the Easel pages and record scores with the dominant hand. It is easier to mark only incorrect responses during the test rather than trying to mark every item. Setting a stopwatch or timer at one minute can help manage the timing.

CAUTION

If Test 7C: Pseudoword Reading was administered and the examinee got fewer than eight items correct, do not administer this test (19C).

≡ Rapid Reference 4.17

Important Administration Points for 19C: Rapid Pseudoword Reading

- Have the necessary materials: TOD-C Easel 2, Record Form, stopwatch.
- Begin with Sample A for all examinees.
- If the examinee pauses for more than three seconds on any item, score the item 0, point to the next item, and say: **Go ahead.**
- If the examinee mispronounces the item, score the item 0.
- Turn the Easel page as soon as the last word on the page is read.
- Stop the test at one minute.
- Do not administer this test if the examinee had less than eight items correct on Test 7C: Pseudoword Reading.

Item scoring: Score correct items as 1 and incorrect or skipped items as 0. If the examinee pauses for more than three seconds on any item, score the item 0. If the examinee mispronounces the word, score the item 0. To be correct, the examinee must pronounce the word as indicated. For example, if the word is san which has a short vowel sound and the examinee says it with a long vowel sound, i.e., sane, score the item as incorrect. The Correct key in the Easel and in the Record Form provides guidance for scoring the responses by listing a rhyming word or breaking the longer words into segments.

Potential administration errors: Administration errors may include not presenting the sample items correctly, not prompting the examinee after three seconds, not turning the Easel page immediately after the last word on that page is read, not scoring the responses correctly, or not adhering to the one-minute time limit.

RAPID IRREGULAR WORD READING (TOD-20C)

TOD-20C: Rapid Irregular Word Reading (See Rapid Reference 4.18) measures basic reading skills and reading rate. The task requires the examinee to read aloud written words that have an irregular element as quickly as possible. There is a one-minute time limit. This test contributes to the Sight Word Acquisition and the Decoding Efficiency composites.

Administration: This test requires the TOD-C Stimulus Easel 2, a Record Form, and a stopwatch or timer. Use the Easel to present all items. Begin with Sample A for all examinees. Read the teal text and follow all pointing directions. If the examinee pauses for more than three seconds or responds incorrectly, provide the correct pronunciation and have them repeat the sample items again. Turn the page and read the teal instructions to introduce the test. After saying **Begin**, start timing for one minute. If the examinee pauses for more than

---

≡ Rapid Reference 4.18

Important Administration Points for 20C: Rapid Irregular Word Reading

- Have the necessary materials: TOD-C Easel 2, Record Form, stopwatch.

- Begin with Sample A for all examinees.

- If the examinee pauses for more than three seconds on any item, score the item 0, point to the next item, and say: **Go ahead.**

- If the examinee mispronounces the word, score the item 0.

- Turn the Easel page as soon as the last word on the page is read.

- It may be easier to score just the incorrect items if the examinee is reading rapidly

- Stop the test at one minute.

- Do not administer this test if the examinee had fewer than eight items correct on Test 11C: Irregular Word Reading.

three seconds, score the item 0, point to the next item and say: **Go ahead.** At the end of one minute say: **Stop.**

> **CAUTION**
>
> If Test 11C: Irregular Word Reading was administered and the examinee responded to fewer than 8 items correctly, do not administer this test (20C).

This test requires the evaluator to multitask. The tasks include paying attention to three-second delays in reading the irregular word, turning the Easel pages immediately after the last item on the page is read, scoring the items, and stopping the test in one minute. The Record Form includes a reminder of when to turn the Easel page. There are eight items on each Easel page and the reminder appears after each group of eight (e.g., after Items 8, 16, 24, 32, and so on). In addition, the test spans three pages in the Record Form, so those pages must be manipulated as well. A few suggestions may help. For example, use the non-dominant hand to turn the Easel pages and record scores with the dominant hand. It is easier to mark only incorrect responses during the test rather than trying to mark every item. Setting a stopwatch or timer at one minute can help manage the timing.

Item scoring: Score correct items as 1 and incorrect or skipped items as 0. If the examinee pauses for more than three seconds on any item, score the item 0. If the examinee mispronounces the word, score the item 0. To be correct, the examinee must read the word aloud correctly.

Potential administration errors: Administration errors may include not presenting the sample items correctly, not prompting the examinee after three seconds, not turning the Easel page immediately after the last word on that page is read, not scoring the responses correctly, or not adhering to the one-minute time limit.

SYMBOL TO SOUND LEARNING (TOD-21C)

TOD-21C: Symbol to Sound Learning (See Rapid Reference 4.19) measures associative memory and retrieval. The task requires the examinee to learn novel associations between a symbol and a sound, store the information, and then blend the sounds into real words. The task is similar to the first stages of learning to read when the association between letters and sounds is formed in order to read a word. This type of learning, symbol to sound or letter to sound, is referred to as paired-associate learning (PAL). This test provides information about the examinee's visual-verbal learning ability.

Administration: This test requires the TOD-C Stimulus Easel 2 and a Record Form. All items are presented from the Easel. There are teaching items, items requiring feedback, response times that are monitored, and items that require pointing coordinated with spoken directions. Practice is required in order to administer this test smoothly without error. In addition, there are consonants (e.g., /m/) and vowels (e.g., /ă/) that must be pronounced correctly. Remember, when a letter is shown between slash marks, say the sound the letter makes, not the letter name. Do not add a schwa sound /uh/ when pronouncing any of the consonants, e.g., /m/ not /muh/. There are three short vowels and one long vowel in the test items. Short vowels include /ă/, /ĭ/, and /ĕ/. The long vowel is /ā/. Review pronunciations and practice in advance before administering this test.

≋ Rapid Reference 4.19

Important Administration Points for 21C: Symbol to Sound Learning

- Have the necessary materials: TOD-C Easel 2, Record Form.
- Begin with Sample A for all examinees.
- Coordinate directions with pointing as indicated.
- Point carefully so the symbol is not covered.
- For letters shown between slash marks, say the sound of the letter not the name.
- Allow 10 seconds for a response on Items 1–38.
- Allow 15 seconds for a response on Items 39–42, the last four items.
- Score as correct self-corrections made within the allowed response time.
- Score as incorrect if no response in the specified timeframe (10 or 15 seconds).

Begin with Sample A for all examinees. Read the teal text and follow all pointing directions. It is important to coordinate the pointing with the directions. For example, when administering Sample A, point to the symbol as directed and read the directions in teal while still pointing to the symbol. Do not point for just a brief second and do not cover the symbol when pointing. Provide the scripted feedback for correct or incorrect responses. If the examinee pauses for more than 10 seconds, the response is incorrect. In either case, continue to Item 1.

For each item, point to the symbol while reading the teal item text aloud. Provide the feedback for correct or incorrect responses and point to the symbol as directed. Allow 10 seconds for the examinee to respond to each item. If there is no response or an incorrect response, score the item 0, and provide the corrective feedback. If the examinee self-corrects within the 10-second timeframe, score the response as correct. Not every item requires corrective feedback, so be careful to provide it only when indicated. For the last four items on the test, allow 15 seconds for a response. Score self-corrections within that time frame as correct. Discontinue the test after 4 consecutive errors.

Item scoring: Score each item during the test to determine when the Stop Rule is met. Score correct responses and self-corrections within the allowed timeframe as 1. Score incorrect responses, or no response in the time allowed, as 0.

Potential administration errors: Administration errors may include not pointing as directed while reading the directions, not providing the correct feedback, not adhering to the response time parameters (i.e., 10 and 15 seconds), not scoring a self-correction as correct if provided within the allowed response time, not pronouncing the letters between slash marks correctly, not presenting items correctly and efficiently, or providing feedback when none is allowed.

CAUTION

This test requires practice in order to administer it efficiently and correctly.

LISTENING VOCABULARY (TOD-22C)

TOD-22C: Listening Vocabulary (See Rapid Reference 4.20) measures receptive vocabulary knowledge and listening comprehension ability. The task requires the examinee to listen to a question and four possible one-word answers. This test contributes to the Vocabulary composite and the Vocabulary and Reasoning 4 composite.

Administration: This test requires the TOD-C Stimulus Easel 2 and a Record Form. All items are presented from the Easel. The four possible one-word answers are displayed on the Easel pages. The evaluator reads the question and the four possible answers aloud. The examinee selects the one word that best answers the question by pointing to the word or saying the word. Begin with Samples A and B for examinees in Grades 1–5 and then proceed to Item 1. Begin with Sample B for examinees in Grades 6–Adult and then proceed to Item 10. Sample A is a demonstration item to illustrate the task. Sample B requires the examinee to listen to a question and then to point to or say the answer. Provide the feedback shown for a correct or an incorrect response. In either case, continue to Item 1 or Item 10 depending on the grade or functional level of the examinee.

The Basal Rule is either Item 1 or 4 consecutive correct responses. The Stop Rule is 4 consecutive errors. Throughout the test, if the examinee does not respond after five seconds, encourage a response, for example, by saying: **Which one?** If there is still no response, score the item 0 and move on to the next item. Each item may be repeated one time if requested.

If an examinee starts at Item 1 and has not made 4 consecutive errors after Item 9 is administered, skip the directions on the next Easel page and go directly to Item 10. Continue until the Stop Rule is met.

If an examinee starts at Item 10 and does not establish a basal (4 consecutive

> ## DON'T FORGET
>
> If an examinee is functioning below or above grade level, a lower or higher Start Point can be selected.

≋ Rapid Reference 4.20

Important Administration Points for 22C: Listening Vocabulary

- Have the necessary materials: TOD-C Easel 2, Record Form.
- Basal Rule: Item 1 or 4 consecutive correct responses.
- Stop Rule: 4 consecutive errors.
- Begin with Sample A for examinees in Grades 1–5.
- Begin with Sample B for examinees in Grade 6–Adult.
- Know the pronunciation of all questions and possible answers.
- When presenting each item, read aloud the question and the four possible answers.
- Accept pointing or oral responses.
- Encourage a response after five seconds. If no response, score the item 0 and move on.

> ## CAUTION
>
> Review the pronunciation of the words before administering this test. As the items progress, the vocabulary becomes more difficult and may not be familiar. Use a standard dictionary to learn pronunciations of any unfamiliar words. The Easel and Record Form do not provide pronunciation guidance for this test.

correct responses, i.e., Items 10–13), test backward beginning with Item 9 until the basal is established or Item 1 has been administered. If the Stop Rule has not been met, resume testing forward until 4 consecutive errors have been made.

Item scoring: Score the items during the test to determine when the Basal and Stop Rules have been met. Score correct responses as 1 and incorrect responses as 0. If the examinee has not responded after five seconds, encourage a response. If there is still no response, score the item 0 and present the next item.

Potential administration errors: Administration errors may include not reading the questions and four possible answers clearly and correctly, not encouraging a response after five seconds, not scoring the item 0 if no response is given after prompting, not accepting a pointing response, not establishing a basal when starting at Item 10, not testing backward if no basal is established, or not resuming testing forward until the Stop Rule is met.

GEOMETRIC ANALOGIES (TOD-23C)

TOD-23C: Geometric Analogies (See Rapid Reference 4.21) measures reasoning abilities. The task requires the examinee to select one of four response options that completes a geometric analogy. The analogies are presented in an A is to B as C is to ? format. This test contributes to the Reasoning and the Vocabulary and Reasoning 4 composite.

> # ≡ Rapid Reference 4.21
>
> ### Important Administration Points for 23C: Geometric Analogies
>
> - Have the necessary materials: TOD-C Easel 2, Record Form.
> - Basal Rule: Item 1
> - Stop Rule: 4 consecutive errors
> - Begin with Sample A for all examinees.
> - Follow all pointing directions carefully.
> - Read all teal text aloud.
> - Accept a pointing or oral response.
> - If necessary prompt for a response by saying: **Which one?**
> - Do not provide any feedback on items.
> - Score items during the test to determine when the Stop Rule is met.

Administration: This test requires the TOD-C Stimulus Easel 2 and a Record Form. All items are presented from the Easel. Begin with Sample A for all examinees. Present Samples A and B following all pointing directions and reading the teal text aloud. Pointing as directed is important to illustrating how the analogy is solved. If the Sample Items are not administered correctly, reading all directions and pointing as indicated, the examinee's chances of understanding and succeeding with this task may be limited. The examinee may point to or say the number of the response option that solves the analogy. As necessary, if there is no response, prompt the examinee by saying: **Which one?** The Basal Rule is Item 1 and the Stop Rule is 4 consecutive errors. Do not provide any feedback on the items. For example, an examinee may be curious about how to solve an analogy. Do not provide that information.

Item scoring: Score the items during the test to determine when the Stop Rule is met. Score correct responses as 1 and incorrect responses as 0.

Potential administration errors: Administration errors may include not administering the Sample Items correctly, not accepting a pointing or oral response, not prompting for a response as necessary, not adhering to the Stop Rule, or providing feedback on items which is not allowed.

⚔ TEST YOURSELF ⚔

1. **Including the three tests of the TOD-S, how many tests are there in total in the TOD-C?**
   (a) 20
   (b) 21
   (c) 22
   (d) 23

2. **Which of the following TOD-C tests does not require a Response Booklet?**
   (a) Silent Reading Efficiency
   (b) Irregular Word Spelling
   (c) Word Pattern Choice
   (d) Listening Vocabulary

3. **Which of the following counts as an error on Oral Reading Efficiency?**
   (a) Repetitions
   (b) Insertions
   (c) Substitutions
   (d) Self-corrections within three seconds

4. **Which tests are required for the Linguistic Processing Index?**
   (a) Tests 4–9
   (b) Tests 4, 6, 8, and 9
   (c) Tests 2, 3, 5, and 7
   (d) Tests 4–7

5. The TOD-C is appropriate for what grade range?

   (a) K–2

   (b) K–12.9

   (c) Grades 1–6

   (d) Grades 1–12.9

6. Which of the following is true about the administration of the TOD-C?

   (a) All of the phonological tests require the digital audio recording.

   (b) There are two Stimulus Easels.

   (c) All tests in the TOD-C must be administered to get the three index scores.

   (d) Use the Response Booklet to score Irregular Word Spelling after the test is completed.

7. If an examinee has fewer than 8 correct on Irregular Word Reading, do not administer Rapid Irregular Word Reading.
True or False?

8. On Rapid Letter Naming, what is the wait time for a response before scoring the item 0 and moving to the next item?

   (a) Three seconds

   (b) Four seconds

   (c) Five seconds

   (d) Wait for a response

9. On which test is the examinee's current grade level used regardless of estimated reading level?

   (a) Irregular Word Reading

   (b) Silent Reading Efficiency

   (c) Oral Reading Efficiency

   (d) Rapid Irregular Word Reading

10. On Word Memory, if an examinee repeats the item as presented, the evaluator should:

   (a) score the item 1.

   (b) say **Remember to say them backward** and re-administer the item.

   (c) score the item 0.

   (d) score the item 0 and say **Remember to say them backward.**

Answers: 1. d; 2. d; 3. c; 4. b; 5. d; 6. b; 7. True; 8. a; 9. c; 10. d

REFERENCE

Hasbrouck, J., & Tindal, G. (2017). An update to compiled ORF norms. (Technical Report No. 1702). *Behavioral Research & Teaching.* University of Oregon.

Five

UNDERSTANDING AND INTERPRETING THE TOD SCORES AND COMPARISONS

Because the TOD offers a number of score options, it is important to become familiar with them and how they are interpreted. The interpretation of TOD scores relies on three hierarchical levels of information, adapted from Woodcock et al. (2001): Level 1 (e.g., qualitative data, such as behavior observations, test scatter, error analysis, and rating scales); Level 2 (age equivalents [AEs] and grade equivalents [GEs]); and Level 3 (standard scores, percentile ranks, and growth scores). In addition, data are provided informing the level of confidence an examiner can place in the scores, performance variability (e.g., strengths/weaknesses), and performance relative to peers expressed as verbal descriptors rather than numbers. The purposes of the assessment and referral question(s) dictate which scores are most appropriate to use.

LEVELS OF INTERPRETATION

The three levels of interpretation offer a framework within which to interpret scores and score profiles and relative differences among scores; information from one level cannot be used interchangeably with information from another. Each level provides unique information about a person's test performance, although information from one level may be consistent with and supportive of hypotheses generated within another level. Typically, information from a higher level builds on information from the previous level. Consider information from all three levels when describing an individual's performance. Rapid Reference 5.1 provides a brief summary of the three levels of information.

Level 1 information: Level 1 information is useful in interpreting results and planning an appropriate instructional program. Informal and qualitative in nature, this information is obtained through behavioral observations during testing, through error analysis of responses to individual items, and from other sources such as the Test Observation Worksheet in the TOD-E and TOD-C Record Forms. The Test Observation Worksheet can be used to help document the examinee's ability to address task demands. This

═ Rapid Reference 5.1

Three Hierarchical Levels of Information

Level	Score or Source of Information	Application
1	Qualitative, error analysis TOD Rating Scales Test session observations	Aids instructional planning Provides support of the direct assessments Describes behavioral observations
2	Age equivalents Grade equivalents	Helps determine level of development Helps determine level of instruction
3	Standard scores Percentile ranks	Defines performance relative to peers

Worksheet is completed by the evaluator and includes questions that may affect performance (e.g., hearing/vision limitations, English language skills, writing skills, presence of any inappropriate behavior, and overall level of motivation). The Worksheet also includes four-point "Strongly Agree" to "Strongly Disagree" items which address levels of the following specific test behaviors: cooperation, confidence, rapport, attention, activity level, oral communication skills, ability to understand the test directions, perseverance, and a characterization of the validity of the results.

Level 1 information can include comments that the examinee makes (e.g., "I really don't like spelling"), as well as behavioral observations (e.g., the student was inattentive during timed tests). It also can help with forming hypotheses about the nature of a problem. For example, Josh, a fourth-grade student, missed several items on both the Irregular Word Reading and Irregular Word Spelling tests. On the Irregular Word Spelling test, he spelled words the way they sound and not how they look. One instructional recommendation was that Josh should be taught to look at the irregular word, cover it, and then write it from memory, saying the word while writing it and underlining the tricky (irregular) part of the word.

Observing how the individual performs the task can also provide insights into instructional recommendations. For example, two ninth-grade students, Judith and Reba, approached the same reading task in different ways. The reading task required word reading within a time limit. Judith was slow and methodical but never made mistakes. Reba pronounced words quickly and made several mistakes. Although both students obtained a similar score, their approaches differed. Consequently, the instructional recommendations would address these differences in approaches. It is possible to record in the margins of the test booklet notes describing problem solving strategies (e.g., impulsive trial and error vs. reflective effort, a pattern of significant scatter, or better performance on items that include visual versus auditory cues).

Finally, qualitative and quantitative information also can be obtained from parents, teachers, and examinees from administration of TOD Rating Scales; this information is often used to supplement and support the results of TOD direct assessments. The TOD Rating Scales include several yes/no questions that focus on risk factors such as family history of reading difficulties and prior instruction, as well as Likert items designed to yield an estimate of dyslexia risk. Rating scale data yielding standard scores from respondents provide an opportunity for the evaluator to determine the extent to which their perspectives agree as to the nature and extent of reading history and limitations. Chapter 6 provides information on the use and interpretation of the rating scales.

> **DON'T FORGET**
>
> Assessment creates opportunity; evaluators have the opportunity to obtain not only quantitative data but also qualitative information from a variety of sources.

Level 2 information: Level 2 information characterizes an examinee's developmental levels and includes AEs or GEs. These equivalents can be used to help estimate an appropriate developmental or instructional level for the individual and are described in some detail in the section on TOD Scores.

Level 3 information: Level 3 information provides a basis for making intra- and interindividual comparisons. For example, in educational and clinical settings, standard scores are commonly used to describe an individual's relative group standing as compared to age or grade peers. In addition, they are often used to describe strengths and weaknesses and are typically required to make placement decisions, such as a need for special education services. Because some parents and teachers are not familiar with test scores, many evaluators include charts in their reports that offer brief explanations of the scores that are used.

> **DON'T FORGET**
>
> The three levels of interpretive information are not interchangeable and provide unique information. Both quantitative and qualitative sources can be helpful in decision-making and planning instruction.

GRADE- OR AGE-BASED NORMS

After calculating the raw score, the first decision is whether to use grade- or age-based norms. The TOD direct assessments provide the option for using either grade- or age-based norms except for adults where only age-based norms are available. Grade-based norms are generally preferable if students are younger or older than their grade-level peers (e.g., in the case of grade retention). Age-based norms are more applicable in clinical settings and should be used when TOD scores will be compared directly to scores obtained on other tests that use age-based norms. In addition, some testing agencies require the use of age-based norms rather than grade-based norms when a student is applying for specific accommodations, such as extended time on exams. Selection of grade- or age-based norms

DON'T FORGET

Remember to indicate in reports which norm group was used for scoring.

CAUTION

Remember, when comparing scores from the TOD to different tests, use the same type of norms, either age or grade.

DON'T FORGET

Grade-based norms can be chosen when interested in comparing performance to grade-level peers and examinees are atypically younger or older than other students in their grade.

does not affect the obtained GEs or AEs, but differences will occur in the other scores obtained (e.g., standard scores, percentile ranks, composites, and indexes). Grade norms are available for examinees in grades K through 12, Fall and Spring, and age norms are available from 5-0 to 89 years. Evaluators select Fall or Spring norms for comparison depending on the time of year.

Calculating Scores

After grade or age norms are chosen, evaluators can calculate all scores manually, but they also can be calculated automatically by the TOD software program. The Score Reports include transformed standard scores and percentiles, composites, indexes, confidence bands (90% or 95% level), and test comparisons. Tables 2.1, 2.2, and 2.3 in the TOD Manual (Mather et al., 2024b) show the transformations and score comparisons that are available for the TOD-S, TOD-C, and TOD-E. The TOD Norms Book contains lookup tables in Appendices A, B, and C. The TOD software program provides raw to standard score/percentile transformations and comparisons. Figures 2.4 and 2.5 in the TOD Manual illustrate a flowchart showing efficient steps for a dyslexia evaluation and which scores are most relevant for decision-making at each step.

TOD SCORES

The TOD offers a variety of scores, each with its own purpose. Evaluators are responsible for understanding these scores and interpreting them correctly. In addition, evaluators must be able to explain the scores to others, including parents and teachers. This section provides a detailed description of each score.

Raw Scores

Scoring the tests begins with obtaining raw scores, which may aid in making some qualitative judgments about performance (e.g., a pattern of scores that may indicate inattentiveness if there is appreciable scatter). Raw scores do not, however, allow for intra- or interperson comparisons. Raw scores must be transformed into standard scores, percentiles, composites scores, and indexes, all of which may be used in intra- and interindividual comparisons. For most tests, the raw score is the number of correct responses among the items administered, plus the number of items below a basal level that were not administered, each receiving one point: this score is then transformed in the Norms Book (or by the TOD software) to standard scores and percentiles. There are two exceptions to this process. The first exception is necessary for timed tests (e.g., TOD-6C: Rapid Letter Naming). For these tests, the raw score is based on the number of correct items within the time limit. The final exception is necessary for the two TOD-S tests that require administration within Item Sets, Picture Vocabulary (1S) and Letter and Word Choice (2S); these tests require an intermediate step between transforming raw to standard scores/percentiles. The raw scores first are converted to Ability scores using the score conversion Tables A.1 and A.2 from the Appendix A in the Norms Book. These scores are then entered on the TOD-S Screener Scoring Sheet. The Ability scores are then transformed to standard scores and percentiles. The TOD software makes these necessary conversions once the raw scores have been entered.

Age and Grade Equivalents

Age equivalent, or age score, reflects performance in terms of the age level in the norm sample at which the average raw score is the same as the examinee's score. For example, if the mean raw score or number correct for an examinee between the ages of 10–0 and 10–5 years in the norm sample is 23 on TOD-5C: Irregular Word Spelling, then any examinee who obtains a raw score of 23 on that test receives an AE of 10–0 to 10–5. The TOD AEs are reported in various age-range categories, beginning with three-month intervals for the youngest examinees (ages 5–0 to 7–11), six-month intervals (8–0 to 12–11), one-year intervals (13–0 to 14–11), and two-year intervals (15–0 to 18–11); AEs are not reported for adults. Note that the <Start Age designation means that the AE is lower than the score range reported for the lowest AE; the >Stop Age means the individual's score on the test was higher than the score range reported for the highest, or top AE. AEs may be more useful in some applications than GEs, especially as they relate to the abilities of young children or older students and adults who are seeking accommodations or not attending school. The AE is useful when attempting to determine an approximate level of development.

Grade equivalent, or grade score, reflects the examinee's performance in terms of the grade level in the norm sample at which the mean raw score is the same as the examinee's score. In other words, if the average raw score on a test for the students in the standardization sample during the Spring of the ninth grade is 32, then an individual who earns a raw score of 32 would receive a GE of Spring, Grade 9. The TOD GEs are reported for Fall and Spring at each grade level through Spring of Grade 12. GEs are not available for adults. Note that the <Start Age designation means that the GE is lower than the score range reported for the lowest GE; the >Stop Age means the individual's score on the test was higher than the score range reported for the highest, or top GE. The GEs on tests like the TOD represent an estimate of the examinee's instructional level and can be used for instructional planning. Because the test includes items distributed over a wide range of difficulty levels (rather than a limited range typically found on group-administered tests), the age and grade scores more accurately reflect the level of task difficulty at which an individual can perform.

Either AEs or GEs can be displayed but not in the same software-generated score

---

DON'T FORGET

The GE can be useful when attempting to determine an appropriate, approximate level for instruction.

≡ Rapid Reference 5.2

Examples of AE and GE Descriptive Statements

- Jimmy's GE score on the Reading Fluency composite indicated that he is reading at approximately a beginning second-grade level (GE = Fall, Grade 2).
- On the Oral Reading Efficiency test, Marisa, a 10th-grade student, scored similarly to the average student in the early seventh grade (GE = Fall Grade 7).
- Dana's listening comprehension as assessed on the Listening Vocabulary test was comparable to the average seven-year-old student.
- The number of items that Terrell, a third-grade student, answered correctly on the Regular Word Spelling test was comparable to the average student in the early second grade (GE = Fall, Grade 2).

report. If grade norms are used, then the score report automatically displays GEs. If age norms are used, then AEs are automatically displayed. If both are needed, select one option and create the report, then select the second option and create a second report. To add in either AEs or GEs, select a new score selection template and choose the AE (or GE) option. Rapid Reference 5.2 shows examples of the types of statements that are used for GE and AE scores.

Percentile Ranks

A traditional percentile rank uses a scale from 1 to 99 and compares the person to peers. This score describes performance relative to a specific age- or grade-level in the norm sample. The examinee's percentile rank indicates the percentage of people in the selected segment of the norm sample who obtained scores the same as or lower than the examinee's score. Percentile ranks are particularly useful for describing a person's relative standing in the population. For example, Tim's percentile rank of 10 on the Reading and Spelling Index (RSI) indicates that his performance was the same as or better than only 10% of the population (age or grade mates), whereas Susan's percentile rank of 90 on this index indicates that her score was the same as or better than 90% of the population. In other words, only 10% of her same age (or grade) peers would have a higher score. Rapid Reference 5.3 provides examples of statements describing percentile ranks.

DON'T FORGET

Percentiles ranks are often easier to understand than standard scores, especially for parents and teachers.

CAUTION

Percentile ranks are not equal interval units. Scores that are around the mean (50) are closer together than the scores at the ends of the bell curve (1–5 or 95–100). Because of this, percentile ranks are not a good metric for determining or inferring growth.

≡ Rapid Reference 5.3

Examples of Statements Describing Percentile Ranks

- Harper's percentile rank of 99 on the Picture Vocabulary test indicates that only one out of 100 of her peers would have a score as high or higher; i.e., her score was as high or higher than 99 out of 100 people.
- Donald's percentile rank of 10 on the Phonological Manipulation test indicates that only 10 out of 100 third-grade students would obtain a score as low or lower. Only 10% of grade-mates scored as low as or lower than Donald.
- On the Vocabulary and Reasoning 2 composite, Nico's percentile rank of 50 indicates that 50 out of 100 of his peers would have a score the same or lower.

Standard Scores

The TOD standard score scale used in the direct assessment tests is based on a population mean of 100 and a standard deviation (SD) of 15; the SD expresses variance around the mean. Standard scores are assumed to be on an interval scale. That is, scores are characterized by equal magnitude between each score. On an interval scale, a minimal score of zero does not indicate a total lack of ability but might mean that an examinee's ability is below the bottom of the test scale. This psychometric scale is the same as most deviation-score scales and is typically available on tests of cognitive abilities and/or achievement. Consequently, this psychometric scale can be used to relate standard scores from the TOD to other test scores from the TOD or other tests that use the same mean and SD. All TOD tests, composites, and indexes use this scale. Tables 1.4 and 1.5 in the TOD Manual, as well as in Chapters 3 and 4 of this book, show the tests, composites, and indexes for the TOD-S and TOD-C and the TOD-S and TOD-E. Rapid Reference 5.4 shows the standard score ranges used in the TOD-C and TOD-E and their corresponding verbal labels; Rapid Reference 5.7 shows those for the TOD-S.

≡ Rapid Reference 5.4

Standard Scores and Corresponding Descriptors

SS Range	Verbal Label
120 and above	Well Above Average
110–119	Above Average
90–109	Average
80–89	Below Average
70–79	Well Below Average
69 and below	Significantly Below Average

As discussed, standard scores characterize performance relative to same age or same grade peers for TOD tests and composites. Although one type of standard score relies on the same psychometric scale as all the others (i.e., mean of 100 and SD of 15), it is somewhat more sophisticated requiring calculations beyond straightforward raw-to-standard score transformations. This type of score is referred to as an Index and is created from a series of multiple regressions equations. The Indexes are powerful global scores; three of them were created specifically to predict either dyslexia *risk* from the TOD-S tests, referenced as the Dyslexia Risk Index (DRI), or diagnostic *probability* from the TOD-E and TOD-C tests, referenced as the Early Dyslexia Diagnostic Index (EDDI), and the Dyslexia Diagnostic Index (DDI). Indexes are perhaps the most critical TOD scores because of their predictive power.

Figures 3.1, 3.2, and 3.3 in the TOD Manual provide checklists, one for each of the TOD batteries. The checklists present several statements to consider when in the process of diagnosing dyslexia. Each statement that is answered "Yes" increases confidence in a diagnosis of dyslexia. The content of the checklists addresses important variables, such as family and intervention/instructional history, early speech and language difficulties, ADHD, and information from the rating scale scores.

The standard score for the TOD Rating Scales relies on a different psychometric scale, specifically a population mean of 50 and SD of 10; it is referenced by the letter "T." (See Chapter 6 for a more detailed description of how to interpret the rating scale T-scores.) Rating scale raw-to-standard score transformations are only available from the electronic software program and are shown on the TOD Rating Scale Report. Rapid Reference 5.5 shows the standard score means and SDs for the two types of TOD standard scores.

DON'T FORGET

Because standard scores are more difficult for parents and other nonprofessionals to understand, many examiners use AE or GE scores or percentile ranks to explain test results.

DON'T FORGET

Any standard score can be converted into a percentile rank and vice versa. Statements describing performance based on standard scores can help place performance in context relative to peers. Rapid Reference 5.6 provides some examples.

≡ Rapid Reference 5.5

Means and Standard Deviations for the Two TOD Standard Scores

TOD	Score	Mean	Standard Deviation
Rating Scales	T	50	10
Indexes, Composites, and Tests	SS	100	15

≡ Rapid Reference 5.6

Examples of Standard Score Descriptive Statements

- Jayden's score on the TOD-5C Irregular Word Spelling test was 72 and fell within the Well Below Average range. This score reflects the difficulty he experiences learning to spell new words.

- Rob's EDDI score was 75 (72–78, 90% Confidence Interval; 5th percentile) and fell within the Well Below Average range. This score is consistent with a Very High Probability of Dyslexia.

- Richard's standard score of 113 (105–121; 90% Confidence Interval; 81st percentile) indicated that his performance on the Picture Analogies Test fell in the Above Average range.

- Joni's DDI score was 61 (57–65, 90% Confidence Interval; percentile rank <1) and fell within the Significantly Below Average range. This score is consistent with an Extremely High Probability of Dyslexia.

Primary Score Relationships and Interpretation

The TOD scores most commonly used by evaluators to represent performance of examinees are the two standard scores shown in Rapid Reference 5.5 and percentile ranks. All direct assessment tests, composites, and indexes use the standard score scale that yields a population mean of 100 and a SD of 15. The TOD Rating Scales use the T-score scale. Both types of standard scores correspond to percentile ranks.

DON'T FORGET

The examples in Rapid Reference 5.6 are based on standard scores and are obtained by comparing the examinee's performance to others of the same age. For school age examinees, however, it is possible to compare an examinee's scores to grade-level peers. As discussed, the choice depends on the referral question.

Figure 5.1 shows the relationships among these three scores and how the scores define ability based on approximate magnitude of the scores across the population. Because the TOD standardization sample closely approximates the U.S. population based on relevant demographics (i.e., gender, race/ethnicities, geographic regions, and SES), performance tends to mimic the normal curve. The height of the graph under the curve corresponds to percentages of the population, linked to standard scores and percentiles, which are shown on the ability dimension, the horizontal x-axis. These scores are nested within SD ranges, specifically within three SDs below and above the population mean.

For example, approximately 34% of the population earns scores from −1 SD to the mean, represented on the graph by the z-score of 0, corresponding to standard scores ranging from 85 to 100, and T-scores ranging from 40 to 50. Similarly, 34% earn scores from the mean to +1 SD above the mean, corresponding to standard scores ranging from 100 to 115 and T-scores ranging from 50 to 60. About 68% of the population falls between −1 and +1 SD around the mean. About 14% falls between −1 and −2 SDs below the mean and because the curve is symmetrical, 14% falls between +1 and +2 SDs above the mean. Approximately 4%

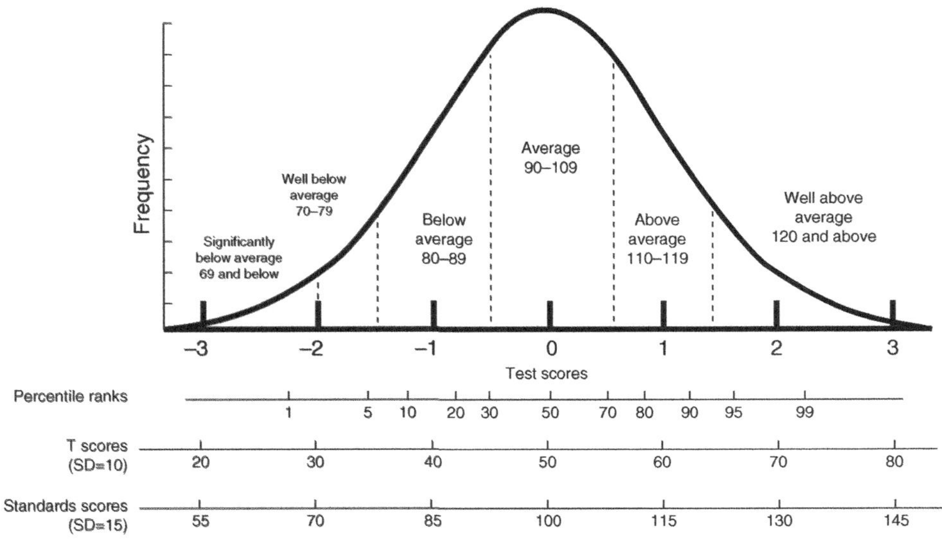

Figure 5.1   Relationship Among Percentile Ranks, T-Scores, and Standard Scores

of the population falls in the extremes: 2% below −2 SDs and 2% above +2 SDs. The graph also shows standard scores that are linked to the TOD descriptive verbal labels shown in Rapid References 5.4 and 5.7. For example, TOD-C and TOD-E test, composite, and index scores between 90 and 109 are designated as Average, those between 80 and 89 as Below Average, those between 70 and 79 as Well Below Average, and those 69 and below as Significantly Below Average. Scores that range from 110 to 119 are Above Average, and those that are 120 and above are Well Above Average. Also, percentages within these categories can be determined by examining the percentile ranks in Rapid Reference 5.7. For example, approximately 10% of the population earns percentile ranks of 90 and above, corresponding to a standard score of 120 and above and designated as Well Above Average, i.e., 100−90% = 10%; about 15% of the population earns percentile ranks between 75 and 90, i.e., 90−75% = 15%, Above Average. Percentages within each of the categories can be determined similarly. About 50% earn percentiles between 25 and 75 and are characterized as Average; about 15% earn percentiles between 10 and 25, Below Average; about 8% earn percentiles between 70 and 80, Well Below Average; and about 2% earn percentile ranks below 2, Significantly Below Average.

Zero Scores

In cases in which an individual receives a zero on any test, it is important to consider whether that score represents a true assessment of ability to perform the task as opposed to lack of understanding of the task demands, inattentiveness, or lack of effort. Also, although unlikely, if the individual has not been exposed to the type of task in question, it may be more appropriate not to score the test rather than interpret a zero raw score. Even when a zero score is considered an accurate reflection of ability and is entered into the scoring program, cautious interpretation is recommended.

Growth Scores

Growth scores are a special transformation of the Rasch ability scale (Rasch, 1960/1980; Wright & Stone, 1979) based on person and ability estimates consistent with the model and implemented for TOD scores using Winsteps (version 5.2.4.0; Linacre, 2023). This scaling process creates equal interval metrics; consequently, using raw to growth conversions, the Growth scores reflect gains across the entire age ranges and can track instructional and developmental progress. Also, growth trajectories can be compared across tests. The Growth scale for each test is centered on a constant unique to each test and 500 is added to the Growth Score equation to eliminate negative numbers. Growth scores were created for all TOD tests except Oral Reading Efficiency; separate Growth score tables were created for the Phonological Manipulation test for both subtests: Substitution and Deletion. Growth scores are included in the Progress Monitoring Report generated by the WPS Online Evaluation System (OES) at platform.wpspublish.com. Tables for determining Raw to Growth scores conversions are available in the TOD Norms Book appendices, Tables A.15, B.18, and C.13, for the TOD-S, TOD-C, and TOD-E.

COMMUNICATING PERFORMANCE LEVELS

When reporting results to parents, teachers, and examinees, the evaluator selects the scores that are most meaningful given the referral question(s) and most easily explained; some metrics are easier to interpret than others. For parents and teachers, AEs and GEs or percentile ranks are often discussed first as they are more easily understood than standard scores. Standard scores are best for discussing intra- and interindividual strengths and weaknesses, typically by comparing scores across tests, composites, or indexes. Evaluators need to consider the audience in order to communicate effectively the purpose and interpretation of each type of score and be able to accurately answer any questions.

Evaluators typically include standard scores, percentile ranks, and AEs or GEs when writing their reports. Alternatively, evaluators may prefer to use verbal labels/categories rather than numbers to describe test performance. This may be especially helpful when interpreting the TOD's Index scores, such as the DRI, DDI, or the EDDI. These Indexes provide information about the individual's risk or probability of dyslexia. The term "risk" is used to characterize the TOD-S DRI, since it is based on only two tests, although both are considered powerful indicators of risk. The third TOD-S test, Picture Vocabulary, is included to provide an estimate of general ability; if it is significantly higher than the DRI, then the pattern reflects the unexpected nature of dyslexia, and more assessment may be warranted. The term "probability" is used with the TOD-C DDI and the TOD-E EDDI because both of these Indexes are more comprehensive.

Exercise care when characterizing an individual at risk for dyslexia and always consider additional information. Also, use person-first language when describing an individual with a high probability of dyslexia (e.g., "an individual with a Very High Probability of dyslexia" rather than "a dyslexic individual"). In general, use cautious language and professional judgment in the selection and application of verbal labels to describe a range of scores.

Rapid Reference 5.7 provides suggested categorical labels to use when describing standard scores and percentile rank ranges for the TOD-S, TOD-E, and TOD-C. In addition, if the DRI, EDDI, or DDI are calculated, then the verbal labels describing the Risk or Probability of dyslexia apply.

≣ *Rapid Reference 5.7*

Verbal Labels for Standard Scores and Percentile Ranks

TOD-Screener

Tests, Composites, Indexes			DRI
Standard Scores	**Percentile Ranks**	**Verbal Labels**	**Risk of dyslexia**
110 and above	Above 75	Above Average	No to Low Risk
90–109	25–75	Average	Possible Risk*
89 and below	Below 25	Below Average	At-Risk

* Lower possible risk at the high end of the average range and higher possible risk at the low end of the average range.

TOD-Comprehensive and TOD-Early

Tests, Composites, Indexes			EDDI or DDI
Standard Scores	**Percentile Ranks**	**Verbal Labels**	**Probability of Dyslexia**
120 and above	90 and above	Well Above Average	Extremely Low Probability
110–119	75–89	Above Average	Very Low Probability
90–109	25–7	Average	Low to Moderate Probability*
80–89	10–24	Below Average	High Probability
70–79	2–9	Well Below Average	Very High Probability
69 and below	Below 2	Significantly Below Average	Extremely High Probability

* Low probability at the high end of the average range and moderate probability at the low end of the average range.

CAUTION

Because the TOD-S is a screener, the verbal descriptors and percentile ranks are not as diagnostic as those for the TOD-C and TOD-E.

Standard Error of Measurement

Every TOD standard score consists of two components: ability and error, and they are inversely related. The less error, the more confidence an evaluator has that the score represents the ability the test is designed to measure. Fortunately, test authors have created a good strategy for determining error, and that strategy results in an estimate referred to as the standard error of measurement (SEM). Every TOD standard score is reported along with a confidence band or interval, created from its corresponding SEM.

To better illustrate the importance of knowing the SEM for any score, perhaps a nontest example of how it applies in our daily lives might be useful. Assume someone wants to buy a new set of scales to determine weight. The goal is to buy scales that are not only accurate but also consistent. That is, if one's weight does not change from day to day, then the scales should reflect no change. So, if a person's weight is 130 pounds and never changes, the scales should show that value each time the person weighs. If it does, scales are consistent, or "reliable." On the other hand, if the person's weight does not change but the scales vary from day to day, the scales are unreliable and not useful. Fortunately, a method exists that scale makers can use to determine the reliability of the scales. The first step is to calculate the amount of variability the scales exhibit. This value is known as the "standard deviation (SD)" and can be obtained by weighing some object of the same weight every day and calculating the variability in the scores using a simple formula. The formula provides an estimate of variability of the scores and may be thought of as the average amount the scores deviate from the mean or average score. The formula requires that each value be subtracted from the mean, squared, and then summed; that value is then divided by the number of scores and the square root of that value obtained. The smaller the SD, the closer the scores are to the average score; the larger the SD, the further the scores typically are from the mean.

The next goal in determining error requires calculation of a numerical representation of it, or the SEM. To calculate the SEM, it is necessary to first use a traditional formula that compares two sets of scores, and for our example of scales, obtained weights across two days, probably alternative days. This formula is defined by a statistical equation referred to as the Pearson Product Moment Correlation Coefficient, usually just represented as "r." In the interest of simplicity, the formula is not provided here, although it is not difficult to calculate, and many hand-held calculators are capable of obtaining it. This value, r, can be used to define reliability, and it characterizes the relationship between two distributions of weights taken, in the above example, on alternate days. The correlation coefficient r always ranges between -1.0 and $+1.0$., and the closer to either extreme value, the stronger the relationship between the two sets of scores (i.e., the more the two numbers within the two sets of scores are similar in magnitude the closer r will be to 1.0). In our example of the scales, the goal is to get a score near $+1.0$, meaning that the scores on alternate days are the same or nearly so. If both sets of scores increase at the same rate, then the r value will be positive; if the scores in one distribution go down and the scores in the other go up by the same or similar magnitude, then the number will be negative and close to -1.0, a very unlikely outcome. Ideally, the numbers would be the same or nearly the same on alternative days, and the r value would be very close to positive 1.0, meaning the scales are useful. These procedures are the same as are used by test authors to define the reliability of a test and the percentage of test error.

Given r, it is possible to obtain an estimate of the similarity of the scores across the two distributions that is easier to understand intuitively. That is, squaring r yields a value called the Coefficient of Determination, and it characterizes the percentage of variance overlap. So, if the r value from the Pearson equation is .90, then the percentage of systematic variance overlap of the two tests is .81; if the r value is .96, then the percentage of systematic variance overlap is .92. At this point, it is simple to get the percentage of error—in this case, 1 minus .92, or 8%, as 1 represents unity, or the total variance a test can possibly contain. Returning to the example with the scales, assuming the r value is .96 and the Coefficient of Determination is .92 the scales have 8% error.

DON'T FORGET

Confidence bands, or intervals, provide a range of standard scores based on the SEM and reflect the confidence that the examinee's true score falls within the identified range.

The SEM for a particular test is obtained by multiplying the standard score SD, 15 for the TOD and most standardized tests, times the square root of 1- reliability. Because errors are assumed to be normally distributed, this value defines the amount of error within one SD below and above the mean of the distribution of errors. For the TOD interpretation (and other tests, typically), the evaluator can choose which level is best for a particular examinee. Fortunately, the TOD software calculates these values.

INTERPRETING STANDARD SCORE OR PERCENTILE RANGES

Each TOD score is presented along with its corresponding estimate of error contained within the confidence band created from the SEM. Interpretation within a confidence band is preferable to interpreting a single score because the band defines error and systematic variance and thus, communicates how much confidence evaluators can have in scores as previously described. The confidence band describes the values that set limits around an examinee's true score. The true score is assumed to represent the examinee's true ability, i.e., without sources of error, such as fatigue, practice, or lack of motivation. The online scoring platform provides an option to select a 90% or 95% level of confidence. A 90% confidence band (±1.65 SEM) represents the region (i.e., range of scores) within which an individual's true ability would fall 9 times out of 10. A 95% confidence band (±1.96 SEM) represents the region within which an individual's true ability would fall 19 times out of 20.

Rapid Reference 5.8 illustrates the standard score confidence bands at the 90% level of confidence based on grade norms for three TOD-C Index scores: the DDI, RSI, and the LPI. As is apparent from this information, the DDI has a smaller range of scores than either of the other two indexes, meaning less error is associated with this score. This pattern is typical as this score is created from more tests and, assuming all other influences are equal, a composite created from more tests is more reliable and, hence, has less error than a composite comprised of fewer tests or an individual test score.

Standard scores and percentiles are important indicators of normative strengths and weaknesses. Because for the standard score ranges the reference point is set to a population mean

≡ *Rapid Reference 5.8*

Standard Score Confidence Bands (90% level)

TOD-C Indexes	SS (90% Confidence Band)
Dyslexia Diagnostic Index (DDI)	93 (89–97)
Reading and Spelling Index (RSI)	87 (80–94)
Linguistic Processing Index (LPI)	101 (95–107)

of 100 (with an associated SD of 15) (a) a standard score of 115 (84 percentile) is one SD above the mean and a score of 115 or above always indicates a normative strength, (b) a standard score of 85–115 often indicates average ability (within one SD below to one SD above the mean), and (c) a standard score of 85 (16th percentile) is one SD below the mean and a score at that level or below usually indicates a weakness.

Not all experts or test developers use the same descriptive ranges to characterize scores below and above the mean. Some recommend that (a) a standard score of 110 (75 percentile) or above should indicate a normative strength, (b) a standard score of 90–110 should indicate average ability (describing 50% of the population), and (c) a standard score of 90 (25th percentile) or below should indicate a weakness. The TOD uses these ranges.

The TOD Score Report shows the most relevant test data, including descriptive ranges, standard scores, confidence intervals, percentile ranks, and either the AE or GE. In addition, test scores that comprise the TOD indexes are graphically profiled so that strengths and weaknesses on these measures can be determined more easily. For example, the profile shows the magnitude of the scores and may inform the selection of interventions from *Dyslexia Interventions and Recommendations: A Companion Guide to the Tests of Dyslexia* (Mather et al., 2024c). Other score comparisons may also be important for determining important variations in the scores and are discussed in more detail in the section on Comparing TOD Scores.

Because a single score on an individual test cannot be assumed to represent a precise description of specific academic skills, a single test score is best used to generate hypotheses about academic performance. Follow-up data from composites and indexes are more reliable estimates of achievement than those derived from individual test scores. In addition, extra test data and observations from the classroom must be considered along with information gleaned from the TOD teacher, parent, and self-rating scales and other relevant academic, medical, and developmental history.

CAUTION

A single score is not a precise representation of a specific skill, ability, or level of performance. Consider the range of scores displayed as confidence bands as well as data from related composites, indexes, and observations to confirm any hypotheses suggested by a single score.

In addition to determining normative strengths and weaknesses, evaluators often discuss "relative" strengths and weaknesses. This concept becomes particularly relevant when analyzing the performance of very low-functioning or very high-functioning students. For example, an examinee may obtain a standard score of 80 in Basic Reading Skills and 58 in Spelling. Although both scores are below average, basic reading could be described as a "relative" strength. A "twice exceptional" student (e.g., a gifted or high ability student who also has dyslexia) may have superior scores in Reasoning (e.g., a standard score of 130), but only average scores in Basic Reading Skills (e.g., a standard score of 95). In this example, basic reading could be described as a relative weakness. The next section describes these types of tests comparisons in more detail.

COMPARING TOD SCORES

In many cases, score comparisons can address referral questions, particularly an individual's pattern of strengths and weakness. For example, when a number of tests are administered, variability will exist among the test scores, and this pattern will inform either normative or within-the-individual ipsative strengths and weaknesses. Observing the score patterns on graphs provided by the TOD software is helpful, but statistical test comparisons often are necessary to determine whether test variability is clinically meaningful. In order to say that one score is meaningfully different than another score, the first step is to determine if the magnitude of difference between the two scores represents chance variation and/or if this difference is rare in the population. For example, the TOD software determines whether a particular test score is statistically significantly different from another, i.e., the magnitude of the difference is so large it would only occur 5 out of 100 times or less ($p < .05$). In addition, the software calculates how rare the difference is in the population of peers and shows the result in the Score Report under the heading, "Percentage of the sample with this difference."

Ultimately, an evaluator must determine whether a statistically significant and rare difference has any practical or educational implications. A difference may exist between measures but have little educational relevance. For example, Serena earned an Average standard score of 98 (45th percentile) on Rapid Letter Naming. This score was significantly lower than her Above Average performance on the Reading Comprehension Efficiency composite standard score of 118 (88th percentile) and rare. Because her Rapid Letter Naming score was within the average range, she probably does not need an accommodation or intervention. In this case, her "average" score is typical of students who are achieving satisfactorily.

Comparisons between the DDI and VR2 and VR4 are printed on the Score Report regardless of significance; all of the others are printed only if the differences reach the $p < .05$ level of significance. Differences that are statistically significant at the .05 level may be "of potential concern" clinically and may be most helpful for creating hypotheses about sources of problems that can be verified by additional data. Differences that are large enough to be significantly different *and* rare should be considered more clinically meaningful and of significant concern.

Finally, a few additional examples can further illustrate how test comparison outcomes can address referral questions. For example, if an examinee was referred because of slow, effortful reading, then it would be helpful to compare the Basic Reading Skills composite to the Reading Fluency composite for statistical significance and frequency of occurrence in the population. This comparison may help to determine if the problem is due to weak basic reading skills or a slow reading rate.

As another example, some examinees who have dyslexia may also have a comorbid developmental language disorder. In this case, the evaluator may begin by determining whether the magnitude of the Reasoning Composite score is significantly higher (and rare) relative to the Vocabulary composite score. If the Vocabulary score is commensurate with reading test scores, but the Reasoning score is much higher, then it is more likely that this pattern reflects a developmental language disorder in addition to or instead of dyslexia. In general, given that dyslexia is often "unexpected" (Catts & Petscher, 2022; S. Shaywitz & Shaywitz, 2020), it is important to compare relevant scores that address the differences between performance on tests assumed to be negatively impacted by dyslexia and those that are not likely to be affected. If an examinee is administered the TOD-E, the first test administered is Picture Vocabulary. Picture Vocabulary is a measure of receptive vocabulary that can then be compared to the TOD-E reading and spelling test scores.

Similarly, if administering the TOD-C Vocabulary and/or Reasoning tests, then these composites can be obtained as an estimate of cognitive ability and compared to the TOD-C

RSI. Alternatively, scores from the TOD-C Vocabulary and Reasoning composites, either the two-test or four-test version, can be compared to the TOD-C Linguistic Processing Index (LPI) to help determine whether certain abilities thought to underlie dyslexia are lower than overall cognitive ability. Chapters 9 and 10 include a number of comparisons within cases and illustrate how the TOD results may help inform diagnosis and interventions. In addition, Table 3.7 in the TOD Manual describes the most critical diagnostic comparisons.

IMPORTANCE OF INSTRUCTIONAL HISTORY IN DECISION-MAKING AND INSTRUCTIONAL PLANNING

In some cases, TOD scores may be influenced by prior instruction. For example, the LPI may be higher than anticipated for students who have a history of systematic basic reading instruction. In these cases, the magnitude of relevant difference scores may not reach statistical significance or be rare, even though the student may have dyslexia. Consequently, it is important to check on the examinee's instructional history through both interviews and data from the TOD Rating Scales.

CAUTION

Do not under interpret test scores for examinees who have a strong history of interventions. They may have dyslexia even though their scores are in the average range, reflecting the efficacy of the interventions.

USING TOD TESTS, COMPOSITES, AND INDEXES TO IDENTIFY DYSLEXIA CHARACTERISTICS AND/OR A SPECIFIC LEARNING DISABILITY IN READING

The TOD-S, TOD-E, and TOD-C test, index, and composite scores, combined with results from the TOD Rating Scales and checklists, can help identify the characteristics of dyslexia. The TOD contains all the direct assessment tests needed to operationalize the constructs most states require to determine dyslexia, including phonemic/phonological awareness, rapid automatized naming, letter/word knowledge, fluency, and spelling.

In addition, TOD data can inform a Specific Learning Disability (SLD) diagnosis in basic reading skills or reading fluency. Figures 3.5, 3.6, and 3.7 from the TOD Manual describe specific steps for identifying an SLD using an Ability-Achievement Discrepancy Model (A-A), a Pattern of Strengths and Weaknesses Model (PSW), or a Response to Intervention (RTI) Model. The following paragraphs describe briefly how scores from the TOD may aid in determining eligibility using these models.

The A-A model relies on establishing a statistically significant and rare difference between an examinee's general cognitive ability and some measure(s) of achievement. Eligibility within this model can be demonstrated by comparing the TOD Vocabulary and Reasoning 4 (VR4) composite score to one or more of the TOD-C reading and/or spelling composites and then determining the difference between VR4 and the relevant composites, using the WPS online scoring system. Those differences can help inform a diagnosis of SLD in the areas of Basic Reading Skills or Reading Fluency.

The PSW model is sometimes referred to as a variant of the A-A model, as both are designed to determine whether there is an unexpected academic weakness given general

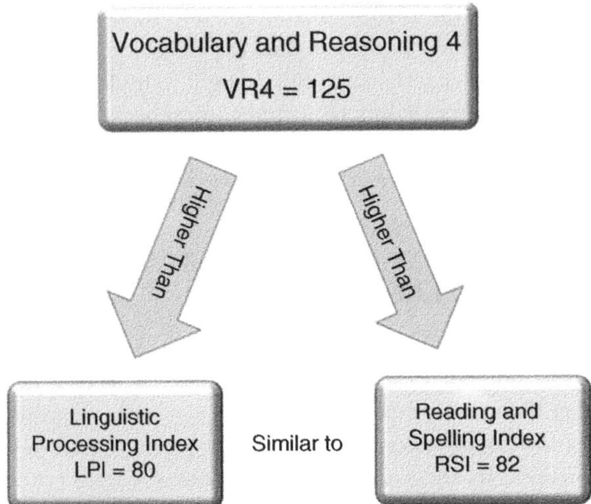

Figure 5.2   Comparison of the TOD-C VR4 Composite to the LPI and RSI Scores to Determine a Pattern of Strengths and Weaknesses

cognitive ability. The PSW model requires that a link be established between the academic weakness (in the case of dyslexia, a weakness in basic reading skills or reading rate) and foundational linguistic processing skills that underlie development of reading and spelling. This link is typically operationalized by similar scores on the weak academic area(s) and the foundational processing skills but higher scores on unrelated academic and cognitive ability measures. Both the A-A and PSW models assume low academic scores in spite of quality instruction, resulting in an unexpected outcome. Tests on the TOD operationalize the relevant abilities. For example, the VR4 composite can be compared to various TOD-C indexes, composites and individual test scores, which may be compared to each other. Figure 5.2 depicts a comparison of the VR4 with the TOD-C LPI and RSI, for an individual with dyslexia.

Finally, the RTI model also requires low scores based on documented universal screening measures combined with lack of adequate progress, despite evidence-based instruction over time. In some cases, at the end of some required period of instruction without evidence of adequate improvement, the likelihood of a SLD eligibility is explored. At this juncture, school systems may require additional psychoeducational assessment (e.g., to rule in or out eligibility based on either the A-A or PSW models).

LINKING TEST SELECTION TO DIAGNOSIS, RECOMMENDATIONS, AND INTERVENTIONS

Evaluators must decide which TOD tests to administer. Particularly important sources are the Test Selection charts that can guide selection beginning on page 11of the TOD Manual. For screening purposes, the TOD-S and the TOD Rating Scales provide reliable estimates of risk of dyslexia. Diagnosis or identification of dyslexia, however, requires more comprehensive assessment with either the TOD-E or TOD-C depending on the age and reading skills of the examinee. The TOD-E EDDI provides a robust measure of the probability that the examinee has dyslexia; it also yields composite scores and individual test scores that can be linked directly to instructional recommendations. Similar to the TOD-E, the TOD-C provides a global score that informs a diagnosis, the DDI, but also numerous composites and individual scores that can aid in selecting instructional recommendations. Many other resources are available in the TOD Manual.

Finally, a good understanding of the TOD constructs and the task demands of the tests that operationalize them is foundational to choosing the most appropriate tests to administer. Of all the TOD direct assessment components, the TOD-C provides the most comprehensive options. Rapid Reference 5.9 lists additional *general* recommendations to guide (TOD-C) test selection. Rapid Reference 5.10 lists recommendations to guide *specific* test selections.

Interventions and recommendations linked to TOD tests can be selected from the print edition of the *Dyslexia Interventions and Recommendations: A Companion Guide to the Tests of Dyslexia (TOD™)* (Mather et al., 2024c). In addition, evaluators can select interventions assumed to be most relevant and include them in a TOD Intervention Report using the TOD software. These interventions and recommendations have empirical support and are written specifically to help teachers/tutors/parents address reading-related limitations. Evaluators can select interventions and/or recommendations specifically for examinees based on their TOD results. Chapters 9 and 10 provide case examples, and many of these incorporate recommendations directly from the guide. Appendix B provides additional practice in interpreting the TOD Score Reports. Appendix C provides copies of the TOD Dyslexia Profiles in which examiners can enter scores from the TOD assessments. Fillable forms can be downloaded from the WPS website.

DON'T FORGET

Appropriate test selection of TOD tests requires knowledge of the constructs, how they are operationalized, and specifically the task demands of the tests selected.

≡ Rapid Reference 5.9

General Recommendations to Guide TOD-C Test Selections

- Obtain composite scores for areas of weakness identified in Tests 1–9.
- Obtain composite scores as needed to determine strengths and weaknesses and to satisfy diagnostic or special education eligibility guidelines.
- Consider the referral question(s)/concerns and choose tests that assess specific skills/abilities of concern.
- Consider areas of weakness as identified by the TOD Rating Scales or from other sources such as student work samples or observations to inform TOD-C test selection.
- Obtain composite scores for major constructs of interest (e.g., phonological awareness, basic reading skills, reading fluency, orthographic processing, and spelling).

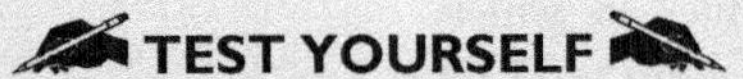

Rapid Reference 5.10

Recommendations for Specific Test Selection on the TOD-C

- In addition to tests 1 through 9, administer 10C: Picture Analogies which allows calculation of the VR2 composite score (a measure of cognitive abilities). The VR2 composite can be compared to the DDI, LPI, and RSI to inform the diagnostic process. For a more robust measure of cognitive abilities, also administer 22C: Listening Vocabulary and 23C: Geometric Analogies to obtain the VR4 composite.

- If an examinee is weak in spelling, administer 15C: Regular Word Spelling in addition to Test 5C: Irregular Word Spelling to form the Spelling composite. Analyze the errors on both tests to guide instructional planning.

- To gain insights into the examinee's decoding skills and to focus instruction, administer 7C: Pseudoword Reading and 11C: Irregular Word Reading to obtain the Basic Reading Skills composite.

- If an examinee performs poorly on 4C: Phonological Manipulation, then administer the more basic phonological awareness tests, 13C: Blending and 14C: Segmenting.

- If reading rate or fluency is a concern, then administer 12C: Oral Reading Efficiency and 16C: Silent Reading Efficiency. In addition, administration of 19C: Rapid Pseudoword Reading and 20C: Rapid Irregular Word Reading may provide helpful information, especially for younger children.

TEST YOURSELF

1. Selecting grade-based norms does not affect

(a) age equivalents.

(b) percentile ranks.

(c) test standard scores.

(d) composite standard scores.

2. The _______ Index is made up of tests of foundational abilities underlying performance of those academic skills most affected by dyslexia.

(a) Reading and Spelling

(b) Linguistic Processing

(c) Early Dyslexia Risk

(d) Vocabulary and Reasoning 2

3. What score is best suited for comparing test and composite scores?

(a) Standard score

(b) Percentile rank

(c) Grade equivalent

(d) Age equivalent

4. **If an examinee received a standard score of 115 on the Reading Fluency test it means**

   (a) the examinee earned a score at the 16th percentile.

   (b) the examinee earned a score at the 55th percentile.

   (c) the examinee scored at the 84th percentile.

   (d) the examinee earned a score at or above 98% of peers.

5. **If an examinee has a percentile rank of 5 on a test, this means**

   (a) the examinee scored the same as or higher than 5 out of 100 people.

   (b) the examinee scored lower than 5 out of 100 people.

   (c) the examinee scored lower than the .5th percentile.

   (d) the examinee scored the same as or better than 5 out of 1,000 people.

6. **The Linguistic Processing Index may be average if an examinee has a history of**

   (a) reading difficulties in the family.

   (b) comorbid language difficulties.

   (c) intensive instruction in reading skills.

   (d) systematic oral language instruction.

7. **The best score on the TOD to operationalize ability for use in an ability-achievement comparison would be**

   (a) Vocabulary and Reasoning 2.

   (b) Vocabulary and Reasoning 4.

   (c) Early Dyslexia Diagnostic Index.

   (d) Dyslexia Diagnostic Index.

8. **If the magnitude of the difference between two tests is significant at the .05 level, it means that**

   (a) the difference is so large that it likely occurred in less than about 5% of the population.

   (b) the difference is so large that it likely occurred in less than about 50% of the population.

   (c) the difference is so small that it likely occurred in more than about 5% of the population.

   (d) the difference is so small that it likely occurred in more than about 50% of the population.

9. **The TOD-S is best for**

   (a) comprehensive assessment.

   (b) qualitative assessment.

   (c) curriculum-based assessment.

   (d) screening assessment.

10. **Standard scores are assumed to be on a (an) _______ scale**

    (a) nominal

    (b) ordinal

    (c) equal interval

    (d) ratio

Answers: 1. a; 2. b; 3. a; 4. c; 5. a; 6. c; 7. b; 8. a; 9. d; 10. c

REFERENCES

Catts, H. W., & Petscher, Y. (2022). A cumulative risk and resilience model of dyslexia. *Journal of Learning Disabilities, 55*(3), 1–14. https://doi.org/10.1177/00222194211037062

Linacre, J. M. (2023). *Winsteps (Version 5.6.0) (Computer Software)*. Retrieved from https://www.winsteps.com/

Mather, N., McCallum, R. S., Bell, S. M., & Wendling, B. J. (2024b). *Tests of Dyslexia (TOD)* [Manual]. Western Psychological Services.

Mather, N., McCallum, R. S., Bell, S. M., & Wendling, B. J. (2024c). *Dyslexia interventions and recommendations: A companion guide to the Tests of Dyslexia (TOD)*. Western Psychological Services.

Rasch, G. (1960/1980). *Probabilistic models for some intelligence and attainment tests*. University of Chicago Press.

Shaywitz, S., & Shaywitz, J. (2020). *Overcoming dyslexia* (2nd ed.). Knopf.

Woodcock, R. W., McGrew, K., & Mather, N. (2001). *Woodcock-Johnson Tests of Cognitive Abilities and Tests of Achievement* (3rd ed.). Riverside.

Wright, B. D., & Stone, M. H. (1979). *Best test designs*. Mesa Press.

Six

USE OF THE TOD RATING SCALES IN THE IDENTIFICATION OF DYSLEXIA

"I was on the whole considerably discouraged by my school days.... It is not pleasant to feel oneself so completely outclassed and left behind at the very beginning of the race."

—Winston Churchill

Many very accomplished individuals have a history of reading-related problems, which includes dyslexia. Evaluators are often responsible for obtaining information about an examinee's performance to inform a diagnosis or determine eligibility for services. In order to do so, test scores obtained from direct assessments are essential. Obtaining additional information about an examinee's history, school and home environment, and perspectives from knowledgeable individuals, including the examinee, is critical as well. A comprehensive evaluation should include both direct assessments and observational rating scales. Fortunately, both are typically used in school and clinical settings as indicators of reading performance and to evaluate risk for reading difficulties.

Direct performance measures, including curriculum-based measures and achievement tests, provide objective assessment of an individual's reading, spelling, and related cognitive and linguistic skills and abilities. The TOD-S, TOD-E, and TOD-C provide direct assessment of the critical skills and abilities related to dyslexia (Mather et al., 2024a). Classroom observational data and teacher reports can provide additional important data. In fact, an extensive body of research affirms the validity of teacher ratings (McCallum & Bracken, 2018). Critical information can also be gathered from review of the individual's history (i.e., family history of reading difficulties, developmental history, medical history, and history of tutorial or remedial support). As part of a comprehensive screening and assessment of dyslexia, rating scales can provide relevant family and developmental history (Pennington et al., 2019; Wagner et al., 2019). Information from multiple informants, including parents/caregivers, teachers, and examinees, is particularly helpful when making screening and diagnostic decisions (Wagner et al., 2019). Rating scales allow for the early identification of reading-related problems, are easy and quick to administer, and add to the diagnostic accuracy of direct assessments.

For individuals with dyslexia, learning to read is very difficult. Rating scales can help gauge that difficulty by eliciting information from the individuals themselves, their teachers, and family members. A young child with dyslexia once said, "I would rather clean mold from the bathtub than read!" (Wolf, 2008).

These reading difficulties often continue into the postsecondary years. A 24-year-old female (pseudonym Sara) underwent a psychoeducational evaluation to procure extended time eligibility and other accommodations in her university setting in relation to her history of struggles with reading and writing. Sara's general intellectual ability was assessed at the 97th percentile. She acquires information almost exclusively through audiobooks. She has a very strong Grade Point Average (GPA) (3.83) and hopes to attend graduate school. She is a dedicated student who spends extensive time studying and preparing for class and tests. Sara describes her reading and spelling skills like this: "I have difficulty reading. I often mistake one word for another. I have cried a river over spelling mistakes by this point in my life. I have an extensive vocabulary, but I cannot spell the majority of words. I have long since accepted these difficulties to be part of who I am and I do not allow them to prevent me from participating" (personal communication, April 24, 2025).

Teachers recognize these struggles and often observe both strengths and weaknesses. When describing a 14-year-old male (Percy F.) with "word blindness" (what we now refer to as dyslexia), Dr. W. Pringle Morgan wrote: "In writing from dictation he comes to grief over any but the simplest words. For instance, I dictated the following sentence: "Now, you watch me while I spin it." He wrote: "Now you word me wale I spin it"; and, again, "Carefully winding the string round the peg" was written: "Calfuly winder the sturng rond the Pag," In writing his own name, he made a mistake, putting "Precy" for "Percy," and he did not notice the mistake until his attention was called to it more than once. . .The schoolmaster who has taught him for some years says that he would be the smartest lad in the school if the instruction were entirely oral" (Morgan, 1896, p. 1378).

Parents and family members are also often aware of the challenges individuals with dyslexia face. In discussing worry about her son, Redford (n.d.), the Education Editor, stated: "I think it is safe to say that parents of dyslexics worry about their children more than most. There is good reason for this: Dyslexic children spend most of their early school dealing with a lot of failure and struggle" (Redford, n.d., Yale Center for Dyslexia and Creativity).

In summary, rating scales are useful when making early screening and identification decisions for those who have reading-related problems, are easy and quick to administer, and have the potential to add to the diagnostic accuracy of the identification of dyslexia. For these reasons, the TOD authors created Parent/Caregiver, Teacher, and Self-Rating Scales that are appropriate for use across the age span. The TOD Rating Scales were co-normed with the TOD direct assessment tests and are designed to be both comprehensive and easy to administer.

DESCRIPTIONS OF THE TOD RATING SCALES

Five forms of the TOD Rating Scales were developed to provide a structured means of collecting relevant information about family history and factors and concerns related to dyslexia: TOD-C Parent/Caregiver, TOD-C Teacher, TOD-C Self-Rating, TOD-E Parent/Caregiver, and TOD-E Teacher. TOD-C Rating Scales assess reading-related skills and history from the perspectives of parents or caregivers, teachers, and the examinee. TOD-E Rating Scales provide perspectives of parents or caregivers and teachers. Although an attempt was made to develop a TOD-E Self-Rating form, the examinees were too young to provide reliable and valid data. Younger children, however, may still be able to provide important qualitative information via an interview format. Rapid Reference 6.1 lists some potential questions that may be useful to ask a young child in order to learn about their experiences with reading and related skills. Table 3.9 in the TOD Manual provides the complete list of questions.

The TOD Rating Scales are available for individuals aged 5 years, 0 months to 89 years, 11 months. Parent/Caregiver forms for TOD-C and TOD-E are available in both English and Spanish. Each of the rating scales contains several yes or no questions related to risk factors for dyslexia. Yes or no questions are followed by a number of items with Likert-like responses ranging from Strongly Disagree (1) to Strongly Agree (4). The number of these types of items ranges from 26 to 35, depending on the rating scale used. Items are designed to elicit relevant background/history and content focusing on: General Reasoning (GR), Verbal Comprehension (VC), Orthographic Processing (OP), Phonological Processing (PP), Rapid Automatized Naming (RAN), Memory (ME), Basic Reading Skills (BRS), Reading Fluency (RF), Reading Comprehension (RC), and Spelling (SP) as well as the contributing factors of Attention (ATT) and Motivation for Reading (MoR). Rapid Reference 6.2 provides examples of possible questions to ask when collecting information related to family history.

≣ *Rapid Reference 6.1*

Sample/Potential Questions to Ask a Young Child

- Do you have a lot of books at home?
- Does anyone at home read books to you?
- Do you like listening to a book when someone reads it to you?
- Do you know the names of the letters in the alphabet?
- Do you know the sounds the letters make?
- Can you say the whole alphabet?
- Do you think it is easy to rhyme words, like dog and log?
- Can you write your name?

≣ *Rapid Reference 6.2*

Family History Related to Dyslexia

- Did anyone in your family have difficulty learning to read or spell?
- Has your child received extra reading support (e.g., tutoring, reading interventions)?
- Did your child repeat a grade?
- Have there been any previous diagnoses?
- Did your child have early difficulties with speech or language?
- Did your child have ear infections/tubes in ears?

≡ Rapid Reference 6.3

Descriptors of TOD-C Rating Scales

- **TOD-C Self-Rating Form:**
  - Number of Items: 35
  - Sample item: *Because I read slowly, I have trouble understanding what I read.*
  - Constructs: Reading Fluency, Reading Comprehension
- **TOD-C Teacher Rating Form:**
  - Number of items: 30
  - Sample item: *Can blend separate sounds together to make a word (e.g., /m/ /a/ /t/ is mat).*
  - Constructs: Phonological Processing, Basic Reading Skills
- **TOD-C Parent/Caregiver Rating Form:**
  - Number of items: 26
  - Sample item: *Gets confused by little words that look alike (e.g., was and saw; who and how).*
  - Construct: Orthographic Processing

≡ Rapid Reference 6.4

TOD-E Rating Scales
- **TOD-E Teacher Rating Form:**
  - Number of items: 26
  - Sample item: *Can write most letters and a few simple words (e.g., A, B, C, I, see).*
  - Construct: Spelling
- **TOD-E Parent/Caregiver Rating Form:**
  - Number of items: 27
  - Sample item: *Has trouble saying the alphabet in order.*
  - Construct: Memory

Rapid Reference 6.3 includes the number of items in each of the three forms of the TOD-C Rating Scales, a sample item, and the reading-related constructs the item addresses. These items require the respondent to choose one of the following choices: Strongly Disagree (1), Disagree (2), Agree (3), and Strongly Agree (4).

Rapid Reference 6.4 includes the number of items in each of the two forms of the TOD-E Rating Scales, a sample item, and the reading-related constructs the item addresses.

CAUTION

Young children may not yet understand the nature and extent of their reading difficulties.

DEVELOPMENT OF THE RATING SCALES

TOD Rating Scales were developed to augment findings from the direct assessments and to assist in the determination of risk for dyslexia and/or diagnosis of dyslexia. They were designed to provide both qualitative and quantitative data to supplement scores obtained from direct administration of the TOD-S, TOD-E or TOD-C. Item development of the TOD Rating Scales was guided by the research literature describing a range of risk factors known to contribute to (or be related to) dyslexia. Some of the content was more suited to a yes or no response (e.g., family history of reading difficulties, history of previous interventions), and some was more suited to a Likert-type scale, ranging from Strongly Disagree to Strongly Agree (e.g., dislike for reading, tendency to confuse similar words). Items were developed and reviewed by all of the authors for redundancy and omissions. The authors engaged in an iterative process, culminating in agreement on the alignment of the Likert-type items to specific categories of interest, as described above (e.g., Orthographic Processing, Spelling, Motivation). Some of the items are linked to more than one category. For example, on the TOD-C Parent/Caregiver Rating Scale, the item *"Has trouble pronouncing some longer words when reading"* assesses both Phonological Processing and Basic Reading Skills.

To avoid respondents developing a response set when answering the items, wording was varied so that difficulty was sometimes indicated by "Strongly Disagree" or "Disagree" and sometimes by "Strongly Agree" or "Agree." These items are reverse scored when raw scores are transformed to T-scores so that the higher the score on the TOD Rating Scales, the greater the risk for dyslexia. For example, on Item 1, *I understand the meaning of most of the words that I hear,4 (1),* selection of 4 (Strongly Agree) becomes a 1. On Item 3, *I sometimes mispronounce words when I am speaking, 4 (4),* a response of 4 (Strongly Agree) stays as a 4 as it is a characteristic of some individuals with dyslexia.

> **DON'T FORGET**
>
> Raw score values in parentheses reflect item input for most items but represent reverse scoring for some items.

Although some of the items are similar in content across the five forms of the TOD Rating Scales, they each have unique content and are designed to elicit specific information from the perspective of the respondent (i.e., Parent/Caregiver, Teacher, Self). All forms of the rating scales include questions about the examinee's verbal and reasoning abilities, attention and motivation for reading, and specific reading and spelling skills. Other questions vary across the rating scales to best elicit information specific to the rater's role and perspective.

Both forms (TOD-E and TOD-C) of the Parent/Caregiver Rating Scale are available in English and Spanish for examinees in kindergarten through Grade 12. Because parents are often the first to notice that their child struggles to learn to read, they can provide valuable information about whether their child has had trouble learning letters and sounds. Parents are typically knowledgeable about whether other family members have or are having difficulty with reading and/or spelling. This information is especially important as family history of reading difficulties is a significant risk factor for dyslexia (Ozernov-Palchik & Gaab, 2006). In fact, children whose parents or siblings have dyslexia are four times more likely to have reading difficulties than their peers without such family history (Snowling et al., 2019). The Parent/Caregiver Rating Scales also include questions related to the examinee's early speech and language development. Generally, early language development predicts reading skills.

Parents of children with dyslexia may note that their child has difficulties with phonological awareness (e.g., understanding rhyming, mispronouncing words) but may not have more general language problems. Some children have both dyslexia and developmental language disorder(s).

DON'T FORGET

Remember to find out if a family history of difficulty learning to read and spell exists. Keep in mind, however, that depending on the age and education of the identified individual family member(s), they may never have been diagnosed with dyslexia.

Both forms (TOD-E and TOD-C) of the Teacher Rating Scales (available for examinees in grades K–12) elicit information from the examinee's teacher about rate of reading progress compared to peers and whether the examinee has difficulty with certain types of reading and spelling skills. The teacher rates other relevant tasks such as note-taking, planning, need for extended time to complete tasks requiring reading, and the examinee's preference for oral versus written exams. This type of information can be helpful in determining appropriate accommodations.

The TOD-C Self-Rating Form (available for examinees in grade 1 through age 89) includes items related to how difficult the examinee finds reading and writing and whether reading is easier for their peers than for them. Even young children are generally aware if reading is unusually difficult for them. The Self-Rating Form also includes questions related to how long it takes the examinee to read and whether they understand what they read.

STANDARDIZATION OF THE TOD RATING SCALES

The TOD Rating Scales were co-normed with the TOD-E and TOD-C (which are inclusive of the TOD-S). Co-norming allows for more accurate comparisons across tests relative to those that rely on different standardization samples, i.e., error is reduced. The TOD-E Rating Scale standardization sample included a total of 211 respondents for grades K–2; 154 completed the TOD-E Parent/Caregiver Rating Scales and 142 completed the TOD-E Teacher Rating Scales. Some of the respondents completed both scales. The TOD-C Rating Scale standardization sample is subdivided into two parts: the Child Sample (Grades 1 through 12) and the Adult Sample (age 18 and above). The TOD-C Child Rating Scale sample (ages 6–18) included a total of 1215 respondents: The Parent/Caregiver Rating Scale had 997 respondents, the Teacher Rating Scale had 448 respondents, and the Self-Rating Form had 1066 respondents. Some of the respondents completed more than one rating scale. The TOD-C Adult Rating Scale sample included only the Self-Rating Form, with 267 respondents.

Tables 4.9 and 4.10 in the TOD Manual provide the demographic characteristics (e.g., age, gender, grade, race/ethnicity, parent's education level, US geographic region) of the TOD-C Rating Scales Child and Adult Samples. Table 4.14 provides the demographic characteristics of the TOD-E Rating Scales. Gender representation is relatively equal across the TOD Rating Scales samples. The TOD-E sample contained approximately equal numbers of participants across grades K–2; the TOD-C sample contained more participants in the age/grade ranges in which children are more likely to be referred for dyslexia assessment (Grades 2–7).

PSYCHOMETRIC PROPERTIES OF THE TOD RATING SCALES

Reliability characterizes the consistency of a measure, while validity refers to the accuracy of a measure. Evidence for the psychometric integrity of the TOD Rating Scales was established by examining internal consistency reliability, cross-form reliability, and content and predictive validity within the standardization samples. Subsequently, additional studies focused on the value of the TOD Rating Scales to contribute to the prediction of dyslexia risk when combined with direct assessment data.

Internal Consistency

Estimates of internal consistency, the extent to which items on a scale are measuring the same construct, are strong and provide evidence of robust reliability of the rating scales. Internal consistency estimates were calculated using Cronbach's alpha for the 1452 individuals in the norm sample who completed the TOD-C Rating Scales. Internal consistency coefficients for TOD-C Self-Rating Form ranged from $r = .91$ to .95. Internal consistency coefficients for the TOD-C Parent/Caregiver Rating Form ranged from $r = .93$ to .96. Internal consistency for the TOD-C Teacher Rating Form ranged from $r = .95$ to .97. Table 5.6 in the TOD Manual reports the TOD-C Rating Scales internal consistency estimates and SEMs. These estimates are strong and indicate little error. Cronbach (1951) characterized reliability estimates as Excellent (.90), Good (.80), and Adequate (.70).

Internal consistency was calculated using Cronbach's alpha for the 211 individuals in the norm sample who completed the TOD-E Rating Scales. Internal consistency coefficients for the TOD-E Parent/Caregiver Rating Form ranged from $r = .95$ to .96 and internal consistency coefficients for the TOD-E Teacher Rating Form ranged from $r = .96$ to .97. Table 5.9 reports the TOD-E Rating Scales internal consistency estimates and SEMs.

Rating Scale Cross-Form Consistency

Cross-form consistency refers to the extent to which the ratings of an individual on two different forms by two different raters are similar (e.g., TOD-C Teacher Ratings and TOD-C Parent/Caregiver Ratings on the same student). Cross-form consistency estimates are typically lower than internal consistency estimates because different raters observe the individual in different settings and under different conditions. For the TOD Rating Scales, cross-form correlational analyses were conducted for all examinees who had at least two completed forms of the rating scales.

Generally, strong correlations between raters were found; most were in the moderate to strong range according to Cohen (1992), who described .30 as weak, .50 as moderate, and .80 as strong/large. For 85 participants, the correlation between the TOD-E Parent/Caregiver and Teacher Forms was $r = .75$. For 880 participants, TOD-C Parent/Caregiver and Self-Rating Forms correlation was $r = .63$. For 344 participants, TOD-C Parent/Caregiver and Self-Rating Forms correlation was $r = .73$ and for 391 participants, TOD-C Self-Ratings and Teacher Forms correlation was $r = .60$. These data indicate that, though the respondents' responses overall were similar, each respondent tends to provide information that contributes uniquely to the overall assessment of the examinee.

Content Validity

The TOD Rating Scales have strong content validity, which is the degree to which an assessment accurately assesses the domain of knowledge it purports to measure. The TOD authors relied on relevant research literature (e.g., Hamilton & Hayiou-Thomas, 2022; Kilpatrick, 2015; Lasnick et al., 2022; Mather & Wendling, 2024; Pennington et al., 2019; Snowling et al., 2019) to inform item development. The Yes/No items were developed to assess research-identified risk areas for dyslexia (e.g., family history of reading difficulty). The Likert-type items were developed to provide a quantitative assessment of the examinee's risk for dyslexia, assessing the examinee's difficulties and perspectives about learning to read/spell as well as the examinee's experiences with reading. During standardization, items that detracted from the internal consistency of each scale were eliminated.

Predictive Validity

Predictive validity, the extent to which a measure accurately predicts the outcome or score on another measure, was established for the TOD Rating Scales by examining the relationships among the TOD Rating Scales results and the results of TOD direct assessments, specifically, the TOD-S Dyslexia Risk Index (DRI), TOD-C Dyslexia Diagnostic Index (DDI), and the TOD-E Early Dyslexia Diagnostic Index (EDDI). For the TOD-C, analyses were conducted for a subsample of the TOD standardization sample ($n = 66$) who had been identified with a reading disability (RD) and who had all three forms of the TOD-C Rating Scales completed (Parent/Caregiver, Teacher, and Self). Logistic regression analyses were conducted to determine the ability of the TOD Rating Scales to predict membership into a group identified with RD or a matched control group. In each case, the TOD-C Rating Scales provided statistically significant improvement (over chance) in predicting RD vs. non-RD group status. Table 6.1 presents the results of the TOD-C Rating Scales logistic regression (Bell, 2022). Percentages of correct diagnostic decisions were: Parent/Caregiver: 77%, Teacher, 82%, and Self-Rating, 83%.

Similar analyses were not conducted for the TOD-E because the TOD-E sample did not have enough participants with a diagnosis of RD. Unfortunately, reading disability is often not identified until students are in grade 3 or beyond. In addition to the logistic

Table 6.1   Logistic Regression Results for TOD-C Rating Scales Prediction of Reading Disability or Non-Reading Disability Status

TOD-C Classification Table for Parent/Caregiver Rating Scale Prediction of Reading LD			
		Predicted	
		No Reading LD	Reading LD	Percentage Correct
Observed	**No Reading LD**	25	8	75.8
	Reading LD	7	26	78.8
Total				77.3

Table 6.1 (Continued)

TOD-C Classification Table for Teacher Rating Scale Prediction of Reading LD

		Predicted		
		No Reading LD	Reading LD	Percentage Correct
Observed	No Reading LD	26	7	78.8
	Reading LD	5	28	84.8
Total				81.8

TOD-C Classification Table for Self-Rating Scale Prediction of Reading LD

		Predicted		
		No Reading LD	Reading LD	Percentage Correct
Observed	No Reading LD	28	5	84.8
	Reading LD	6	27	81.8
Total				83.3

≡ Rapid Reference 6.5

Correlations between the TOD Rating Scales and TOD Direct Assessments

TOD-S DRI	r	TOD-C DDI	r	TOD-E EDDI	r
TOD-C Parent/Caregiver	−.71	TOD-C Parent/Caregiver	−.69		
TOD-C Teacher	−.65	TOD-C Teacher	−.64		
TOD-C Self	−.70	TOD-C Self	−.65		
TOD-E Parent/Caregiver	−.33			TOD-E Parent/Caregiver	−.51
TOD-E Teacher	−.40			TOD-E Teacher	−.55

regression predicting group membership as RD or non-RD by the TOD-C Rating Scales, analyses were conducted to determine the strength of the relationship between the TOD Rating Scales and scores on the TOD direct assessments. Rapid Reference 6.5 summarizes these relationships. Most of the correlations are moderate to moderately strong, providing support for predictive validity.

Additional Evidence of TOD Rating Scale Validity

McCallum and Bell (2025) investigated the ability of the TOD Rating Scales to improve prediction accuracy of the DRI, obtained from administration of the TOD-S. Based on results of a logistic regression for 261 participants with dyslexia and 261 matched controls, the DRI alone predicted group membership with 75% accuracy. Further logistic regression analyses indicated that prediction accuracy improved to 80–82% depending upon which of the three rating scales was added (i.e., Self, Teacher, or Parent/Caregiver). When all three rating scales were added, prediction accuracy increased to 91%. The results indicated that dyslexia probability has increased accuracy when all three TOD Rating Scales *and* the TOD-S direct assessment data are considered.

> **DON'T FORGET**
>
> Evidence for the TOD Rating Scales reliability and validity indicates that they are effective measures of dyslexia risk that can be used alone or in conjunction with the TOD direct assessments. They are particularly well-suited for use with the TOD because they are co-normed.

ADMINISTRATION, SCORING, AND INTERPRETING THE TOD RATING SCALES

The TOD Rating Scales are easy to administer and score. A unique feature of the TOD Rating Scales is that one form is used across the entire age or grade span for which it was designed. During development of the rating scales, means were calculated by year/grade and did not differ. Consequently, the same form of the TOD-E Parent/Caregiver is used across all ages. Similarly, the same TOD-E Teacher Rating Scale is used for all examinees in grades K–2. The same is true of the TOD-C Parent/Caregiver, Teacher, and Self-Ratings; the forms do not vary by age or grade.

Administration

TOD Rating Scales are available electronically from the publisher, WPS. They are designed to be administered online, either in a face-to-face situation (particularly desirable for young examinees completing the TOD-C Self-Rating Form) or remotely. In either case, the evaluator starts administration of the appropriate form of the rating scale on the WPS OES platform. The evaluator is prompted to indicate whether the respondent is "in person" or needs to receive an emailed link to complete the scale. Alternatively, evaluators have the option to download and print the rating scales, allowing respondents to complete the scales on paper. In this case, the evaluator enters the responses in the WPS OES system to generate a Score Report. Respondents are directed to respond Yes or No to each of the background questions and, if requested, provide specific information in an open-ended format (e.g., nature of extra reading support). Then, they are asked to read each question and choose the answer that best describes the examinee's current behaviors, or if a Self-Rating, their own behaviors: Strongly Disagree, Disagree, Agree or Strongly Agree. They are encouraged to respond to all items. Whether the rating scale is completed electronically by the respondent or is initially completed on paper by the respondent with the evaluator later entering the responses electronically, the rating scales are scored online, and a three-page Score Report is generated.

> **DON'T FORGET**
>
> The rating scales can be completed online or on a paper form.

Scoring and Interpretation

The TOD Rating Scales yield a T-score, which is a type of standard score with a population mean of 50 and standard deviation of 10. Like other types of standard scores, T-scores provide a comparison of the examinee to their peers in the norm group. The TOD Rating Scales are designed to identify areas of difficulty for examinees suspected of having dyslexia; thus, higher scores are more indicative of risk for dyslexia. Rapid Reference 6.6 shows the Risk Levels associated with TOD Rating Scale scores.

> **DON'T FORGET**
>
> Higher T-scores on TOD Rating Scales indicate greater risk for dyslexia.

Note that scores in the Low to Moderate Risk range may still be indicative of dyslexia when considered with other data. Scores at the low end of this range suggest Low Risk, whereas scores at the high end of this range suggest Moderate Risk.

As with the TOD-E and TOD-C direct assessments, evaluators must determine whether to administer the TOD-E Rating Scales or the TOD-C Rating Scales for examinees who are in Grades 1 and 2. If the evaluator also plans to administer direct assessments, then the rating scales should be selected to correspond to the direct assessments administered. When deciding between the TOD-E and TOD-C, consider whether the child is able to read connected text. If so, then the TOD-C is likely more appropriate, especially for students in second grade. If the rating scales are being used as stand-alone screeners, then either the TOD-E or TOD-C Rating Scales can be used for children in Grades K–2; however, there is no Self-Rating Form for children in Grade K. Although the TOD-C Self-Ratings Form can be used with children as young as first grade, the examiner would need to read the items to the examinee. An alternative is simply to ask a younger child questions, such as those described in Rapid Reference 6.1.

≡ Rapid Reference 6.6

Levels of Risk Based on TOD Rating Scale Scores

Risk Level	T-Ranges	Percentage in Population
Very High Risk	70 and above	Less than 2%
High Risk	60–69	About 14%
Low to Moderate Risk	59 and below	About 84%

Once the TOD Rating Scales have been scored electronically, the Score Reports can be downloaded in either Microsoft Word or PDF format. The Score Report contains a graph depicting the T-score and risk level as well as information about the degree of difficulty noted in the various categories assessed by the rating scale. Figure 6.1 illustrates the completed and

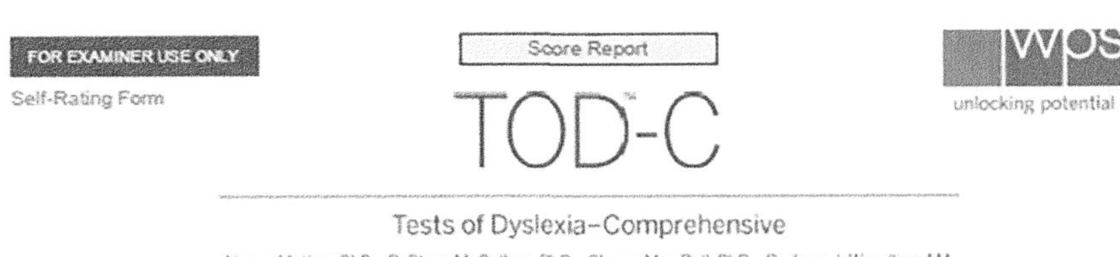

Tests of Dyslexia–Comprehensive

Nancy Mather, PhD   R. Steve McCallum, PhD   Sherry Mee Bell, PhD   Barbara J. Wendling, MA

Examinee Information

Name	Date of birth	Age at testing
Mella Carr	02/10	9 years 4 months
School	Grade	Administration date
Sweetgrass Elementary	4th	06/16

Score Profile

TOD Total Score Results

Total Raw Score: 100

T-score: 65

- ≥70T: Very High
- 60T–69T: High
- ≤59T: Low to Moderate

Confidence Interval: 90%	%ile	Risk Level
61 – 69	93	High Risk

Category	Degree of Difficulty			
Vocabulary and Reasoning	None	Minor	Some	Major
VC – Verbal Comprehension		X		
GR – General Reasoning		X		
Linguistic Risk Factors				
PP – Phonological Processing			X	
OP – Orthographic Processing			X	
RAN – Rapid Automatized Naming *				
ME – Memory				X
Reading and Spelling				
BRS – Basic Reading Skills			X	
RF – Reading Fluency			X	
RC – Reading Comprehension			X	
SP – Spelling				X
Contributing Factors				
MoR – Motivation (for Reading)			X	
A – Attention *				

Note: Category not measured on this form.

The Rating Scale *T*-score indicates a High Risk for dyslexia. Considerable specific difficulties in reading, spelling, and related skill areas are likely present. Item-level responses, as well as additional data from TOD tests, will be helpful in understanding the specific areas of difficulty.

Figure 6.1   Melia's Completed and Scored TOD-C Self-Rating Form Report Page 1

scored page 1 of the TOD-C Self-Rating Form score report for Melia, a fourth-grade student. She perceives that she has some difficulty with reading, but her greatest difficulties are with memory and spelling.

The second and third pages of the Rating Scales Score Reports provide Melia's responses to each item. Qualitative analyses of these responses can yield useful information for planning interventions and accommodations. For example, Melia noted that she has a hard time spelling new words as well as words that are not spelled like they sound. Figures 6.2 and 6.3 present the completed and scored pages 2 and 3 of the score report.

As another example, William, a 15-year-old sophomore, completed a Self-Rating Form as part of a reevaluation. William began receiving special education services for reading difficulties in second grade. Now, as a high school student, he no longer has an IEP but has a 504 Plan that provides accommodations, such as extended time on tests, access to audiobooks, and use of a reading pen. Figure 6.4 presents his Score Profile. William noted that he has major difficulties in the linguistic risk factors of phonological processing, orthographic processing, and memory and the reading and spelling areas of basic reading skills, reading fluency, and spelling, all primary characteristics of dyslexia. His results indicated a High Risk for dyslexia.

His answers to the background questions in Figure 6.5 indicated a family history of dyslexia (both reading and spelling), ear infections, and extra support for reading in both the home and school. When asked about family members, William reported both his father and his sister in fourth grade had been diagnosed with dyslexia.

His responses to the items involving reading and spelling further supported his difficulties. Figure 6.6 illustrates a few examples.

Results from both the Self-Rating Form and the TOD-C supported a need for additional intervention and continued use of accommodations.

Rater Comparison Report

A unique feature of the TOD Rating Scales is that evaluators can create a Rater Comparison Report when multiple forms of the rating scales have been completed for an individual. Specifically, the Rater Comparison Report function summarizes the scores from up to three different forms for the same examinee and determines the extent to which the scores are (statistically) significantly different from each other across Parent/Caregiver and Teacher (TOD-E Rating Scales) and across Parent/Caregiver, Teacher, and Self-Ratings (TOD-C). Further, the Rater Comparison function can be used to summarize rating

DON'T FORGET

The WPS Online Evaluation System (OES) provides the option to create a Rater Comparison report when more than one rating scale has been completed for the same examinee.

DON'T FORGET

Rating scales provide essential information that goes beyond the direct assessment test scores. Rating scales help document the examinee's history, school and home context, and multiple perspectives on the examinee's reading and spelling abilities. When incorporated with direct assessment data, rating scales enhance the predictive accuracy of the test results alone.

Background Information

		Response
1.	One or more of my family members has/had difficulty with reading.	Yes
2.	One or more of my family members has/had difficulty with spelling.	Yes
3.	I have had ear infections or tubes in my ears.	No
4.	I receive/received extra help with reading.	Yes
	If yes, please specify:	in school, testing kind of like this and with my group teacher

Item Responses

		Response	(Score)	Category
1.	I understand the meaning of most of the words that I hear.	3	(2)	VC
2.	I can tell others what I am thinking.	4	(1)	VC
3.	I sometimes mispronounce words when I am speaking.	3	(3)	PP
4.	I like to figure out how to do new things.	4	(1)	GR
5.	I sometimes cannot think of the word I want to say.	4	(4)	VC
6.	I enjoy reading.	1	(4)	MoR
7.	I have many books at home.	3	(2)	MoR
8.	Other people my age are better readers than I am.	3	(3)	MoR
9.	It takes me longer to read than other people my age.	4	(4)	RF
10.	I have trouble pronouncing some longer words when I am reading.	3	(3)	BRS, PP
11.	I would rather listen to a book than read one.	2	(2)	MoR
12.	I sometimes get confused by little words that look alike (for example, *was/saw* or *who/how*).	3	(3)	OP
13.	It helps me if I get extra time on tests that require reading.	3	(3)	RF
14.	I would rather work on math problems than read a book.	4	(4)	MoR
15.	I would rather take an oral exam than a written exam.	1	(1)	MoR
16.	I read for pleasure.	1	(4)	MoR
17.	Because I read slowly, I have trouble understanding what I read.	3	(3)	RC, RF
18.	I try to avoid reading aloud.	4	(4)	MoR
19.	Reading makes me feel tired.	3	(3)	MoR

Figure 6.2   Melia's Completed and Scored TOD-C Self-Rating Form Page 2

20.	I prefer activities that do not require reading (for example, sports, music art).	3	(3)	MoR
21.	I have trouble keeping my place when reading.	4	(4)	OP, RF
22.	I am good at reading words.	2	(3)	BRS
23.	Reading is hard for me.	3	(3)	BRS
24.	I usually understand what I read.	2	(3)	RC
25.	I recognize many words automatically and don't have to try to sound them out.	3	(2)	RF
26.	It is easy for me to tell others about what I have read.	1	(4)	ME, RC
27.	I pay attention to punctuation marks when I read.	1	(4)	RF
28.	I like writing.	4	(1)	MoR
29.	I have trouble spelling words that are not spelled like they sound, such as "once."	4	(4)	ME, OP, SP
30.	It is hard for me to learn how to spell new words.	4	(4)	ME, OP, SP
31.	It takes me a long time to copy things from a book or a board.	1	(1)	OP
32.	No matter how hard I try, reading is hard for me.	3	(3)	BRS, MoR
33.	People sometimes tell me that I just need to try harder.	2	(2)	MoR
34.	I am good at thinking about how things are alike or different.	3	(2)	GR
35.	I can repeat back information I have just heard, such as a telephone number.	2	(3)	ME

Item Response Key:
1 = Strongly Disagree
2 = Disagree
3 = Agree
4 = Strongly Agree

Missing response
Default value was used for missing response.

Note: Raw Score values in parentheses reflect item input for most items, and represent reverse scoring for the following items: 1, 2, 4, 6, 7, 16, 22, 24, 25, 26, 27, 28, 34, 35.

VC = Verbal Comprehension
GR = General Reasoning
PP = Phonological Processing
OP = Orthographic Processing
RAN = Rapid Automatized Naming
ME = Memory
BRS = Basic Reading Skills
RF = Reading Fluency
RC = Reading Comprehension
SP = Spelling
MoR = Motivation (for Reading)
A = Attention

Figure 6.3   Melia's Completed and Scored TOD-C Self-Rating Form Page 3

scales scores from two raters on the same examinee on the same form (e.g., if both parents independently completed a Parent/Caregiver Rating Scale or if two different teachers completed a Teacher Rating Scale). Although T-scores are shown, the Report does not indicate whether the scores differ significantly. Figure 6.7 shows a completed Rater Comparison Report for Melia with TOD-C Parent/Caregiver, Teacher, and Self-Ratings. In this example, the differences among the raters were not significant.

Score Profile

TOD Total Score Results

Total Raw Score: 105

T-score: 68

- ≥70 T: Very High
- 60 T-69 T: High
- ≤59 T: Low to Moderate

Confidence Interval: 90%	%ile	Risk Level
64 - 72	96	High Risk

Category	Degree of Difficulty			
Vocabulary and Reasoning	None	Minor	Some	Major
VC = Verbal Comprehension		X		
GR = General Reasoning	X			
Linguistic Risk Factors				
PP = Phonological Processing				X
OP = Orthographic Processing				X
RAN = Rapid Automatized Naming *				
ME = Memory				X
Reading and Spelling				
BRS = Basic Reading Skills				X
RF = Reading Fluency				X
RC = Reading Comprehension			X	
SP = Spelling				X
Contributing Factors				
MoR = Motivation (for Reading)			X	
A = Attention *				

* **Note:** Category not measured on this form.

The Rating Scale *T*-score indicates a High Risk for dyslexia. Considerable specific difficulties in reading, spelling, and related skill areas are likely present. Item-level responses, as well as additional data from TOD tests, will be helpful in understanding the specific areas of difficulty.

Figure 6.4 Willliam's Completed and Scored TOD-C Self-Rating Form Page 1

Background Information

		Response
1.	One or more of my family members has/had difficulty with reading.	Yes
2.	One or more of my family members has/had difficulty with spelling.	Yes
3.	I have had ear infections or tubes in my ears.	Yes
4.	I receive/received extra help with reading.	Yes
	If yes, please specify:	Accommodations, tutors, special school, IEP

Figure 6.5 William's Completed Background Information

8.	Other people my age are better readers than I am.	4	(4)	MoR
9.	It takes me longer to read than other people my age.	4	(4)	RF
10.	I have trouble pronouncing some longer words when I am reading.	4	(4)	BRS, PP
11.	I would rather listen to a book than read one.	4	(4)	MoR
21.	I have trouble keeping my place when reading.	4	(4)	OP, RF
22.	I am good at reading words.	1	(4)	BRS
23.	Reading is hard for me.	4	(4)	BRS
29.	I have trouble spelling words that are not spelled like they sound, such as "once."	4	(4)	SP, OP, ME
30.	It is hard for me to learn how to spell new words.	4	(4)	SP, OP, ME
31.	It takes me a long time to copy things from a book or a board.	4	(4)	OP
32.	No matter how hard I try, reading is hard for me.	4	(4)	MoR, BRS

Figure 6.6   Examples of William's Responses to Items on the Self-Rating Form

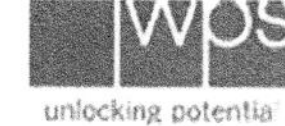

FOR EXAMINER USE ONLY

Rater Comparison Report

TOD™

Tests of Dyslexia

Nancy Mather, PhD   R. Steve McCallum, PhD   Sherry Mee Bell, PhD   Barbara J. Wendling, MA

Individual's name	Current age	Report date
Mella Carr	9 years 4 months	06/20

Compare Scores From Multiple Raters

Rater 1	Rater 2	Rater 3
Form	**Form**	**Form**
Parent/Caregiver Rating Form	Teacher Rating Form	Self-Rating Form
Administration date	**Administration date**	**Administration date**
06/16	06/17	06/16
Age at testing	**Age at testing**	**Age at testing**
9 years 4 months	9 years 4 months	9 years 4 months
Grade	**Grade**	**Grade**
4th	4th	4th
Rater's name	**Rater's name**	**Rater's name**
Carrie Carr	Stephanie Lynn	
Relationship to individual	**Relationship to individual**	**Relationship to individual**
Parent	General education classroom teacher	Self

Rater 1 T-Score	Rater 2 T-Score	Rater 3 T-Score	Difference in T-scores	Significant difference	% of sample
65	64		1	No	
	64	65	1	No	
65		65	0	No	

Figure 6.7   Completed TOD-C Rater Comparison Report

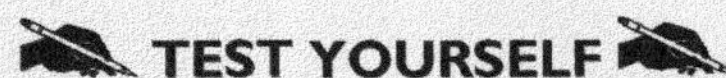

TEST YOURSELF

1. **What is the benefit of co-norming the TOD Rating Scales and the TOD direct assessments?**
   (a) They provide a combined risk score.
   (b) Error is reduced when comparing scores from different tests.
   (c) They all yield the same type of standard score.
   (d) They all provide a dyslexia diagnosis.

2. **Which of the following is not a strong risk factor for dyslexia?**
   (a) Family history of dyslexia
   (b) Delays in speech and language development
   (c) Left handedness
   (d) History of previous reading interventions

3. **The TOD Rating Scales yield**
   (a) T-scores with a mean of 50.
   (b) standard scores with a mean of 100.
   (c) grade equivalents.
   (d) age equivalents.

4. **The TOD Rating Scales can be administered in a paper-and-pencil format. True or False?**

5. **A T-score of 70 and above on the TOD Rating Scales means that the examinee is**
   (a) at Low Risk for Dyslexia.
   (b) at Moderate Risk for Dyslexia.
   (c) at Risk for Dyslexia.
   (d) at Very High Risk for Dyslexia.

6. **Which of the following is not included in the TOD-Early Rating Scales?**
   (a) Parent/Caregiver Form
   (b) Teacher Form
   (c) Self-Rating Form
   (d) None of the above

7. **The TOD Rating Scales contain Likert-type items? True or False?**

8. **Qualitative information from the TOD Rating Scales can be used to**
   (a) make a dyslexia diagnosis.
   (b) help determine appropriate interventions and accommodations.
   (c) create a dyslexia probability score.
   (d) create a dyslexia risk score.

9. **TOD Rating Scale reports provide all but which of the following?**
   (a) Graph depicting the T-score and level of risk
   (b) Items related to motivation, attention, and reasoning

   (c) Levels of difficulty in key areas of reading, spelling and other key areas

   (d) Correlation with TOD-S, TOD-E, and/or TOD-C direct assessment results

10. The TOD-C Rating Scales Rater Comparison Report determines statistical differences between which of the following?

   (a) TOD-C Rating Scale results and TOD direct assessment results for the same examinee

   (b) Results of TOD-C Rating Scales completed on the same examinee by both parents

   (c) Results of TOD-C Rating Scales completed on the same examinee by a parent/caregiver, teacher, and/or by the examinee

   (d) Results of TOD-C Rating Scales completed on the same examinee by two different teachers

Answers: 1. b; 2. c; 3. a; 4. True; 5. d; 6. c; 7. True; 8. b; 9. d; 10. c

REFERENCES

Bell, S. M. (2022, November). *Advances in diagnostic and progress monitoring assessments for students with dyslexia. Using rating scales: An under-studied method for screening and identification of dyslexia.* [Conference session]. Annual Conference of the International Dyslexia Association, San Antonio, TX, United States.

Cohen, J. (1992). Statistical power analysis. *Current Directions in Psychological Science, 1*(3), 98–101.

Cronbach, L. J. (1951). Coefficient alpha and the internal structure of tests. *Psychometrika, 16,* 297–334.

Hamilton, L. G., & Hayiou-Thomas, M. E. (2022). The foundations of literacy. In M. J. Snowling, C. Hulme, & K. Nation (Eds.), *The science of reading: A handbook* (pp. 125–147). Wiley-Blackwell. https://doi.org/10.1002/9781119705116.ch6

Kilpatrick, D. (2015). *Essentials of assessing, preventing, and overcoming reading difficulties.* Wiley.

Lasnick, O., Feng, J., Quirion, A., Hart, S., & Hoeft, F. (2022). The importance of family history in dyslexia. *Reading League Journal, 3*(2), 35–40.

Mather, N., McCallum, R. S., Bell, S. M., & Wendling, B. J. (2024a). *Tests of Dyslexia.* Western Psychological Services.

Mather, N., & Wendling, B. (2024). *The essentials of dyslexia: Assessment and intervention* (2nd ed.). Wiley.

McCallum, R. S., & Bell, S. M. (2025, February). *Advances in using data: Efficient and equitable dyslexia screening.* [Poster presentation]. National Association of School Psychologists. Seattle, WA, United States.

McCallum, R. S., & Bracken, B. (2018). *The universal talented and gifted administration manual.* Prufrock Press.

Morgan, W. P. (1896). A case of congenital word blindness. *British Medical Journal, 2,* 1378.

Ozernov-Palchik, O., & Gaab, N. (2006). Tackling the dyslexia "paradox": Reading brain and behavior for early markers of developmental dyslexia. *WIREs Cognitive Science, 7*(2), 156–176. https://doi.org/10.1002/wcs.1383

Pennington, B. F., McGrath, L. M., & Peterson, R. L. (2019). *Diagnosing learning disorders: From science to practice* (3rd ed.). Guilford.

Redford, K. (n.d.). *Mother worry: Academic support away from home.* The Yale Center for Dyslexia and Creativity. https://dyslexia.yale.edu/resources/parents/stories-from-parents/

Snowling, M. J., Nash, H. M., Gooch, D. C., Hayiou-Thomas, M. E., & Hulme, C. (2019). Developmental outcomes for children at high risk of dyslexia and children with developmental language disorder. *Child Development, 90*(5), 548–564. https://doi.org/10.1111/cdev.13216

Wagner, R. K., Edwards, A. A., Malkowski, A., Schatschneider, C., Joyner, R. E., Wood, S., & Zirps, F. A. (2019). Combining old and new for better understanding and predicting dyslexia. *New Directions for Child and Adolescent Development, 165*, 11–23. https://doi.org/10.1002/cad.20289

Wolf, M. (2008). *Proust and the squid: The story and science of the reading brain*. HarperCollins.

Seven

PSYCHOMETRIC PROPERTIES OF THE TOD

The TOD components were developed to operationalize the reading, spelling, linguistic processes, and vocabulary and reasoning domains that are most relevant for identifying dyslexia. Ultimately, results from administration of the TOD-S, TOD-C, and TOD-E help identify an examinee's strengths and weaknesses within reading and spelling, linguistic processing abilities, and cognitive abilities. These assessments provide an estimate of dyslexia risk and the probability associated with a diagnosis, consistent with the theoretical literature, neurobiological foundations, and identification models used in schools and clinics. Items were written and tests created to align with these goals. Much of the evidence for technical adequacy reported in this chapter is taken from the TOD Manual, although some additional results are reported from analyses conducted after the manual was written. Finally, the results of an independent review from the *Journal of Psychoeducational Assessment* are described (Pena & Villarreal, 2024). It will help to have the TOD Manual close by when reading this chapter (Mather et al., 2024b). All of the tables that are referenced in this chapter are in the TOD Manual.

PILOT STUDIES

Three direct assessment batteries were deemed most appropriate for assessing dyslexia for the range of grades (K–12) and ages (5–80+) and included a 23-test comprehensive instrument, the TOD-C; a 9-test early assessment instrument, the TOD-E; and a screener, the TOD-S, which comprises the first three tests in the TOD-C and TOD-E. In addition, rating scales were developed for parents, teachers, and examinees. Chapter 6 describes the

DON'T FORGET

The purpose of a pilot study is to try out the research design, the methods, and the instruments before undertaking the main study, in this case standardization. For example, pilot data can inform test quality (e.g., if items should be added, refined, or eliminated). In addition, a pilot study can help estimate the administration time and sample size needed.

development history, standardization, reliability and validity data, and implications for using the TOD Rating Scales.

TOD-C

The TOD-C pilot data were obtained for 24 tests from a sample of 220 individuals in second grade through college. The sample was 20% Hispanic, 2% Asian, 11% Black, 62% White, and 6% other; 44% of sample participants were male, and 56% were female. Item data were analyzed and order determined by using traditional classical test theory criteria (e.g., difficulty and discrimination indices) and the one-parameter Rasch model statistics based on item difficulty and person ability parameters. Goodness-of-fit of items to scales guided item selection as did differential item functioning between groups of interest. Items that displayed evidence of bias, identified by a bias expert and Rasch analysis, were dropped. Based on the pilot data, items were dropped, modified, improved, and rearranged. Finally, 23 tests were retained for standardization, the first three of which were designated for the TOD-S.

TOD-E

Pilot data for the TOD-E sample included 66 prekindergarten through first-grade participants. Thirty-eight percent were in prekindergarten, 29% in kindergarten, and 33% in first grade; 15% were Hispanic, 11% Asian, 11% Black, 54% White, 9% other, 50% male, and 50% female. Eight tests were piloted, and items were retained or eliminated, modified, improved, and/or rearranged based on a review of item statistics from passing rates, examiner feedback, and item-response theory statistics. Three tests performed poorly and were dropped. Two other tests were added for standardization, along with the three tests designated for the TOD-S. Ultimately the nine tests shown in Table 1.5 of the TOD Manual were retained.

STANDARDIZATION

Data collected for standardization relies on a stratified random sampling technique and requires selection of participants to match population demographics such as gender, race/ethnicity, socioeconomic status (SES), and geographic region. TOD data were collected based on these demographics from 2019 through 2021. The COVID-19 pandemic occurred near the end of this period and affected data collection, although most of the data were obtained face-to-face under pre-pandemic conditions. A few cases were collected in person using personal protective equipment, primarily masks worn by the examinee and the evaluator; 19 additional cases were collected remotely using digital easels. Based on an equivalency study and scrutiny of means by age, no evidence of differential performance was found; consequently, these cases were included in the standardization sample.

One hundred and six evaluators from 39 states administered the TOD to examinees, typically at schools or community organizations. Oversampling occurred, and some cases were deleted to obtain accurate representation of the sample to population parameters of gender, race/ethnicity, SES defined by parental education, and region. To ensure adequate representation of the school-age population, those attending schools with high-incidence disabilities (e.g., specific learning disabilities, attention-deficit hyperactivity disorder [ADHD]) were included. Those with low-incidence disabilities (e.g., moderate intellectual disability [ID], autism spectrum disorders [ASD]) and other relevant clinical conditions were excluded but included in the clinical studies to be reported later in the validity section of this chapter. Altogether, a total of 2,518 examinees ranging in age from 5 to 89 years were included in the TOD standardization and validity studies.

Because representation of the standardization sample to a target population is critical, evidence of the match is typically shown in test manuals. This goal is also supported by a recent study designed to investigate the extent to which demographics affect dyslexia identification from TOD-C data; results from this study provided some evidence that they can (Bell & McCallum, 2023). According to results from a binary logistic regression equation, gender and SES statistically significantly ($p < .05$) predicted group membership into one of two groups—one group consisted of 261 participants who had previously been identified as having dyslexia and a second group of 261 participants who had not been diagnosed with dyslexia. Participants in the two groups had been matched on relevant demographic variables. The final predictive model explained 21.5% (Nagelkerke R2) of the variance in dyslexia identification. Race/ethnicity did not enter the predictive equation. These results provided evidence that certain demographics of participants that comprise standardization and clinical samples can influence identification of dyslexia. Consequently, evaluators need to have demographic information available.

DON'T FORGET

All of the tables that are referenced in this chapter are in the TOD Manual.

TOD-S

The TOD-S standardization sample consisted of all the participants who were administered the TOD-C or TOD-E, for a total of 2,070 examinees, and then divided into a child and an adult sample. The child sample included all those from kindergarten through 12th grade who were administered both the TOD-C and TOD-E, totaling 1,723; of these, 337 had a high-incidence clinical diagnosis and/or a reading disability. The percentage of those who had a reading disability is consistent with population percentages. Table 4.1 shows the match of the TOD-S child sample percentages to the U.S. Census percentages based on gender, SES defined as parent educational level, race/ethnicity, and geographic region.

In general, the matches are very close; for example, the TOD-S sample percentages for males and females are 49 and 50.9, respectively, as compared to the U.S. Census percentages of 51.1 and 48.9; 1 (.1%) was classified as other. Children whose parents characterized themselves as having no high school diploma were under-represented in the TOD-S sample by 3%, those with high school diplomas were over-represented by 1.6%, those with some college were under-represented by 2.1%, and those with at least a bachelor's degree were over-represented by 3.5%. The White subsample was under-represented by 1.9%, the Black subsample was over-represented by .7%, and the Hispanic subsample was over-represented by .9%. As is true for all of the TOD standardization sub-samples, other race/ethnicities categories are represented but comprised relatively small percentages: 4.8% Asian (over-represented by .1%), 1.5% American Indian/Alaska Native (over-represented by .8%), .9% Native Hawaiian/Pacific Islander (over-represented by .7%), and 3.3% Other/Multiracial (under-represented by 1.3%).

The greatest disparity occurred in the geographic region category; the Northeast was under-represented by 6%, the Midwest was under-represented by 2.2%, the South was over-represented by 8.9%, and the West was under-represented by .8%. Tables 4.2 and 4.3 show the age and grade breakdown of the child sample; the sample is more heavily concentrated in the elementary and middle school years when children develop the relevant reading-related skills more rapidly and are more likely to be referred.

The TOD-S adult sample included 347 participants; this sample provided data for both the TOD-S and TOD-C and closely matched the U.S. Census data, as shown in Table 4.4. For example, 162 (46.7%) participants were male, 183 (52.7%) were female, and 2 (.6%) classified themselves as other. As far as SES, determined by the educational level of the participants, those who characterized themselves as having no high school diploma were under-represented in the TOD-C sample by 5.3%, those with high school diplomas were over-represented by 1.2%, those with some college were over-represented by 3%, and those with at least a bachelor' degree were over-represented by 1%.

The percentage of Whites was slightly under-represented (3.4%), the percentage of Blacks was slightly over-represented (1.1%) and those with Hispanic origin were over-represented by 1%. The percentages represented by participants from other race/ethnicities are small, very similar to those reported previously for the TOD-S child sub-sample. Because this pattern exists across all TOD standardization subsamples, only the percentages for White, Blacks, and Hispanic sub-samples are reported for other sub-samples. The Northeast was under-represented by 8.1%; all the other regions were over-represented, the Midwest by 5.2%, the South by 2.1%, and the West by .8%. Table 4.5 shows the age breakdown; relatively more of the participants were in the college-age category (33%) and, in general, the numbers decreased as a function of age.

TOD-C

Two subsamples of participants contributed to the standardization data pool for the TOD-C:1,401 participants in grades 1 through 12 comprised the first sample, referred to as the child sample, and 272 of these had a high-incidence clinical diagnosis or reading disorder; 347 participants of post-high-school age comprised the adult sample, some of whom were enrolled in college. Table 4.6 shows the match of the TOD-C sample percentages to the U.S. Census percentages for the child sample based on gender, parent educational level, race/ethnicity, and geographic region. In general, the matches are very close; for example, the TOD-C sample percentages for males and females are 49 and 50.9 compared to the U.S. Census percentages of 51.1 and 49.9; 1 (.1%) was classified as Other. Percentages differed by only .2, .3, and .4 for the White, Black, and Hispanic categories.

As far as SES, which was determined by the parental educational level, parents who characterized themselves as having no high school diploma were under-represented in the TOD-C sample by 3.1%, those with high school diplomas were over-represented by 1.6%, those with some college were under-represented by 2.4%, and those with at least a bachelor's degree were over-represented by 3.8%.

The greatest disparity occurred in the geographic region category; the Northeast was under-represented by 7.6% and the South was over-represented by 11.6%. The disparities between the percentages in the Midwest and West were 3.3 and .8. Tables 4.7 and 4.8 show the age and grade breakdown of the child sample; the sample is more heavily concentrated in the elementary and middle school years, when children are developing the relevant reading-related skills more rapidly and are more likely to be referred for an evaluation. The TOD-C adult sample closely matched the U.S. Census data, as shown in Table 4.4; this same sample provided the basis for the TOD-S adult scores. Consequently, the demographics for the sample are described in the TOD-S standardization section.

TOD-E

The TOD-E sample consisted of 342 individuals in kindergarten through second grade; 70 had a clinical diagnosis of a high-frequency condition (e.g., reading disability). Table 4.11 shows the match of the TOD-E sample percentages to the U.S. Census percentages based on gender, parent educational level, race/ethnicity, and geographic region. In general, the matches are very close; for example, the TOD-E sample percentages for males and females are 49.7 and 50.3, compared to the U.S. Census percentages of 51 and 49.

As far as SES, which was determined by the educational level of parents, parents who characterized themselves as having no high school diploma were under-represented in the TOD-C sample by 2.7%, those with high school diplomas were over-represented by .8%, those with some college were under-represented by .2%, and those with at least a bachelor's degree were over-represented by 2%. The percentage of Whites was under-represented (7.8%), the percentage of Blacks was slightly over-represented (2.3%), and those with Hispanic origin were over-represented by 2.1%. Little disparity existed across geographic regions; disparities ranged from .6% over-representation in the Northeast to 4.1% under-representation in the South; the Midwest is over-represented by 1.6% and the West by 1.9%. Age and grade break-downs are shown in Tables 4.12 and 4.13, with approximately 36% in K, 34% in Grade 1, and 30% in Grade 2.

CAUTION

When selecting a test, examine the match between the demographics reported in the standardization sample(s) and the U.S. census data. The sample demographics should reflect closely those of the population, neither under- nor over-represented, as either leads to scores that are less likely to reflect the performance of the population of interest. Consequently, interpret tests that report significant discrepancies more cautiously.

Clinical Samples

Tables 4.15 and 4.16 show the demographics of the TOD-S child clinical samples; Tables 4.17 and 4.18 show the TOD-S/TOD-C demographics for the adult clinical sample. Tables 4.19 and 4.20 show the demographics for the TOD-C child clinical samples, and Tables 4.21 and 4.22 show the demographics for the TOD-E child clinical samples. The demographic data include the same categories used for the standardization of the TOD-S, TOD-C child, and TOD-E clinical samples. Although the number of participants within some of the various categories within these sub-samples appears roughly similar to the demographics reported for the standardization sub-samples, there are a few notable exceptions. For example, males outnumbered females for the TOD-S child sample (17.4%), TOD-C child sample (17.2%) and TOD-E (20.2%); however, females outnumbered males (21.1%) for the TOD-S/TOD-C adult clinical sample.

For a variety of reasons, the results from clinical samples are much less likely to represent the overall U.S. population. Clinical samples often reflect selective referral rates. More boys than girls are referred (and evaluated) for externalizing behavior problems, as well as learning difficulties. On the other hand, females are more likely than males to be referred for internalizing problems, such as anxiety and depression. Similarly, clinical samples are not expected to reflect a geographic match to the U.S. population. Clinical samples are difficult to obtain, and availability is a function of various factors (e.g., willingness of schools and other institutions to share these data, incidence rates are not constant across the country). Finally, selection of clinical samples also depends on the goals of the authors, and certain populations may be targeted. For example, the TOD authors were particularly interested in reporting data from participants who presented with reading-related difficulties/diagnoses, and the clinical sample reflects this over-representation. For these reasons and more, the TOD Manual does not compare percentages of participants within the clinical samples to the U.S. Census figures.

The overall clinical sample is a heterogeneous collection of individuals with various diagnoses: ID, developmental delay (DD), ASD, ADHD, developmental language disorder, speech disorder, emotional or behavioral disorder, visual impairment, hearing impairment, other health impairment, and reading disability. For example, in the TOD-S clinical sample, children with a reading disability comprised the largest sub-sample (73.6%); 28% had a diagnosis of ADHD, 19% a speech disorder, 12.5% a developmental language disorder, 11.1%, a developmental delay, and 10.3% were identified as having ASD. Participants within the other diagnostic categories reported percentages well below 10. The percentages do not add to 100 because some of the participants reported co-morbid diagnoses. In summary, percentages within the demographic and diagnostic categories varied as a function of the sample under study. The Validity section of this chapter presents the results from the clinical studies.

RELIABILITY

The term "reliability" was coined by poet Samuel Taylor Coleridge in 1816 (see Salen & Marais, 2006) and has been celebrated over the years as a commendable attribute in a person or a product; one that users can trust. In the psychometrics/statistics world, it has come to refer to consistency of a test to yield stable scores that users can have confidence in. Importantly, as reliability increases in magnitude, test error decreases (an inverse relationship). A number of methodologies are available to obtain reliability estimates, as described in this section of the chapter. Reliability estimates are typically operationalized by either Pearson Product Moment Correlation coefficients or from other similar correlational equations (e.g., the Spearman-Brown formula) and range from 0 to 1; the closer the estimate is to 1, the greater confidence the evaluator has in the score.

DON'T FORGET

The reliability of a test indicates how consistently the test measures an ability or trait. It is often represented by the letter "r" or "rel" depending on the statistical equation used to obtain it. It is a number ranging from 0 (no reliability) to 1.00 (perfect reliability), although no test ever has perfect reliability. Cronbach (1951) characterized reliability estimates for tests as Excellent (.90), Good (.80), and Adequate (.70).

Reliability estimates can be transformed into another statistic, the standard error of measure (SEM). The SEM defines the probability (68%) that the obtained score corresponds to the examinee's true (ability) score. Another simple process can then be used to create confidence bands with particular levels, typically 90% or 95%. Chapter 5 of this text and the Reliability chapter in the TOD Manual describe the relationship between reliability and error and the development of the confidence bands. Because reliability and errors are inversely related, some experts recommend that placement/eligibility decisions be based on scores characterized by high reliability estimates, .90 or greater, and screening decisions be based on estimates of at least .80 (Bracken, 1987).

In this section, evidence for reliability estimates is reported for the TOD tests, composites, and indexes. These estimates have been computed from standardization and/or from clinical samples. Reliability coefficients are derived from various methodologies.

DON'T FORGET

Ensure that confidence bands that correspond to TOD tests, composites, and indexes are reported to parents, teachers, and examinees as appropriate. The range of standard scores within the confidence band indicates the "confidence" one can have that the individual's true score falls within that range.

CAUTION

When possible, base screening and eligibility decisions on scores characterized by reliability estimates of .80 and .90 respectively.

Internal Consistency

Internal consistency defines the extent to which all of the items within a test consistently assess the same ability/trait. Test authors rely on several internal consistency formulae to operationalize reliability for direct assessment measures. The TOD authors used the Split-Half method, the Rasch-Based method, and for composite and indexes, the Reliability of Linear Combinations. Coefficient Alpha is also commonly used to estimate reliability for measures that do not rely on a developmental gradient, such as the TOD Rating Scales. Chapter 6 in this text describes those estimates.

Tables 5.1 and 5.2 show internal consistency reliability estimates and SEMs of the TOD-S Tests and DRI Index by grade for the child sample and by age ranges for the adult sample. Tables 5.3 through 5.5 show reliabilities and SEMs for the TOD-C indexes and composites by age and grade; Tables 5.7 through 5.9 show internal consistency for the TOD-E indexes, composites, and tests.

TOD-S reliability estimates for the three tests and the Dyslexia Risk Index (DRI) are reported in Tables 5.1 (by grade for children) and 5.2 (by age range for adults). A review of Table 5.1 shows reliabilities for the DRI are generally greater than .90 (9 out of 13 grade levels), and the remaining 4 grade levels are equal to or greater than .81. For Test 1S: Picture Vocabulary, all reliabilities are equal to or greater than .70 and six are equal to or greater than .80. For Test 2S: Letter Word Choice, 11 of 13 grade levels have reliabilities equal to or greater than .80. For the remaining two grade levels, Grades 8 and 9, the reliability coefficient was .78. For Test 3Sa: Word Reading Fluency, the estimate for K is .93

and .95 for Grade 1. For Test 3Sb: Question Reading Fluency, the estimates range from .97 to .99. Table 5.2 illustrates a similar pattern for adults; all estimates are at least .70, and most are in the .80s and .90s for the three TOD-S tests. The DRI reliability for adults ranged from .85 to .94, with four of the six age ranges equal to or greater than .90.

Table 5.3 shows internal consistency estimates/SEMs (361 coefficients) for TOD-C tests for the child and adult standardization samples. Internal consistency could not be calculated for the Oral Reading Efficiency test as it functions more like a single "item." The majority of the reliability coefficients are ≥ .90, almost all are > .80, and only .02% are less than .70.

Tables 5.4 and 5.5 show the TOD-C internal consistency estimates/SEMs for the Dyslexia Diagnostic Index (DDI), the Reading and Spelling Index (RSI), the Linguistic Processing Index (LPI), and the composites by grade for the child sample (Table 5.4) and by age range for adults (Table 5.5). All index reliabilities are equal to or greater than .94 for Grades 1–12 and .92 for the adult age ranges. All composites for Grades 1–12 have a reliability equal to or greater than .81 with most being greater than .90.

Tables 5.7 and 5.8 display internal consistency reliabilities/SEMs for the TOD-E tests and the composites, respectively. Table 5.7 shows coefficients for the six TOD-E tests by age. Of the 24 coefficients, 23 were greater than .90; the remaining one, Sounds and Pseudowords at ages 8–9:3, was .87. Table 5.8 shows index and composite coefficients by grade (K, 1, and 2), and all are equal to or greater than .90 with most being greater than .95.

Test–Retest

Test–retest reliability (temporal stability) operationalizes the extent to which scores of the same individual remain the same over time, assuming the underlying ability does not change. Calculation of this reliability estimate requires that the same test be administered two times, typically over a period of two to three weeks. The coefficient is actually a correlation coefficient, as described in Chapter 5 of this text, and is obtained from the two distributions of scores obtained from multiple participants (one set of scores from Time 1 and one from Time 2). According to Cohen (1992), .30 represents a weak strength of association, .50 is moderate, and .80 is strong/large. Correlation coefficients from TOD-S data were obtained from 81 participants ranging in age from 5 to 54 (M = 14.37, SD = 10.93), with an equal number of males and females. TOD-C data were obtained from 61 participants who ranged in age from 8 to 64 years (M = 17.43; SD = 11.71). TOD-E data were obtained from 30 individuals ranging in age from 5 to 8 (M = 6.38; SD = .92). Tables 5.10 to 5.12 display the means at Time 1 and Time 2, reliability coefficients, SEM, and effect sizes for the TOD-S, TOD-C, and TOD-E samples. Across all three, the coefficients ranged from .70 to .97 (median of .88). Most are .80 and above, and all of the indexes are .90 and above except two, one of which is .88 (DRI, calculated for older examinees with the Question Reading Fluency test) and the other is .89 (Linguistic Processing Index). These tables report the obtained coefficients and those corrected for restriction or expansion in range, represented by standard deviations. Corrected coefficients aid interpretation when the standard deviations do not reflect the expected population standard deviation (i.e., 15), either because they are larger or smaller.

Effect sizes also inform temporal stability/reliability and are calculated by subtracting the mean standard score obtained on Time 1 from Time 2 then dividing that value by the pooled standard deviation. The effect size then shows the change from the two administrations in SD units, so the smaller the effect size, the less change from Time 1 to Time 2. According to Cohen (1992), .2 is considered a small effect size, .5 is considered a medium effect size, and .7 is large. The effect sizes ranged from .01 to .48 (median = .18) across all TOD tests, composites, and index scores; most are small. Larger effect sizes characterize tests more sensitive to practice effects. In general, these results support the stability of the TOD scores over time. Nonetheless, a small-to-medium practice effect may exist for some tests, particularly timed tests; consequently, if a second administration is needed, then it is best to delay the administration for at least three months to limit practice effects.

As is apparent from the various reliability estimates, strong evidence supports the basic integrity and stability across all TOD tests, composites, and indexes. Evaluators can have confidence that TOD scores reflect solid estimates of examinees' abilities. Rapid Reference 7.1 provides a summary of reliability information for the TOD tests, composites, and indexes.

DON'T FORGET

Typically, a moderate (.50) correlation coefficient is required for evaluators to have confidence in the strength of association between two variables, but the larger the better. The two variables in a test–retest study are two administrations of the same test to the same group of people, which typically occur over two to three weeks. The higher the correlation between the two sets of scores, the higher the reliability. High reliabilities mean that results can be reproduced under the same conditions over time, and any variations are not due to measurement inconsistencies/error.

DON'T FORGET

A small effect size between two test administrations shows that little difference exists between the scores on Time 1 and Time 2.

DON'T FORGET

Practice effects can occur in a retest situation. Effect sizes of .2 are considered small, .5 are medium, and .7 are large. Large effect sizes indicate that a test is vulnerable to practice effects. The TOD effect sizes range from .01 to .48, indicating small to medium practice effect for some tests. Allowing a minimum of three months between administrations can limit practice effects.

≡ *Rapid Reference 7. 1*

Summary of Reliability Information

- Almost all of the reliability estimates are considered either Excellent (in the .90s), Good (in the .80s), or Adequate (in the .70s).
- All TOD-S tests have adequate to excellent reliability for children in Grades K–12. The DRI has excellent reliability at 9 of the 13 grade levels and good reliability at the remaining four grade levels. The adult sample has similar reliabilities.
- All TOD-C indexes have excellent reliabilities that are equal to or greater than .94 for Grades 1–12 and .92 for the adult age ranges.
- All TOD-C composites for Grades 1–12 have a reliability equal to or greater than .81 with most being greater than .90.
- All TOD-E tests have reliabilities equal to or greater than .90 at all ages with one exception: Sounds and Pseudowords had a reliability coefficient of .87 for ages 8–9:3.
- All TOD-E composites and indexes have reliabilities equal to or greater than .90. Most were equal to or greater than .95.
- Test–retest reliability coefficients and low mean differences from Test 1 to Test 2 (i.e., small effect sizes) indicate the TOD's scores remain stable over time. The tests are characterized by very little measurement inconsistencies.
- Strong evidence exists for the reliability of the TOD-S, TOD-C, and TOD-E tests, composites, and indexes.

CAUTION

When comparing tests to inform strengths and weaknesses, limit the risk of over-interpretation of significant and rare differences by carefully choosing only those needed to address the referral question. Because all tests have error, as reflected in the size of confidence bands, with multiple comparisons a test may be significantly different from another based on chance alone.

VALIDITY

The term "validity" originates from the Latin word "validus," meaning strong or powerful. In the measurement world, it has evolved to signify the degree to which a test measures what it was developed to measure. Although this definition of validity is generally accepted, it is not one-dimensional. Determining the validity of a test requires evidence in support of its ability to assess a construct: (a) for carefully defined purpose(s), (b) under specified conditions, and (c) for a target population. The TOD Manual describes multiple methodologies designed to provide such evidence, including content description validity; construct validity; convergent validity; clinical group or diagnostic validity, which is based in part on the ability of TOD scores to reflect weaknesses for those predicted to have limitations; and predictive validity.

DON'T FORGET

The validity of a test refers to the extent to which it measures the intended content/construct. It indicates how confident evaluators can be in deriving conclusions from the test scores. Although adequate reliability is a prerequisite of validity, it does not guarantee that a test is valid.

Content Description Validity

Content description validity of a test requires that items be developed in sufficient quantity and of adequate psychometric quality to represent the target construct. The authors created a conceptual framework that guided TOD development in Rapid Reference 7.2 that was adapted from Figure 1.1 in the TOD Manual (p. 2).

The TOD tests, composites, and indexes were created to directly assess those constructs listed in the first three columns. The last column shows related factors that are assessed by the TOD Rating Scales. The test blueprint in Table 1.2, the TOD Test Descriptions in Table 1.3, and the Test Selection Charts shown in Tables 1.4 and 1.5 of the TOD Manual provide

Rapid Reference 7.2

Comprehensive Dyslexia Assessment Components

Reading and Spelling Domain	Linguistic Processing Domain	Vocabulary and Reasoning Domain	Factors That May Contribute to a Diagnosis of Dyslexia
Sight Word Acquisition	Phonological Awareness	Vocabulary Reasoning	Family history of reading/spelling difficulties
Phonics Knowledge	Rapid Automatized Naming		Co-morbid Disorders (e.g., ADHD, Developmental Language Disorder, dyscalculia)
Basic Reading Skills	Auditory Working Memory		Motivation
Decoding Efficiency	Orthographic Processing		
Spelling	Visual-Verbal Paired Associate Learning		
Reading Fluency			
Reading Comprehension Efficiency			

elaborations of the assessment options by listing all of the available tests, composites, and indexes. These Test Selection Charts are also in Chapters 3 and 4 of this text.

The clinical pattern of dyslexia shown in Table 1.1 provides a brief description of how the TOD content and related components can be used to assess dyslexia by showing examinee characteristics most likely to be affected. Examinees who have dyslexia will likely exhibit significant difficulties in one or more of the following skill areas: (a) ability to read nonsense words, (b) ability to read irregular words, (c) reading at a pace consistent with typical development, and (d) spelling words consistent with typical development. These individuals will also likely have low performance on one or more linguistic processing abilities: (a) phonological awareness, (b) rapid automatized naming, (c) auditory working memory, (d) orthographic processing, and/or (e) visual-verbal paired associate learning.

Because dyslexia is often unexpected, individuals with dyslexia will likely also have average or better cognitive abilities, assessed by the TOD vocabulary and reasoning tests. Finally, internal and external influences are assessed on the TOD Rating Scales, such as family history of dyslexia and early speech and/or language difficulties. There may also be environmental limitations, such as poor instructional history or poor parental support for learning to read.

DON'T FORGET

Although the TOD batteries contain many tests, only eight are required to obtain the more critical indexes for making a diagnosis of dyslexia based on reading, spelling, and linguistic processing measures: the DDI and the EDDI; however, evaluators will likely administer additional tests, such as the vocabulary and reasoning tests and the rating scales to obtain more definitive information.

Construct Validity

Construct validity is defined as the extent to which a test accurately measures a theoretical construct. The construct validity of the TOD has been operationalized by evidence obtained from a variety of methodologies, all of which assess the relevant constructs or sub-constructs related to dyslexia.

One of the most critical sources of evidence for construct validity is provided by scrutiny of the developmental progression of the TOD tests. Developmental progression is assumed for all TOD tests because the abilities assessed by them increase as a function of increasing chronological age. Evidence for developmental progression can be obtained from correlational data taken from the standardization sample showing the relationship between age and ability, with ability defined by the raw score progression. This relationship can be characterized by simple graphs showing ability on the ordinate, or vertical axis, and chronological age on the horizontal axis, the abscissa (see Figures 5.1 through 5.5 in the TOD Manual).

As an example, Figure 5.1 shows a steady increase in raw scores across ages from 5 to 23 years for the Picture Vocabulary test from the TOD-S. Although vocabulary development continues to grow through adulthood, several of the academic constructs measured by the TOD-E plateau during the late elementary ages (e.g., Letter and Sound Knowledge, Phonological Awareness, Rhyming), or in some rare cases, even earlier. In the measurement world this phenomenon is referred to as a "ceiling effect," and is defined by the link to a specific chronological age at which even average or slightly above average ability examinees can earn the highest possible score. For the Rhyming tests (5E) typically developing eight-year-old examinees earn the highest score reflecting the fact that rhyming is a skill that most individuals have mastered at this young age; typically, examiners will simply say that examinees tend to "ceiling out." Only those with dyslexia or some other reading-related condition have significant difficulty on such tests. All of the TOD-E tests show a similar developmental progression plateau. Typically, these tests initially show rapid development, as they were created to be sensitive to reading-related skills development within grades K through 1. TOD-C tests that tend to show this ceiling effect in middle school include Phonological Manipulation, Blending, Segmenting, and Symbol to Sound Learning. TOD-C tests that tend to ceiling out during high school include Word Memory, Letter Memory, Rapid Letter Naming, Rapid Number and Letter Naming, Word Pattern Choice, Pseudoword Reading, Rapid Pseudoword Word Naming, and Oral Reading Fluency. Other TOD-C tests tend to plateau after high school.

> **CAUTION**
>
> Abilities plateau at different ages/grades. Don't assume that a low test ceiling is a psychometric problem. It may simply show that most people have acquired that skill by a certain age or grade.

Test intercorrelations also provide sensitive indicators of construct validity. Tables 5.14 to 5.18 show intercorrelations of TOD-S, TOD-E, and TOD-C tests from the standardization sample. Correlation coefficients range from .08 to .84, although most are in the modest to moderate range. Lower coefficients are expected between tests of divergent skills that have little variance in common. For example, Phonological Manipulation and Rapid Number and Letter Naming only correlate at .31 in the TOD-C child sample and .30 in the adult sample. Skills that share more theoretical and actual statistical variance, like Regular Word Spelling and Irregular Word Spelling, correlate at .81 in the TOD-C child sample and .78 in the adult sample. These tables show higher correlations among the tests that are similar in purpose and lower correlations between tests with little in common. The authors of the TOD purposely created this pattern and specifically created highly correlated test pairs that would form composites. Similarly, the TOD authors also created even more global scores consisting of several tests that share significant variance, referred to as the DDI on the TOD-C and the EDDI on the TOD-E. These indexes are described in more detail in the next paragraph, along with an explanation of how they provide evidence of construct validity. Also, in a later section, evidence is presented and describes how these indexes contribute to predictive validity.

Tables 5.14 and 5.18 present correlational coefficients that illustrate the relationships among the tests. Patterns can also be determined from factor analytic methodology, relying on complex statistical equations. Factor analytic models are referred to as either Exploratory (Exploratory Factor Analysis, EFA) or Confirmatory (Confirmatory Factor Analysis, CFA). EFA is typically more useful in the preliminary stage of test development when the number of factors is unknown. EFA creates factors consisting of like tests, but it does not offer statistical tests of a hypothesized factor structure. CFA is typically chosen to determine factorial structure of tests that comprise a battery when there is theoretical or empirical evidence to support structures of interest. The goal is to compare the fit of these multiple structural models to data. Consequently, CFA was chosen for these analyses. Table 5.19 displays results that explore the model fit for the TOD-C tests most predictive of dyslexia—the tests that comprise the RSI and tests in the LPI. When these eight tests are combined, they form the DDI.

Table 5.20 shows confirmatory factor analytic results from the TOD-E tests that were most predictive of dyslexia, the Early Reading Spelling Index (ERSI) and the Early Linguistic Processing Index (ELPI), both consisting of multiple tests; when all of these tests are combined, they comprise the TOD-E EDDI. Because existing theoretical evidence provides support for interpretation based on two models, they were compared: a one-factor model, i.e., based on the DDI for the TOD-C and the EDDI for the TOD-E, and a two-factor model, based on the RSI/LPI scores for the TOD-C and the ERSI/ELPI scores for the TOD-E. CFA output compares the models using a number of statistical tests of models fit to the data (e.g., chi-square, Tucker Lewis Index, TLI). Results from Tables 5.19 and 5.20 in the Manual confirm that both the one-factor and the two-factor models result in a good fit to the standardization data. Consequently, evaluators can have confidence interpreting the DDI and the EDDI as well as the RSI, LPI, and the ERSI and ELPI scores. CFA data from the clinical sample shown in Tables 5.21 and 5.22 in the TOD Manual also support both the one-test and two-factor models.

Concurrent/Convergent Validity

The concurrent/convergent validation method relies on examining the relationship between a test of interest and other tests that purport to assess the same or similar constructs. Moderate (r = .50) to strong (r = .80) correlation coefficients support the construct validity of the target test. Several tables in the TOD Manual provide convergent validity data. They present pairwise comparisons for tests within the combined TOD-S/TOD-C and combined TOD-S/TOD-E batteries and related tests within other batteries. Table 5.23 shows the sample sizes and demographics for the TOD-S/TOD-C and the following 7 batteries: WJ IV COG (Schrank et al., 2014a), WJ IV ACH (Schrank et al., 2014b), CASL-2 (Carrow-Woolfolk, 2017), CTOPP-2 (Wagner et al., 2013), TOWRE-2 (Torgesen et al., 2012), TOC-2 (Mather et al., 2022), and the UNIT GAT (Bracken & McCallum, 2019). Table 5.25 shows the sample sizes and demographics for the TOD-S/TOD-E tests for the following 3 batteries: WJ IV ACH, CASL-2, and the CTOPP-2. Correlation coefficients between the TOD-S/TOD-C tests and tests of similar abilities on the seven batteries ranged from .30 to .91, as shown in Table 5.24. Most are in the moderate range; in fact, 27 of the 41 coefficients are .50 and greater. Correlation coefficients between the TOD-S/TOD-E tests and tests of similar abilities from 3 batteries ranged from .52 to .91 and are shown in Table 5.26. Most are in the moderate to strong range; in fact, 7 of the 10 coefficients are .71 and greater. Chapter 5 in the TOD manual provides detailed descriptions of the relevant comparisons.

> **DON'T FORGET**
>
> Data from studies demonstrate converging validity from the comparisons between the TOD tests and several other tests that have typically been used to assess dyslexia. Consequently, evaluators can now adequately diagnose dyslexia using one battery of tests—the TOD.

Diagnostic/Clinical Validity

Evidence for validity may also be obtained by comparing the performance of individuals who are typically developing to those who are expected to perform differently in the abilities being measured (i.e., those with a relevant clinical diagnosis). Specifically, tests that are developed to identify/diagnose those with limited skills in a particular area should do so. The TOD was created to help identify/diagnose those with limited reading and spelling skills who exhibit the characteristics of dyslexia. In order to obtain this type of validity evidence, it is important to obtain data from those who have been previously identified as having dyslexia and then determine if the TOD differentiates between those individuals and those who do not have dyslexia. To investigate this hypothesis, conditional probability analyses yielding receiver operating characteristic curves (ROC) were obtained at various standard score levels. Specifically, students who had been identified as having a specific learning disability in reading were compared to typically developing students in reading matched on relevant demographics from the TOD standardization sample. Because the TOD-S DRI, TOD-C DDI, and the TOD-E EDDI were created by the TOD authors to differentiate those who have dyslexia or are at risk for dyslexia and those with typical reading skills, each index was entered into the analysis. Each provided statistically significant improvement over chance in detecting dyslexia status: TOD-S (area under the ROC curve = .97, $p < .001$); TOD-C DDI (area under the curve = .99, $p < .001$); and TOD-E EDDI (area under the curve = .99, $p < .001$). Tables 5.27, 5.28, and 5.29 show sensitivity and specificity values that correspond to various TOD-S, TOD-C, and TOD-E standard scores. Sensitivity indicates the capacity to detect true positive cases, i.e., in this case, those who have dyslexia. Specificity refers to the extent to which the predictor scores exclude true negative cases, i.e., in this case, those who do not have dyslexia (Betz et al., 2013). Higher sensitivity will result in lower specificity, and higher specificity will result in lower sensitivity.

As cut scores increase in magnitude, sensitivity goes up, and specificity goes down, although the progression is not obvious until the cut scores get very high. As an example, for the TOD-S, a cut score of 70 yields a sensitivity value of .40 and specificity of .99; a cut score of 80 yields a sensitivity value of .80 and specificity of .99; a cut score of 90 yields a sensitivity value of .99 and specificity value of .87. The pattern is the same for the TOD-C and TOD-E, and the magnitude of the three values is similar. According to the TOD Manual, a cut score of .80 is reasonable to use. This means that 80% of those with characteristics of dyslexia will have standard scores less than or equal to 80; 99% of those without characteristics of dyslexia will have scores greater than 80. The TOD index scores can help evaluators identify those with dyslexia, although other data should be considered (e.g., rating scales, classroom work samples).

The TOD Manual provides additional evidence of construct validity based on a

DON'T FORGET

Test sensitivity (true positive) is the probability that a positive test result indicates that an individual has the condition (dyslexia), whereas test specificity (true negative) is the probability that a negative test result indicates that an individual does not have the condition.

DON'T FORGET

Identification of dyslexia may be most accurate when adopting a DDI cut score of 80, as it provides the best estimate given the balance between sensitivity and specificity.

CAUTION

Examinees who are intellectually gifted/high ability may achieve a DDI higher than 90 and still have dyslexia.

number of clinical studies documenting differential performance of those with diagnostic conditions that likely limit performance on reading-related tasks compared to typically performing individuals from the standardization sample. Means and effect size differences on the TOD-C and TOD-E tests, composites, and indexes are shown.

The total TOD-C child clinical sample included 511 participants ages 6 to 18. Table 5.30 shows the results from perhaps the most critical data set. In this study, TOD-C test, composite, and index means of 278 individuals who had previously been identified as having dyslexia or a learning disability in reading were compared to a matched control group. The mean and effect size differences between the two are large, supporting the hypotheses that the TOD-C components yield mean differences in the predicted direction, i.e., means are lower for the clinical group. For example, the effect size differences for the reading and spelling tests are typically > 1.0; those from the linguistic processing, vocabulary, and reasoning tests are typically < 1.0, reflecting the unexpected nature of dyslexia and the fact that individuals with dyslexia may not earn relatively low scores on all linguistic processing measures. The effect sizes for the DRI and DDI are 1.42 and 1.41; these large effect sizes reflect the ability of these indexes to differentiate between these two groups. Similarly, the effect size for the Reading and Spelling Index is 1.71.

As shown in Table 5.31, effect size differences for 33 individuals diagnosed with a language disorder and a matched sample range from medium to large and range in size from .62 to 1.17 for the reading and spelling tests and from .20 to 1.0 for the linguistic processing, vocabulary, and reasoning tests. Effect sizes for the DRI and DDI are large, .70 and .93. Those for the composites and indexes for reading and spelling scores are also large, ranging from .78 to 1.01. Effect sizes for some of the other skill areas range from .49 to .84. Again, these results reflect an expected pattern given the heterogeneity of this group and provide evidence of construct validity.

Table 5.32 shows a sample of students with ADHD ($N = 118$) compared to a matched control group. Given the heterogeneity of this group, the results are as expected. Effect sizes between the groups are medium to large and range from .53 to .90 for the reading and spelling tests and from .00 to .79 for the linguistic processing tests, vocabulary, and reasoning tests. The effect size for the mean DRI and DDI differences are large, .79 to 1.0, respectively. Those for the composites and indexes for reading and spelling are medium to large; the RSI is .90, although effect sizes for some of the other skills ranged from .42 to .81, a bit smaller in magnitude. All of the effect sizes reflect the same pattern for all the test/index composites and show that individuals with ADHD did not perform as well as the matched controls on all measures, with one exception. One effect size was .00, indicating that the means for the Segmenting test are virtually the same (100.04 for the ADHD sample and 100.00 for the matched sample). In general, these results provide evidence that the TOD-C can help detect dyslexia within the ADHD population.

Table 5.33 shows descriptive statistics for 49 participants with ASD and a matched sample. Findings reflect the fact that many within this population have difficulties in language and related skills. Effect sizes between the groups reflect a similar pattern across TOD-C test scores and are small to large (from .31 to .1.02 for the reading and spelling tests and, for the linguistic processing tests, vocabulary, and reasoning tests, .33 to .87). The effect sizes for the mean differences for the DRI and DDI are .68 and .80, and, for the composites, .45 to .76. These results provide evidence that the TOD-C is sensitive to limitations that are characteristic of dyslexia for many within the ASD population.

Table 5.34 shows results for 34 individuals diagnosed as having an ID or a developmental disability compared to a matched sample. As expected, most test and index means are well below the population mean of 100 and range from 63.31 to 82.24; the matched sample means range from 89.35 to 100.41; the effect sizes are equally telling, ranging from .69 to 1.89 for all TOD-C tests, composites, and indexes. These results indicate that the TOD-C is capable of distinguishing between typically developing individuals and those with ID or DD.

Table 5.35 shows descriptive statistics for a TOD-E clinical sample, 31 children with dyslexia or a learning disability in reading and a matched control group from the standardization sample. The effect sizes of the differences between group means are large, ranging from .91 to 1.21 for the spelling and reading tests; those of the linguistic processing, vocabulary, and reasoning tests are medium to large, ranging from .59 to 1.23. The effect sizes for the DRI and EDDI are large (.83 and 1.20). Mean differences and effect sizes for the index and composite scores measuring reading and spelling are also large, ranging from 1.03 to 1.38, and are similar to effect sizes of the other related skills, .94 to 1.14. These scores provide additional construct validation for the TOD, as evidenced by its ability to distinguish between those who have dyslexia or a learning disability in reading and typically developing young students.

Because the TOD-E covers only a very limited age/grade range, the number of individuals with a clinical diagnosis is small. Consequently, all those with diagnoses (N = 80) were combined, including students with DD, ID, language disorders, ASD, and ADHD; these students were compared to a matched sample from the standardization sample. Table 5.36 in the TOD Manual shows the descriptive statistics for this combined group and the matched controls. Effect size differences for the TOD-E tests ranged from .46 to 1.08 and for the composites and indexes from .69 to .99. These comparisons provide evidence that the TOD-E can discriminate between typically developing young students and those with a variety of clinical diagnoses.

Predictive Validity

Evidence for predictive validity was obtained by examining the power of the TOD-C DDI score to assign membership of individuals into two groups, one consisting of 261 individuals previously diagnosed with dyslexia and a matched control group also consisting of 261 participants from the standardization sample without the diagnosis (Castleman et al., 2023). Two binary logistic regression analyses were conducted. The first required the use of four TOD tests to operationalize the Simple View of Reading (SVR), described by Gough and Tunmer (1986), using the following formula: Decoding X Language Comprehension = Reading Comprehension. The tests Irregular Word Reading and Pseudoword Reading define "decoding" and Picture Vocabulary and Listening Vocabulary were used to define "language comprehension." Individuals with dyslexia were 3.44 times more likely to be predicted to have dyslexia than those without the diagnosis when the SVR score alone was included in the regression equation. Individuals with dyslexia were 9.29 times more likely to be predicted to have dyslexia than those without when the model included the TOD-C DDI scores. These results contribute to validity as they reflect the strong ability of the DDI to accurately predict dyslexia.

Results of a recently conducted study using standardization data show the predictive power of combining direct assessment and rating scale data (McCallum & Bell, 2025).

Specifically, TOD-S DRI scores and scores from three rating scales were obtained for participants comprising two groups, one of individuals with dyslexia and one of individuals without dyslexia; however, these groups were matched on relevant demographic variables: age, race/ethnicity, SES, and region. Scores were entered into a logistic regression analysis. The DRI alone predicted group membership with 75% accuracy; accuracy improved from 80% to 82% depending upon which rating scale also entered into the equation. When all three rating scales were entered, accuracy improved to 91%. These results suggest that combining the direct assessment and rating scale data provides the best prediction of dyslexia.

> **DON'T FORGET**
>
> Validity is never demonstrated by a single study and never proved conclusively; rather, the collection of evidence is ongoing, accrues over time, and is obtained from multiple sources.

In summary, data from several studies addressing the validity of the TOD provide strong evidence of its ability to operationalize and predict dyslexia. Supportive evidence was obtained from various psychometric methodologies, including those investigating construct validity, content validity, concurrent validity, predictive validity, and diagnostic/clinical validity. Rapid Reference 7.3 reviews the various types of validity. Rapid Reference 7.4 presents a summary of the validity evidence.

INDEPENDENT RESEARCH

This chapter ends with findings from an independent research study published in the *Annals of Dyslexia* (Ho et al., 2025) and observations from an independent review of the TOD-C that appeared in the *Journal of Psychoeducational Assessment* (Pena & Villarreal, 2024). Ho et al. (2025) examined the effects of orthography, phonology, semantics and working memory on the reading comprehension of children aged 8 to 11 without ($n = 575$) and with dyslexia ($n = 143$), using selected tests from the TOD-C). They found that the performance

≡ *Rapid Reference 7.3*

Different Types of Validity

- **Content validity**: the extent to which a test represents a target domain of interest.
- **Construct validity**: the extent to which a test measures some hypothetical construct of interest.
- **Concurrent/convergent validity:** the extent to which a test is related to and shares content in common with other tests designed to measure similar content.
- **Clinical validity:** the extent to which a test distinguishes typically developing individuals from those who are expected to perform differently.
- **Predictive validity:** the power of a test to predict performance on an outcome of interest.

≡ Rapid Reference 7.4

Summary of Validity Evidence

- **Content validity:** Related research and theoretical literature guided the development of the TOD conceptual framework, and the selection of the skills and abilities included. Vocabulary and Reasoning tests were included to help document the sometimes unexpected nature of dyslexia.

- **Construct validity:** Developmental progression of the various skills and abilities is documented as are intercorrelations among the tests. Tests that measure similar skills or abilities have higher inter-correlations than tests that measure different skills or abilities. Results from confirmatory Factor Analyses (CFA) document construct validity.

- **Concurrent/convergent validity:** TOD tests were compared to tests in 7 batteries that purport to measure similar constructs: WJ IV COG, WJ IV ACH, CASL-2, CTOPP-2, TOWRE-2, TOC-2, and the UNIT GAT. Most of the correlation coefficients were in the moderate ($r = .50$) to strong ($r = .80$) range providing evidence of concurrent validity.

- **Clinical validity:** Studies were conducted to compare TOD scores between typically developing individuals and those with a relevant clinical diagnosis (e.g., dyslexia, ADHD, ASD, ID, and DD). The results indicate that the TOD can differentiate those with dyslexia from matched controls within clinical populations.

- **Predictive validity:** Results from ROC Curve analyses confirmed the power of the TOD-C DDI and TOD-E EDDI to predict dyslexia. Results of a second study provided evidence that the TOD-S DRI predicted group membership with 75% accuracy. Prediction improved to more than 80% accuracy when information from one TOD Rating Scale was added and up to 91% when information from all three rating scales were included.

of typically developing children on all of the selected TOD-C tests was significantly higher than that of the children with dyslexia ($p < .001$). They also found that the selected TOD-C tests were all at least moderately correlated with the TOD-C reading comprehension measure for both groups. These findings lend independent support to the validity of the TOD-C tests.

Comments by Pena and Villarreal are included in this chapter because these authors examined the technical adequacy of the TOD-C, including psychometric features such as test development procedures, standardization process and data, reliability, and validity. According to Pena and Villarreal, the reliability estimates are "excellent" and "satisfactory," for internal consistency and test–retest. They conclude that "content and construct validity seemed appropriate" and that interpretation of both the one-factor and two-factor models based on the DDI "is appropriate using either model." They report evidence for convergent validity from comparisons with several other tests of cognition and academics and share predictive validity data from the manual (e.g., sensitivity, specificity) demonstrating that the DDI is capable of differentiating between at-risk and typically performing individuals. Finally, they noted that data from the TOD Manual demonstrate how clinical group members with dyslexia or other reading disabilities scored lower on the TOD-C than examinees from other clinical groups that are less affected by dyslexia. Pena and Villarreal summarized their review with the following selected comments: "The TOD-C is a technically sound measure of the characteristics most often associated with dyslexia... the TOD-C distinguishes itself as it allows for a specific focus on dyslexia, particularly through the DDI which represents a unique index score that demonstrates appropriate validity... allows for a comprehensive evaluation...can yield significant information for identifying examinee strengths and weaknesses...for aiding examiners in interpretation and offering specific recommendations... includes a recommendations guidebook...the recommendations seem to be evidence based...”

TEST YOURSELF

1. The reliability estimate experts recommend for screening is ___.

(a) .60

(b) .70

(c) .80

(d) .90

2. The reliability estimate experts recommend for diagnostic eligibility is ___.

(a) .60

(b) .70

(c) .80

(d) .90

3. Collection of standardization data typically relies on selection of participants based on all of the following demographics except ____.

(a) age

(b) gender

(c) race

(d) county of origin

4. Factor analytic data are used to determine ________ validity.

(a) content

(b) construct

(c) concurrent

(d) predictive

5. Test error is based on the magnitude of the ________ estimate.

(a) validity

(b) reliability

(c) logistic binary

(d) multiple regression

6. According to Cohen, a strong/robust strength of association based on a correlation coefficient is _____.

(a) .20

(b) .40

(c) .60

(d) .80

7. **The ability of a test to detect individuals "true positives," those who have a diagnosis from those who do not is referred to as ________.**
   (a) specificity
   (b) sensitivity
   (c) diagnostic index
   (d) risk index

8. **The statistic that defines the difference between two means based on standard deviation units is the ______.**
   (a) difference size
   (b) standard size
   (c) deviation size
   (d) effect size

9. **The TOD score that most accurately predicts a dyslexia diagnosis is the ______.**
   (a) SVR
   (b) DRI
   (c) DDI
   (d) EDDI

10. **The geographic region most over-represented in the TOD-C child standardization sample was the South.**
    True or False?

Answers: 1. c; 2. d; 3. d; 4. b; 5. b; 6. d; 7. b; 8. d; 9. c; 10. True

REFERENCES

Bell, S. M., & McCallum, R. S. (2023, November). *Do demographics affect dyslexia identification? Current perspectives.* Paper presented to the annual convention of the International Dyslexia Association, Columbus, OH.

Betz, S. K., Eickhoff, J. R., & Sullivan, S. F. (2013). Factors influencing the selection of standardized tests for the diagnosis of specific language impairment. *Language, Speech, and Hearing Services in Schools, 44*(2), 133–146. https://doi.org/10.1044/0161.1461(2012/12-0093)

Bracken, B. A. (1987). Limitations of preschool instruments and standards for minimal levels of technical adequacy. *Journal of Psychoeducational Assessment, 4,* 313–326.

Bracken, B. A., & McCallum, R. S. (2019). *Universal Nonverbal Intelligence Test-Group Abilities Test (UNIT-GAT).* PRO-ED.

Carrow-Woolfolk, E. (2017). *Comprehensive Test of Spoken Language-2 (CASL-2).* Western Psychological Services.

Castleman, D. M., McClurg, V. M., McCallum, R. S., Bell, S. M., & Mather, N. (2023, February). *Predicting dyslexia: Contributions of demographic information.* [Poster Presentation]. National Association of School Psychologists Annual Convention. Denver, CO: United States

Cohen, J. (1992). Statistical power analysis. *Current Directions in Psychological Science, 1*(3), 98–101.

Cronbach, L. J. (1951). Coefficient alpha and the internal structure of tests. *Psychometrika, 16,* 297–334.

Gough, P. B., & Tunmer, W. E. (1986). Decoding, reading, and reading disability. *Remedial and Special Education, 7*(1), 6–10. https://doi.org/10.1177/074193258600700104

Ho, J. C., Reed, D. K., & McBride, C. (2025). The effects of orthography, phonology, semantics, and working memory on the reading comprehension of children with and without reading dyslexia. *Annals of Dyslexia, 75*(5), 225–240. https://doi.org/10.1007/s11881-025-00322-5

Mather, N., Roberts, R., Hammill, D. D., & Allen, E. A. (2022). *Tests of Orthographic Competence-2 (TOC-2)*. PRO-ED.

Mather, N., McCallum, R. S., Bell, S. M., & Wendling, B. J. (2024b). *Tests of Dyslexia (TOD)* [Manual]. Western Psychological Services.

McCallum, R. S., & Bell, S. M. (2025, February). *Does combining direct assessment and ratings scores improve dyslexia screening?* [Poster Presentation]. National Association of School Psychologists Annual Convention, Seattle, WA.

Pena, L. M., & Villarreal, V. (2024). Test review: Tests of Dyslexia-Comprehensive. *Journal of Psychoeducational Assessment, 42*(8), 1042–1048. https://doi.org/10.1177/07342829241273227

Salen, J. H., & Marais, K. (2006). Highlights from the early (and pre-) history of reliability engineering. *Reliability, Engineering and System Safety, 91*(2), 249–256.

Schrank, F. A., Mather, N., & McGrew, K. S. (2014a). *Woodcock-Johnson IV Tests of Achievement (WJ IV ACH)*. Riverside.

Schrank, F. A., McGrew, K. S., & Mather, N. (2014b). *Woodcock-Johnson IV Tests of Cognitive Ability (WJ IV COG)*. Riverside.

Torgesen, J. K., Wagner, R. K., & Rashotte, C. A. (2012). *Test of Word Reading Efficiency-2 (TOWRE-2)*. PRO-ED.

Wagner, R. K., Torgesen, J. K., Rashotte, C. A., & Pearson, N. A. (2013). *Comprehensive Tests of Phonological Processing-2 (CTOPP-2)*. PRO-ED.

Eight

USING THE TOD RESULTS TO INFORM INTERVENTIONS

"The most notable factor that can have a positive impact on risk for dyslexia is instruction."
(Catts & Petscher, 2022, p.176)

Administration of the *Tests of Dyslexia*™ (TOD) often reveals weaknesses in phonological awareness and reading and spelling skills that require intervention; the findings may indicate that an individual has weaknesses in phonological awareness, basic reading skills, structural analysis, reading fluency, and/or spelling and requires specific interventions and accommodations. A resource that accompanies the TOD is *Dyslexia Interventions and Recommendations: A Companion Guide to the Tests of Dyslexia* (Mather et al., 2024c). This guide provides numerous examples of instructional recommendations that evaluators can include in assessment reports. In addition, the University of Florida Literacy Institute has numerous free resources, including tutorials, sample lessons, and a scope and sequence chart. Under the Virtual Teaching Resource hub, there is a Dyslexia Resource Hub (https://ufli.education.ufl.edu/resources/teaching-resources/instructional-activities/connected-text/).

STRUCTURED LITERACY

In 2019, the International Dyslexia Association (IDA) coined the term *structured literacy* to describe systematic approaches to reading instruction that emphasize the structure of language and the key principles of instruction. Although all students can benefit from a structured literacy approach, this type of instruction is critical for students with dyslexia (Moats, 2019; Odegard, 2020). The content of instruction addresses the production of language at all levels: speech sounds, spelling and syllable patterns, syntax (the rules of combining words into sentences), morphology (meaningful units of language), and semantics (the meaning that language conveys). In a Fact Sheet, IDA (2019) summarized that instruction should be (a) explicit, and the teacher should explain concepts directly and provide guided practice; (b) systematic, cumulative, and follow a scope and sequence of skills; (c) engaging, multimodal, and include hands-on learning activities; and (d) diagnostic and prescriptive, where each student's progress is monitored and lessons are adjusted as needed.

Explicit instruction is sometimes referred to as the "I do. We do. You do." model (Archer & Hughes, 2011). In the "I do" phase, the teacher demonstrates the task while thinking aloud to support the student's initial learning of the task. In the "We do" phase, the student practices the task with teacher supervision, and the teacher provides cues, prompts, and feedback as necessary; immediate corrective feedback is key to this phase. In the "You do" phase, the student works independently. The student should participate in the "You do" phase only after the target task is completely understood by the student. Nothing is left to chance.

CAUTION

Many popular reading programs that are used in schools are ineffective for students with dyslexia because they are not sufficiently explicit and systematic.

Although structured literacy addresses the full spectrum of language development, including syntax and reading comprehension, this chapter focuses on the major areas of difficulty for individuals with dyslexia: phonological awareness, basic reading skills, structural analysis, reading fluency, and spelling. The chapter concludes with information regarding the selection of appropriate accommodations for individuals with dyslexia.

PHONOLOGICAL AND PHONEMIC AWARENESS

Phonological awareness is an umbrella term that refers to the oral language abilities to hear and manipulate sounds in words and word parts, such as rhyming words, deleting a syllable from a word, or identifying the first sound of a word. Phonemic awareness refers to the ability to hear and manipulate individual phonemes in words, such as deleting the first or last sound in a word. The TOD-E contains two phonological awareness tests: TOD-5E Rhyming and TOD-8E Early Segmenting. The TOD-C contains three phonological awareness tests: TOD-4C Phonological Manipulation, TOD-13C Blending, and TOD-14C Segmenting. Rapid Reference 8.1 provides examples of phonological and phonemic awareness tasks.

≡ Rapid Reference 8.1

Examples of Phonological and Phonemic Awareness Tasks

- Rhyming: Tell me a word that rhymes with dog.
- Blending: What word is this… /m/ /e/? (me)
- Phoneme Counting: How many sounds do you hear in the word "ship"?
- Phoneme Segmentation: Tell me each of the sounds you hear in the word "bus."
- Phoneme Deletion: What word is left if the /t/ sound is taken from "cart"?

Both phonological and phonemic awareness develop early in school for most children. Typically, students in kindergarten and first grade can rhyme, blend, and segment compound and multisyllabic words. By the end of kindergarten, most children can blend and segment words with three to four phonemes, particularly if they have received effective instruction (Moats, 2020). By first and second grade, most children can usually blend and segment phonemes and manipulate the initial, final, and lastly the middle sounds of words. Acquisition of these skills is often more difficult, however, for children with dyslexia. Explicit instruction is most effective in kindergarten and first grade but also benefits older students (Rehfeld et al., 2022).

When providing instruction in phonological awareness, consider the difficulty level of the task and the student's developmental level. It is easier to identify rhymes than to produce them. It is easiest to identify the initial sound of a word, then the final sound, and then the medial sound. It is easier to blend and segment speech sounds than to manipulate them. Rapid Reference 8.2 provides a typical sequence of phonological awareness development.

Teachers often wonder: How much time should I spend on phonological awareness instruction? Although the amount of time depends upon the student, results from a meta-analysis indicated that from preschool to first grade the optimal cumulative dosage of early phonemic awareness instruction was approximately 11 hours for students with reading difficulties (Erbeli et al., 2024). Moats (2020) suggested that 5–10 minutes a day for about

DON'T FORGET

Analyzing errors on the relevant TOD-E and TOD-C tests can help determine where to begin instruction. A number of tests cover the developmental sequence for the targeted skill area. For example, TOD-8E Early Segmenting and TOD-14C Segmenting require first segmenting compound words, then words into syllables, and then words into phonemes. An error analysis helps inform where to begin instruction.

CAUTION

Be careful not to waste instructional time on phonological awareness skills that the examinee has already mastered.

⚏ *Rapid Reference 8.2*

Example Sequence of Phonological Awareness Development

- Discriminate rhymes
- Produce rhymes
- Identify the initial and final sounds in words
- Identify the middle vowel sound
- Blend sounds (two sounds, three sounds)
- Segment sounds (VC, CVC words)
- Manipulate sounds (e.g., delete and substitute)

12–20 weeks is typically sufficient for enhancing phonemic awareness in young children but that older students with reading difficulties will need more prolonged instruction.

Sound Blending and Segmentation

The TOD-13C: Blending and the TOD-14C: Segmenting tests measure the two most important early phonemic awareness tasks. Blending speech sounds provides the basis for learning phonics, and segmenting speech sounds provides the basis for spelling words. When teaching both blending and segmenting, begin instruction with phonemes. If a child cannot blend and segment phonemes, then start instruction with syllables, and if that is still too difficult, then start with compound words.

- If I put these sounds together, what would the word be? /t/ /o/ /p/? (top)
- If I put these syllables together, what would the word be? pen-cil
- If I put these words together, what would the word be? rain . . . coat

Initially, with a few children, it is necessary to employ visual supports with compound words until they understand the concept that words can be broken apart and then put back together again. The ultimate goal, however, is to ensure that the child can blend and segment phonemes. Incorporating graphemes is particularly beneficial for teaching blending and segmentation as it facilitates orthographic mapping (Rehfeld et al., 2022).

Rapid Reference 8.3 provides a simple sequence for teaching blending of phonemes. Rapid Reference 8.4 provides a simple sequence for teaching segmenting of phonemes.

An alternative procedure that may be more effective for younger children is segmented phonation. Segmented phonation methods teach students to convert graphemes to phonemes by segmenting the sounds ("mmm–aaa–nnn"). Connected

DON'T FORGET

TOD-13C: The test presents three tasks: blending compound words, blending syllables, and blending phonemes to make whole words. An error analysis helps to pinpoint instruction.

≡ Rapid Reference 8.3

Simple Sequence for Teaching Blending of Phonemes

- Begin the instruction with continuous consonant sounds where the sound can be prolonged (e.g., /s/, /f/, /m/). The glide into the next sound makes it easier to blend the sounds.

- Present words with two sounds, three, and then four (e.g., /m/ /e/, /f/ /a/ /t/, /s/ /a/ /n/ /d/).

- Initially, present the sounds in a continuous stream with no pauses between the phonemes (e.g., /mmmaaaattt/).

- Introduce a short interval between the sounds. Gradually increase the interval between the sounds from 1/4-second to 1-second break.

≡ *Rapid Reference 8.4*

Simple Sequence for Teaching Segmenting of Phonemes

- Start the instruction with stop consonant sounds that are said with a puff of air (e.g., /b/, /d/, /t/). The break after the sound makes it easier to segment the sounds.
- Say the word and move the blocks: Place two (or three) blocks or chips on the table and push each block forward for each sound in the word (e.g., /d//o//g/; "dog").
- Present words with two sounds, three, and then four (e.g., be, bed, best).
- Students may also clap or tap on a table to count the number of sounds in a word.

phonation techniques teach students to convert graphemes to phonemes by holding continuant sounds ("mmmaaannn") without breaking the speech stream. Some evidence suggests that, for beginning instruction, connected phonation techniques are more effective than segmented phonation methods (Gonzalez-Frey & Ehri, 2021). In teaching blending, one would continue to present the sounds in a continuous stream rather than breaking apart the sounds.

Phonemic Manipulation

The TOD-4C Phonological Manipulation test consists of two measures: Subtest 1: Substitution and Subtest 2: Deletion. These subtests measure the abilities to substitute sounds in words and delete sounds from words to form new words. Proficient reading and spelling require the ability to combine and manipulate phonemes quickly and with ease (Kilpatrick, 2015). These types of tasks involve moving or rearranging the phonemes within a word. They are more difficult than blending and segmenting as they also involve working memory and require a more detailed analysis of words (Kilpatrick, 2015). The tasks require holding a word in memory and then altering the word in some way. Rapid Reference 8.5 provides several examples of phonemic manipulation tasks.

≡ *Rapid Reference 8.5*

Examples of Phonemic Manipulation Tasks

- Deletion: Say *cart* without /t/.
- Addition: Say *at* with /k/ at the front.
- Substitution:
  - → Initial: Change the /s/ in sun to /f/.
  - → Final: Change the /t/ in cat to /b/.
  - → Medial: Change the /i/ in hit to /a/.
- Reversal: What is the new word, if you say the sounds in the word *nap* backward?

DON'T FORGET

TOD-4C Phonological Manipulation: Substitution requires the examinee to change a word, syllable, or phoneme to create a new word. The Deletion subtest requires the examinee to remove a word, syllable, or phoneme to make a new word. Both subtests present tasks that follow a developmental sequence. An error analysis provides information on an examinee's developmental stage and helps guide instruction. Rapid Reference 8.6 lists examples of a few programs that provide a sequence for teaching phonemic awareness.

CAUTION

Research suggests that it is important to introduce graphemes (letters) into instruction as early as possible.

DON'T FORGET

The alphabetic principle is the basic understanding that spoken language is made up of speech sounds (phonemes) that can be represented by a letter or letter group (graphemes).

BASIC READING SKILLS

Once students have a clear concept of speech sounds (phonemes), teach them how letters and letter combinations represent these sounds. The basic understanding that alphabetic letters represent speech sounds and how speech sounds are represented in print is referred to as the alphabetic principle. Moats (2020) suggested that speech sounds can be described as the "parking spots" for the letters and letter groups (graphemes) that the sounds represent. Conversely, one could say that graphemes are the parking spots for phonemes. The TOD-E contains two tests of basic reading skills: TOD-4E Sounds and Pseudowords and TOD-9E Letter and Sound Knowledge.

The TOD-4E Sounds and Pseudowords has three sections designed to measure the examinee's developmental knowledge of sound-letter correspondences. First, the examinee identifies a picture that starts with the sound the evaluator says; next, the examinee produces the sound for a letter; and, finally, the examinee reads aloud phonically regular nonsense words.

TOD-9E Letter and Sound Knowledge measures phoneme–grapheme knowledge by asking the examinee to point to or say the letter or letters that represent the first, last, or middle sounds in words that the examiner presents orally. Do examinees only know initial sounds? Or do they struggle with final or medial sounds? This type of information informs targeted instruction.

≋ Rapid Reference 8.6

Examples of Instructional Programs for Enhancing Phonemic Awareness

Road to the Code (Blachman et al., 2000)

Equipped for Reading Success (Kilpatrick, 2016)

Heggerty Phonemic Awareness Curriculum (https://heggerty.org/programs/phonemic-awareness/)

The TOD-C contains two tests of basic reading skills: TOD-7C Pseudoword Reading and TOD-11C Irregular Word Reading. Pseudoword Reading measures the ability to use phonics to pronounce nonsense words. Irregular Word Reading requires the examinee to recognize words that have an element that cannot be read using phonics, such as pronouncing the sound for the "ai" in the word *said*.

Phonics and Orthographic Mapping

The starting point in learning to read and spell is first learning a few letters and their sounds and then forming the connections between the phonemes (sounds) and the graphemes (the letters or letter groups that represent the sounds). This process is referred to as orthographic mapping as it requires mapping the speech sounds to the print and then blending the sounds together to read a word. The TOD-21C: Symbol to Sound Learning Test was designed to mimic this initial process of learning to read. It requires learning the sounds for symbols and then blending the sounds together to form words.

Developing mapping skills involves using both phonic decoding (applying phonics to pronounce unfamiliar words) and orthographic mapping. This process of assigning individual speech sounds to the letters that represent those sounds bonds the spelling, pronunciation, and meaning of a specific word in memory and explains how children learn to read sight words (Ehri, 2022). Kilpatrick (2015) explained that orthographic mapping is ". . . the process readers use to store written words for immediate, effortless retrieval. It is the means by which readers turn unfamiliar written words into familiar, instantaneously accessible sight words" (p. 81). Figure 8.1, adapted from Mather and Wendling (2024), illustrates the relationship between these two strategies.

Provision of a comprehensive phonics program provides children with the foundational skills they need to learn sight words (Ehri, 2022). Once they know a

DON'T FORGET

Tests provide much more than scores. The examinee's responses, especially the errors, are keys to planning an appropriate place to begin instruction.

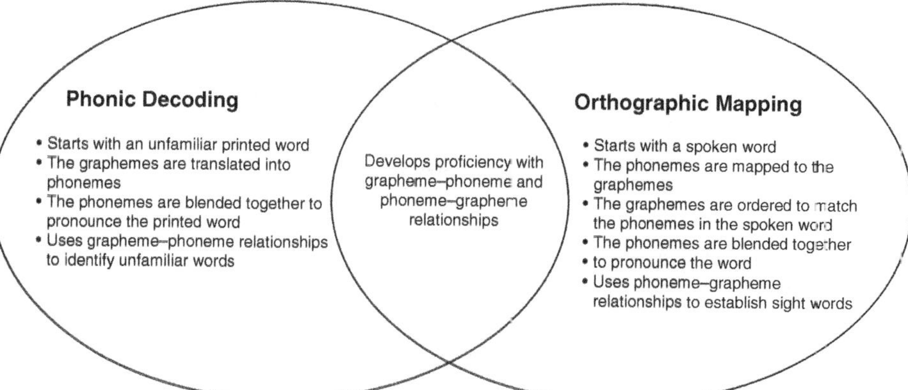

Figure 8.1   The Relationship Between Phonic Decoding and Orthographic Mapping

small set of grapheme–phoneme relationships (e.g., a, m, s, p, f, o, t), they can begin to read and spell words (e.g., mat, mop, pot).

The instructor should:

- Teach phoneme–grapheme relationships guided by a scope and sequence chart. It may prove helpful to use picture mnemonics (e.g., the letter "s" represented as a snake).
- Teach how to segment spoken words into phonemes.
- Teach how to accurately sound out graphemes and then blend the sounds together. Begin the instruction with vowel-consonant (VC-am, at) and then CVC words (e.g., bit, ham, ten).

Snow and Juel (2005) noted that a wide range of studies support the conclusion that attention to small units of language in early reading instruction is helpful for all, harmful to none, and crucial for some. This type of explicit instruction is crucial for individuals with dyslexia.

DON'T FORGET

Teach a small set of phoneme–grapheme relationships, such as m, a, s, p, f, o, t, and segmentation and blending of these sounds in words. Then read and write simple VC and CVC words using these letters (e.g., am, at, mat, pot, mop) (Ehri, 2022).

Because many individuals with dyslexia have difficulty forming orthographic images, they are often particularly slow to develop sight vocabulary. Willows and Terepocki (1993) explained: "When a reader who has a limited sight word vocabulary is asked which word looks right, the response is likely to be, 'Words never *look right* to me'" (p. 35).

Teaching Orthographic Mapping

The process of teaching orthographic mapping is often done using chips or tiles and word boxes. Interventions using word–sound boxes are highly effective for improving phonemic awareness, phoneme–grapheme relationships, and spelling (Aspiranti et al., 2024; Ross & Joseph, 2019). Rapid Reference 8.7 describes a simple procedure adapted from Elkonin (1973).

≡ Rapid Reference 8.7

Adapted Elkonin Procedure

1. Show the child a simple picture of the word.
2. Place a rectangle for the word under the drawing divided into the number of squares equal to the number of phonemes.
3. Have the child say the word slowly and push a chip forward into the square for each sound.
4. Next, color-code the chips to differentiate between vowel and consonant sounds (e.g., red chips for vowels and blue chips for consonants).
5. Once the above steps are mastered, have the child use letter tiles to push into the squares.

In her book, *Phonics and Spelling Through Phoneme–Grapheme Mapping,* Grace (2022) provides a more detailed procedure for teaching phoneme–grapheme mapping. The teacher begins with regular words where the number of phonemes equals the number of graphemes, then introduces blends, consonant digraphs, words with silent letters, and finally vowel digraphs. The rules for mapping include:

- Vowel and consonant digraphs go in one box with an additional box drawn around the digraph.
- Consonant blends go in separate boxes with a circle drawn around each individual blend.
- The letter *x* goes on the line between the two boxes because it makes two sounds.
- CVCe words: the last consonant and small *e* go in one box with an arrow pointing to the long vowel.
- Double consonants go in one box.

Figure 8.2 illustrates these rules for orthographic mapping.

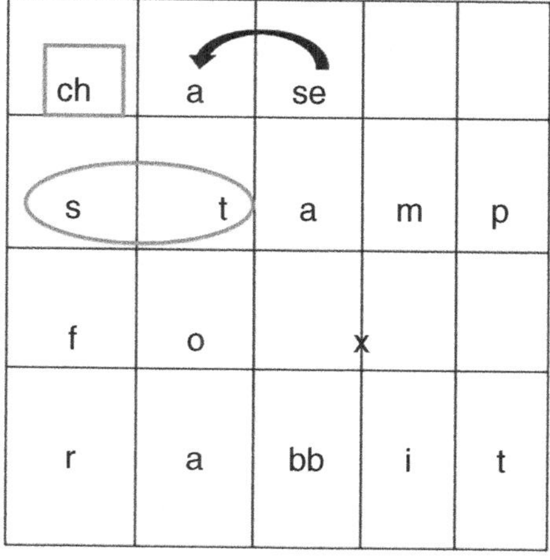

Figure 8.2   Rules for Orthographic Mapping

Decodable Books. As students learn the rules of phonics, they can practice these newly acquired skills by reading decodable books. Decodable books help students learn to accurately pronounce words by applying phonics. These books systematically introduce new sounds in accordance with a careful review of previously learned sounds. All exceptions or irregular words are introduced with considerable review. Rapid Reference 8.8, adapted from Mather and Wendling (2024), provides examples of sources for and brief descriptions of decodable books. In addition, textproject.org includes free decodable and other books for K–1, grades 2–5, middle school, and high school.

≡ *Rapid Reference 8.8*

Examples of Sources for Decodable Books

Beanstalk Books: Beanstalk Books has over 400 titles of decodable books for students in PreK–2nd grade. The Letters & Sounds Decodable Readers are 100% decodable, and each story has been written with a strictly controlled text. Children are only exposed to words and text based on their knowledge of letter-sound correspondences. Available at www.beanstalkbooks.com.

Bob Books: Bob Books offers decodable texts and practice workbooks for emerging to advanced beginner readers. Uses word families and compound words. Emergent readers begin with text that uses only the letters M, A, T, and S and then move toward long vowels. Available at www.scholastic.com and most major bookstores.

Developing Decoders: Developing Decoders is a series of decodable stories designed to help beginning or struggling readers acquire phonics skills. Each book contains fifteen stories that focus on a specific phonics pattern. Available at www.developingdecoders.com and www.amazon.com.

Dog on a Log Decodable Books and Chapter Books: These books start with fun, easy activities for phonological awareness. The first decodable book has six letters and two sight words. The first chapter book has 260 words. By Step 10, books include over 8,000 words. Available at Amazon and major online booksellers. Free printable Parent and Teacher Guides, board games, D'Nealian Letter Tracing Cards, and letter/sound cards are available at www.dogonalogbooks.com.

Express Readers: These decodable books are designed for students in PreK–3rd grade. The stories are engaging and humorous. They include "slow down sounds" that are tricky or being practiced for the first time and sticky words that are high-frequency or irregular words. The website allows the user to download and print some of the books and to flip through the ones in color. Available at www.expressreaders.org.

Flyleaf Publishing: Flyleaf's decodable books provide beginning and struggling readers with opportunities to apply their phonics knowledge in meaningful, colorful books. Their decodable books stress both foundational skills and reading comprehension. Available at www.flyleafpublishing.com.

High Noon Books: High Noon Books offers a large variety of decodable books, including the "Sound Out Chapter Books Kit" and "Phonetic Fiction." These series can be used for both adult and adolescent struggling readers. Available at www.highnoonbooks.com.

J and J Language Readers: A set of 36 decodable books for beginner, intermediate, and advanced students. Content advances to spark interest from young readers at the lower levels to older readers at higher levels. Available at www.amazon.com.

Just Right Reader: Just Right Reader offers an array of research-based, phonics-aligned texts designed to support early literacy development (pre-emergent to second grade). These engaging books follow a structured scope and sequence, allowing students to practice specific phonics skills in context. Ideal for classroom and home use, they help build confident, independent readers by providing meaningful repetition, controlled vocabulary, and diverse, inclusive storylines that reflect students' lives and interests. Books are available in both English and Spanish. Available at www.justrightreader.com.

Merrill Reading Program: This catalog of decodable books is designed for children in first through third grade and may be used to support any phonics program. Each book covers specific phonic skills and provides high-frequency word practice. Available at www.mheducation.com.

Open Court Reading: Open Court Reading offers multiple series of decodable books that are separated by grade level. Available at www.mheducation.com. Free resources are available at www.opencourtresources.com/teaching/OCRunits/decodable_books/decodables.html.

Pat & Pals Decodable Graphic Novels: Pat & Pals Decodable Graphic Novel series combine the excitement of graphic novels with research grounded in the Science of Reading to support phonics and decoding development. A laugh-out-loud series with mature, high-interest content that is accessible for beginning and striving older readers, such as those with dyslexia. The series was created by Sue Marasciulo, a retired special education teacher certified in Wilson Reading. Visit suemarasciulo.com for info about her Discounted Price List.

Pioneer Valley Books: Pioneer Valley Books offers high-quality decodable books that support early reading through systematic phonics instruction. Their Phonics Storybooks and MyCodables series are aligned with the Science of Reading and follow a clear scope and sequence. The texts feature diverse characters and relatable stories to motivate young readers. The books build decoding skills and confidence by reinforcing phonics patterns in meaningful contexts and are ideal for both classroom and home use. Available at www.pioneervalleybooks.com.

PLD (Promoting Literacy Development): PLD's range of decodable reading books align with PLD's Structured Synthetic Phonics (SSP) sequence. The type of words, word count, and amount of high-frequency words gradually become more complex as more phonic concepts are introduced. Set 1 starts with VC and CVC words with no high-frequency words. Gradually, as new phonic concepts are introduced, length progressively increases. The first 11 books introduce approximately a quarter of the alphabet sounds. Available at www.pld-literacy.com.

Power Readers and Supercharged Readers: Power Readers has 28 related decodable stories with recurring characters and includes activity pages aligned with the story and the phonics concepts presented. The stories begin with simple, one-syllable short vowel words (sat) and gradually progress to simple, two-syllable words (rabbit, ringing). Supercharged Readers builds upon the skills that readers gain from the Power Readers series and presents 37 decodable chapter books. Available at www.voyagersopris.com.

Reading A–Z: A yearly membership includes access to over 1,500 decodable texts in addition to supplemental materials, including instructions, printable and projectable resources, lesson plans, and teaching tools. Available at www.readinga-z.com.

Reading Universe: Reading Universe offers a collection of 80+ free decodable texts. Texts are clearly organized and presented based on the phonics skill being taught. Additional resources, such as interactive phoneme cards and a Word Recognition Continuum scope and sequence chart, are available to guide and enrich instruction. Available at www.readinguniverse.org.

Simple Words Books: This series of engaging books is written for upper elementary and more advanced readers. There are stand-alone books, as well as series that follow the same characters. The website provides additional resources for parents and teachers, including free webinars. Available at: www.simplewordsbooks.com.

(continued)

SPELD SA: SPELD SA Phonic Books follow a structured synthetic phonics approach. The books support the learning of letter-sounds and blending in a sequential order, helping students to develop decoding skills. A few high-frequency words are taught before reading each book. Several book sets are available at no cost and may be downloaded as a pdf or a powerpoint. Available at www.speldsa.org.au.

S.P.I.R.E.® Decodable Readers: This library contains 120 decodable readers that cover a wide range of topics in science, social studies, and literature. The texts provide practice for every concept, allowing students to apply new phonics skills to connected text. The texts include a variety of genres, including biographies, poetry, Greek myths, and science and social studies articles. Available at www.epslearning.com.

Whole Phonics™: This series contains stories that are of high interest to beginning readers. The stories follow a systematic approach to teaching phonics. High-frequency words are introduced carefully. The program includes accompanying workbooks, games, and other teaching tools. Available at www.whole-phonics.com.

Wright Skills Decodable Books: This series offers comprehensive phonemic awareness, phonics, and word study resources for reading instruction. Available at www.mheducation.com.

Youkan Decodable Books: These funny, engaging, and whimsical books are designed for early elementary children. Each series has multiple stories with colorful illustrations on each page. The series follows a structured, sequential phonics scope and sequence, and there is a chart included at the beginning of each story to help identify the sounds and concepts needed to be able to decode the story with independence. Available at www.youkanpublishing.com.

Many of the programs for teaching basic reading skills are based on the principles and sequence of Orton-Gillingham (OG) instruction (Gillingham & Stillman, 1956; Orton-Gillingham Academy, 2020). Rapid Reference 8.9 reviews the main steps in the sequence of OG instruction. Rapid Reference 8.10 provides examples of commercially available programs for teaching basic skills.

≡ Rapid Reference 8.9

Overview of the OG Instructional Sequence

1. The student is shown a letter and told its name and repeats the name.

2. The teacher demonstrates how to form the letter, and the child traces over the model. The child then copies the letter and writes the letter from memory.

3. Each phonic unit is present on individual cards with consonant letters on white cards and vowel letters on salmon-colored cards. The sound is introduced with a key word. The student repeats the key word before providing the sound (e.g., a. . .apple. . ./æ/).

4. The letter sounds are taught in groups as rapidly as they can be learned. The first letters are: a (short sound/æ/as in "cat"), b, f, h, j, k, m, p, t.

5. After the names and sounds of letters are learned, blending is introduced. The teacher presents a consonant, vowel, and consonant, and the student provides the sounds rapidly until the student can produce the whole word.

6. The teacher pronounces a word slowly and separates the sounds. The teacher then asks the child to: repeat the word, name the letters, write the word while naming each letter, and then read back the word.

7. Once mastery is assured, additional phoneme–grapheme correspondences are introduced. The manual provides the following sequence: g (go), o, initial r and l, n, th (this), u, ch, e, s, sh, d, w, wh, y, v, z.

8. Consonant blends are introduced and then the following phoneme–grapheme correspondences: qu, x, y, ph, s, and z.

9. The long sounds of all vowels are introduced and the vowel consonant –e spelling pattern (e.g., a–e, safe).

10. The student practices reading material that has a controlled vocabulary (decodable text) to practice this alphabetic approach to words.

≡ *Rapid Reference 8.10*

Examples of Instructional Programs for Enhancing Basic Reading Skills

Fundations: *Wilson Fundations®* is a structured literacy classroom program for grades K–3 that provides foundational instruction in reading. Based on the *Wilson Reading System®* *(WRS)*, *Fundations* is explicit, systematic, cumulative, interactive, and data driven. Skills are presented across four levels: K, 1, 2, and 3, with a Pre-K Activity Set also available. *Fundations* Ready to Rise® is a summer or early fall acceleration program that helps teachers instruct rising first and second graders. *Fundations* focuses extensively on phonemic awareness, decoding, spelling, and handwriting, using an integrated approach. Fundations® K–5 is an expansion of the Fundations® K–3 program. It directly extends Wilson's Structured Literacy framework through fourth and fifth grades, providing a focus on advanced and essential literacy skills. In addition, FUN HUB® is an online extension of *Fundations* that provides a digital platform for both teachers and administrators that supports literacy instruction. Available from Wilson Language Training (www.wilsonlanguage.com).

Phonic Reading Lessons: Skills, Phonic Reading Lessons: Practice: This program is appropriate for all ages of individuals who need direct and explicit phonics instruction. The Skills book teaches short vowels, CVC words, CVCe and consonant blends and digraphs, r-controlled vowels, vowel digraphs, common word endings and spellings, affixes, and Latin and Greek roots. These phonics skills are then reviewed with reading text in the Practice book. Available from Academic Therapy, 800-422-7249.

Take Flight: Take Flight is an adaptation of the OG method written by the staff of the Luke Waites Center for Dyslexia and Learning Disorders of Scottish Rite for Children and published since 2006. The program was designed for use by dyslexia therapists for students with dyslexia from ages 7 and up. The two-year program is designed to be taught four days per week (60 minutes per day) or five days per week (45 minutes per day) for 230 hours of direct instruction. It is intended for one-on-one or small group instruction with no more

(continued)

than six students per group (Ring et al., 2017). Take Flight contains the five components of effective reading instruction identified by the National Reading Panel (phonemic awareness, phonics, fluency, vocabulary, and reading comprehension). Training and descriptions of additional programs (Bridges, Jet) are available from https://scottishriteforchildren.org/research-and-education/education/dyslexia-educator-center.

Wilson Reading System: The *Wilson Reading System® (WRS)* is an intensive, diagnostic, structured literacy approach for students in grades 2–12 and adults who are making insufficient progress in their current intervention or who may require intensive reading language instruction due to dyslexia. *WRS* is widely used with elementary students, adolescents, and adults who have not been successful learning how to read and write. *WRS* directly teaches English language structure at both the word and text levels using an integrated instructional approach to phonology, morphology, and orthography (internalizing the rules that govern written English). It provides extensive instruction in phonemic awareness, phonics, word automaticity, fluency, vocabulary, and comprehension. Comprehensive support and professional learning for *WRS* include *WRS* Level I and Level II Certifications that incorporate coursework and supervised practicums, including observations. Wilson Language Training also offers a Wilson® Credentialed Trainer Development Program, which includes a year-long internship, requiring an application and acceptance. Information available from Wilson Language Training (www.wilsonlanguage.com).

ONLINE INSTRUCTION AND TEACHER TRAINING

Evidence-Based Literacy Instruction

Evidence-Based Literacy Instruction (EBLI) is a comprehensive framework for both teacher training and student instruction. Grounded in research, EBLI delivers integrated, systematic, and explicit literacy instruction designed to accelerate reading, spelling, and writing acquisition for all learners, including those with dyslexia. Each instructional activity incorporates between four to eight of the following key components of literacy development: phonemic awareness, phonics, vocabulary, fluency, comprehension, handwriting, spelling, and writing. The literacy skills, concepts, and knowledge taught through EBLI's explicit methodology are immediately reinforced and applied through authentic reading and writing tasks. Available from https://eblireads.com/.

MindPlay Education

MindPlay Education's reading intervention software is appropriate for individuals of all ages. The program provides instruction based on Orton-Gillingham's structured language approach with content created by speech-language and reading experts. The reading coaches provide instruction in phonemic awareness, phonics, vocabulary, comprehension, fluency, and grammar. Students begin with an embedded Universal Screener. The screener quickly and carefully identifies each student's individual student needs. The program further provides a customized lesson plan and differentiated instruction for each student. Each student is assigned only the lessons that are required to fill in missing gaps in their overall skills. The students' interest level remains high because they quickly see improvement in their skills. The instructional software enables every learner to receive individualized instruction with explicit, systematic, and individualized formative feedback. Available from https://mindplay.com/mindplay-reading-coach/.Individual subscriptions are available from https://parents.mindplay.com/account/plans.

In addition, MindPlay offers a 3-hour course that provides an overview of dyslexia and a 40–45-hour course (i.e., the Comprehensive Reading Course) that provides comprehensive professional development for teachers and professionals who work with developing or struggling readers. Available from https://mindplay.com/academy/.

Read, Write, and Type

Designed for students ages 6–9, this program teaches phonics, spelling and keyboarding skills via an engaging game format. A student can complete the first eight lessons at no charge. There are 40 lessons designed to be done 15 minutes a day. Available from https://www.talkingfingers.com/shop/category/read-write-type-online/.

Dyslexia on Demand

Dyslexia on Demand provides high-quality, virtual dyslexia therapy and testing to students worldwide, removing barriers caused by geography or limited local resources. Their services are built on a four-pronged philosophy: individualized one-on-one therapy led exclusively by Certified Academic Language Therapists (CALTs), data-driven instruction tailored to each student's unique profile, intentional support for the social–emotional needs of every learner, and a strong focus on advocacy and education for families. Using evidence-based, structured literacy programs grounded in the science of reading, their CALTs deliver personalized, multisensory lessons that build essential language skills and foster long-lasting success. Students are formally assessed by educational diagnosticians at intake and key milestones throughout therapy, allowing measurement of progress with precision and ensuring instruction remains responsive to each learner's needs. Outcome data consistently show that Dyslexia on Demand students achieve gains in reading accuracy, fluency, comprehension, and spelling that are commensurate with the research findings of high-quality, in-person dyslexia therapy. In addition to quantitative academic growth, students develop confidence, resilience, and self-advocacy skills—empowering them to thrive in school and beyond. More information is available at: www.dyslexiaondemand.com.

STRUCTURAL ANALYSIS

Most multisyllabic English words consist of a prefix, root, and/or a suffix. Structural analysis refers to the ability to analyze a word and break it down into its main parts. Operating with chunks or word parts makes it easier to decode and encode (spell) multisyllabic words (Ehri, 2000). Once readers have mastered phoneme–grapheme correspondences, attention to word parts (prefixes, roots, and suffixes) and syllable patterns can facilitate reading and spelling development. Learning about word parts also helps one understand the meaning of the word and how the addition of affixes (prefixes and suffixes) alters a word's meaning.

As with the ability to identify phonemes, students need to be able to identify the syllables within words. An easy way to help students detect the number of syllables in a word is to say the word with your hand on your chin and count the number of chin drops (Moats, 2020). One rule of English spelling is that all syllables contain a vowel. Pronouncing a vowel in each syllable makes your mouth open and your chin drop. Rapid Reference 8.11 presents basic tips for teaching structural analysis.

≡ Rapid Reference 8.11

Tips for Teaching Structural Analysis

- Teach how to break a word into syllables.
- Teach that a rule of English spelling is that each syllable contains a vowel.
- Teach common prefixes and suffixes (affixes).
- Teach common roots and their meanings and show how words are formed using affixes and roots.

One effective commercial program for teaching students how to pronounce multisyllabic words and build academic vocabulary is REWARDS° for students in grades 4–12. There are two levels: intermediate for grades 4–6 with 25 lessons (50–60 minutes each) and secondary for grades 6–12 with 20 lessons (50–60 minutes each). REWARDS Plus provides practice decoding words in science and social studies context (https://www.voyagersopris.com/produ cts/reading/rewards/overview).

The strategy taught in REWARDS is relatively simple. The teacher writes a multisyllabic word and then circles the prefix(es), circles the suffix(es), underlines the vowel in the root word, draws scoops under the parts, and says: What part? What part? What part? What word? Figure 8.3 illustrates the marking of the word *prescription*.

Wilson Just Words° is a word-level structured language intervention program for students who need additional support learning to read and spell at grade level. *Just Words* is "just the word study" part of the intensive *Wilson Reading System* program and focuses on decoding and spelling instruction. The program is appropriate for students in grades 4–12 and adults who have mild-to-moderate gaps in their decoding and spelling proficiency but do not require intensive intervention. The program reviews the six English syllable types: sound-symbol correspondence as related to syllable patterns; reading and spelling phonetically regular and high-frequency irregular words; spelling rules; and prefixes, suffixes, and common Latin roots.

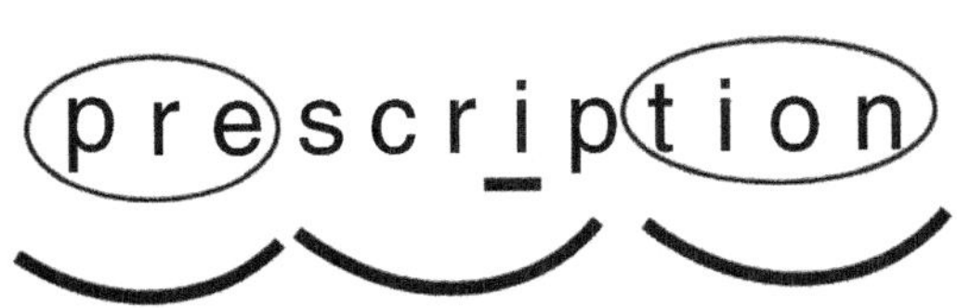

Figure 8.3   Markings for the Word "Prescription"

READING FLUENCY

The key to efficient reading is the ability to read words automatically by sight. Automaticity allows readers instant access to words in text without having to pay conscious attention to the words (Ehri, 1998). This frees the reader's working memory and fosters comprehension. Accuracy underlies comprehension and leads to fluent reading. The TOD contains several measures of reading rate and fluency. The TOD-3S includes Word or Question Reading Fluency and the TOD-C includes: TOD-12C, Oral Reading Efficiency; TOD-16C, Silent Reading Efficiency; TOD-19C, Rapid Pseudoword Reading; and TOD-20C, Rapid Irregular Word Reading. These timed measures can help identify students who read both words and text slowly.

The following short tale reminds us that we should not ask students to do something quickly if they are not yet accurate with the skill.

Day 5 of kindergarten, and after her students were screened in their abilities to name letters quickly, the classroom teacher is told that a full one-third of her class is performing below expectations as they cannot identify letters rapidly. As she struggled to explain to a young mother how her child was one who needed extra help, I witnessed the most insightful response from the mother. She replied, "How with only five days of formal schooling and his first time not home, not taking a nap, and not playing during the day can you tell he is behind? He's still adjusting to a new routine! How can this be a good thing to put children through their first week of school?" The teacher replied, "No one said it was a good thing". (Provided by Dr. Annmarie Urso, personal communication, September 5, 2025).

As children enter kindergarten, it would be appropriate to determine what letters and sounds of letters each child already knows but not to ask them to do this task quickly. Drs. Hasbrouck and Glaser (2011) remind us that "Accuracy is first, foremost, and forever the foundation of fluency."

Repeated Reading. To date, repeated reading remains the most effective intervention for improving fluency in students with reading disabilities (Stevens et al., 2017). Samuels (1979) explained that repeated reading is designed for children who read slowly, despite adequate word recognition. Stevens et al. suggested teachers should (a) provide a model of fluent reading prior to repeated reading practice and (b) establish a performance criterion of how fast the student should read. They also found that the use of easier-level text produced greater gains in accuracy, fluency, and comprehension for most students and that correction, feedback, and practice reading with peers can also enhance performance. For improving reading fluency for students with dyslexia, a listening passage preview in combination with repeated reading (reading the passage at least four times) was most effective (Lee & Yoon Yoon, 2017). Rapid Reference 8.12 reviews the steps for repeated reading, and Rapid Reference 8.13 provides examples of several instructional programs for building fluency.

CAUTION

Do not ask students to read fast if they are struggling with decoding.

DON'T FORGET

Fast mapping of print to speech is the hallmark of efficient reading (Moats, 2020).

≣ *Rapid Reference 8.12*

Steps for Repeated Reading

- Create a graph with Words per Minute on one side and the Number of Errors on the other side.
- Select a passage from 50 to 100 (or 100–200 for older students) words long from a book that is slightly above the student's reading level.
- Read the passage to the student as the student follows along with the text.
- Have the student read the same passage four to five times.
- Provide a performance goal of how fast they should read.
- Time each reading and count the number of errors.
- Provide feedback on errors between each reading.
- Record the reading time and the number of errors for each reading.
- On the graph, use two different colored pencils for recording time (blue) and errors (red), or make time a circle and errors an "X" or square. Draw lines to connect the points for four to five readings.

≣ *Rapid Reference 8.13*

Examples of Instructional Programs for Enhancing Reading Fluency

Great Leaps: Three versions of this program are available: grades K–5, grades 6–8, and grades 9–12. The program develops reading fluency through daily work (about 15 minutes) in three timed sessions that include Phonics, High-Frequency Word Phrases, and Grade-Appropriate Stories that are followed by comprehension questions. Print, online subscriptions, and online tutoring are all available. Available from greatleaps.com.

RAVE-O: RAVE-O is appropriate for students in first through fourth grade. It is delivered in half-hour sessions individually or to small groups. The program has three modules that have about 50 lessons each. RAVE-O helps develop fluency by integrating strategies in word recognition, vocabulary, morphology, and parts of speech. Available from https://www.nidolearning.com/rave-o.

Read Naturally®: Read Naturally is appropriate for beginning readers through adults. It includes both print and online instruction. Students read high-interest nonfiction stories designed to improve fluency, vocabulary, and comprehension. The program includes teacher modeling of the passage, repeated reading of the passage, and progress monitoring where the student uses graphs to track performance. Available from readnaturally.com.

Wilson Fluency® Basic: This program may be used with individuals K–Adult. It provides fluency practice at a student's instructional level. It can supplement any reading program that begins with words with short vowels. It can also be used in conjunction with the Wilson Reading System (WRS), Just Words, and/or Fundations. Available from wilsonlanguage.com.

SPELLING

Accurate spelling requires (a) phonemic awareness (segmenting the sounds and writing them in order); (b) orthographic awareness (recalling the graphemes that are used to spell the phonemes); and (c) morphological awareness (learning affixes, roots, and how spelling changes when these morphemes are added to words). Some vocabulary knowledge is needed when deciding how to spell homophones, that is, words that differ in meaning or spelling yet sound the same (e.g., rain, reign, and rein). The TOD includes several measures of spelling: TOD-2S, Letter and Word Choice; TOD-5C, Irregular Word Spelling; and TOD-15C, Regular Word Spelling. The Irregular Word Spelling test measures orthographic knowledge as the individual must recall the spelling pattern that does not conform to English spelling rules. The Regular Word Spelling test measures knowledge of common sound-symbol correspondences and the ability to sequence these sounds in the correct order.

> ### DON'T FORGET
>
> After administering the TOD-5C Irregular Word Spelling and TOD-15C Regular Word Spelling tests, analyze the errors to determine where to focus instruction. Did the examinee do well on the phonically regular words but not on the irregular words? Did the examinee struggle on both spelling tasks? Are there certain sounds or spelling patterns that were most problematic?

Spelling is very difficult for students with dyslexia. Cleary (1979) explained how Ramona was extremely puzzled by the television commercial: How do you spell relief? R-o-l-a-i-d-s

Ramona said: "Spelling was full of traps—blends and silent letters and letters that sounded one way in one word and a different way in another, and having a man stand there on television fooling children was no help" (p. 105). As Ramona observed, spelling is full of traps. Because of weaknesses in several aspects of language, learning to spell words is particularly difficult for individuals with dyslexia. Students with dyslexia tend to have weaknesses in the recall of spelling patterns and spell words the way they sound rather than the way they look (e.g., egzact for exact). Even adults with dyslexia have difficulty memorizing orthographic patterns in words (Kemp et al., 2009).

Matthew is in fifth grade. His teacher is trying to help him learn some irregular words that he always misspells. She shows Matthew the correct spelling and, when he says he's ready, she covers it up for him to write the word. Figure 8.4 provides his spellings. His spelling shows that he is not retaining a visual orthographic image of the words and so has to rely on sounds, spelling the word *once* as "wuns."

Because learning to spell words is so difficult for students like Matthew, these students often develop a negative attitude regarding both spelling books and instruction. Kevin, an eighth-grade student with dyslexia, had the following entries in his daily journal, presented in Figure 8.5.

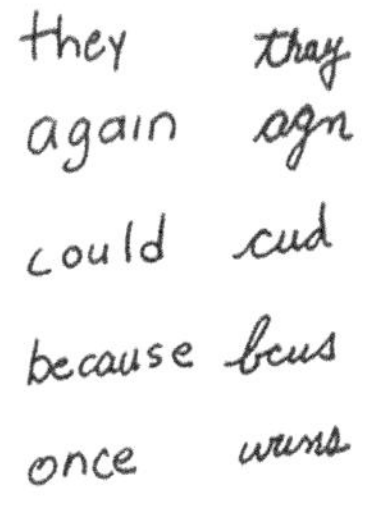

Figure 8.4   Matthew's Spellings

Today I worked on my science fair project. It is coming along nicely. I hat the Spelling Book!

The rabbet cage is almost finished. I hate the spelling Book alot more.!!

Figure 8.5   Kevin's Journal Entries about his Spelling Book

DON'T FORGET

Accurate spelling requires phonemic awareness, orthographic awareness, and morphological awareness.

Rapid Reference 8.14 reviews general principles of spelling instruction for individuals with dyslexia.

Cody is in fifth grade. Figure 8.6 shows his recent spelling test. One can see by looking at his spellings that the words are too hard for him. One also has to laugh a bit at the teacher's comment in reference to the holes on the paper: "Cody, the holes should be on the other side." Of greater concern than the holes is his difficulty with spelling. For some words, he is not even putting sounds in order, spelling the word *street* as "serthest."

≡ Rapid Reference 8.14

General Principles of Spelling Instruction for Individuals with Dyslexia

- Select words at the instructional level.
- Only count off for spelling errors on spelling tests.
- Don't ask students to write their spelling words five times each. Instead have them write words from memory.
- Mark the number of words spelled correctly, not the number wrong on spelling tests.
- Don't assign students words to spell that they can't read or don't use in their writing.
- Change the difficulty level of the words when a student is missing too many.
- Don't ask students to edit their own work. Provide students with feedback to help identify and correct any errors.
- Focus on ideas and treat spelling as part of the editing process.

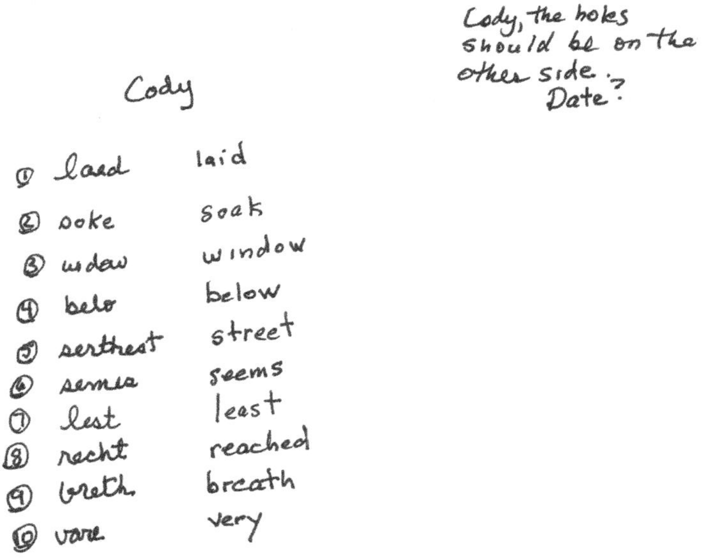

Figure 8.6 Cody's Spelling Test

Irregular words are words that contain one or more elements that do not conform to standard English spelling rules. Active processing of a word's orthography is crucial for learning irregular words (Colenbrander et al., 2022). This can be accomplished by having students spell words and discussing the irregular element(s). The University of Florida Literacy Institute describes several procedures for teaching irregular words (https:// ufli.education.ufl.edu/resources/teaching-resources/instructional-activities/irregular-and-high-frequency-words/). Rapid Reference 8.15 presents ideas for teaching spelling patterns and the spelling of irregular words.

Many of the instructional techniques for helping individuals to spell irregular words involve tracing words. Tracing words can be effective because it requires the individual to pay close attention and carefully look at each letter. Because the word is pronounced while tracing, the connections between the phonemes and graphemes are reinforced. Once the word has been traced several times, the individual covers the word and attempts to write the word from memory. A teacher can follow these steps:

- Select a word and write it on a card.
- Pronounce the word and have the individual look at and say the word.
- Have the individual pronounce the word while tracing it as many times as needed until the individual can write the word from memory.
- Have the individual write the word correctly three times from memory and then file the word in a word bank.
- Review the word periodically to ensure the individual can read and spell the word with ease.

≡ *Rapid Reference 8.15*

Teaching Spelling Patterns and Irregular Words

- Introduce a few words at a time.
- Provide frequent review.
- Provide a personal spelling list for a student or have high-frequency words posted on a word wall.
- Teach related spelling patterns in families when possible (e.g., would, could, should).
- For spelling irregular words, point out the regular parts of the word and highlight the irregular element(s). Draw a heart around the irregular element (s) and say: "This is the part you have to memorize by heart." The University of Florida Literacy Institute suggests mapping the word by putting different color blocks under the regular sounds and drawing a heart under the irregular part like this:

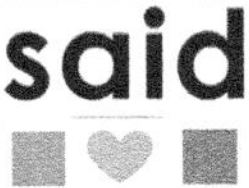

A similar procedure is referred to as cover–copy–compare (CCC). CCC has students look at the spelling of a written word, cover the word, write the word, and then compare the word to the original. The CCC strategy can be used to review learned words, as well as to learn new words. A teacher can follow these steps:

1. Select up to 10 words and write them in the left column of a piece of lined paper that has three columns.
2. Ask the individual to study the first word, cover it, write it in the adjacent column, and then compare the word for accuracy.
3. If the word is correct, then the individual moves on to the next word.
4. If the word is incorrect, then the individual erases the word in the third column, repeats the first two steps, writes the word in the third column, and checks for accuracy again. (Adapted from Skinner et al., 1997).

Another easy approach to target several irregular words at a time is to use a spelling flow list that involves daily testing of select words from the target word list. A target word is kept on the list until it is spelled correctly three days in a row and then it is put it a word box. Words are reviewed weekly, and if a word is incorrect, then it is added back to flow list for more practice. Words may be selected from a student's writing samples or a high-frequency word list.

Spelling instruction can also support structural analysis. Wong (1986) suggested drawing a spelling grid with about 6–8 columns. The first and last columns should be large enough to write a multisyllabic word. The steps include

- Write the first word in the column, pronounce the word, and discuss the meaning.

- Count and write the number of syllables in the second column.
- Write each syllable in the next columns.
- Write the word again and pronounce it.

As a final step, the individual could turn over the paper, pronouncing and writing the word syllable by syllable. Rapid Reference 8.16 lists a few commercial programs for spelling instruction that are particularly appropriate for students with dyslexia.

Of utmost importance is that teachers and parents are supportive and understanding of how difficult it is for individuals with dyslexia to spell all words correctly. Let us consider contrasting cases. Jamie has dyslexia and is in high school. His teacher's comments on his paper (Figure 8.7) reveal that she has little understanding of dyslexia and how difficult spelling can be. In contrast, see the supportive comment from Melissa's third-grade teacher on her spelling test (see Figure 8.8). Although she has dyslexia, Melissa will keep trying.

ACCOMMODATIONS

Individuals with dyslexia often require accommodations and modifications in the curriculum throughout their years in school. Accommodations adjust the demands to allow the person to perform the task (e.g., listen to rather than read a book). Modifications alter the task so that students can perform some aspect of the task (e.g., make it easier, make it shorter, or provide a different assignment). Accommodations are reasonable and possible within the environment, do not alter the fundamental requirements, and are supported by both the student and teacher.

≡ Rapid Reference 8.16

Examples of Structured Spelling Programs

CASL Handwriting and Spelling Program (Grade 1): The CASL Handwriting and Spelling Program was designed to teach young children basic sound/letter combinations and spelling patterns. The program also teaches letter formation and handwriting. Available from the author: steve.graham@asu.edu.

Zaner-Bloser Spelling Connections, Grades 1–6: Spelling Connections teaches students common spelling and syllable patterns. Each unit includes approximately 15 minutes of instruction per day supplemented with student-directed work. Teachers can follow a three- or five-day plan. Learn more at https://www.zaner-bloser.com/spelling/spelling-connections/index.

Spellography, Grades 3–5, and older students in need of spelling instruction: Spellography teaches spelling concepts to help students understand why words are spelled the way they are. It does not require memorization or weekly spelling tests but rather emphasizes the history, sound, and meaning of words. Learn more at https://www.95percent group.com/spelling/.

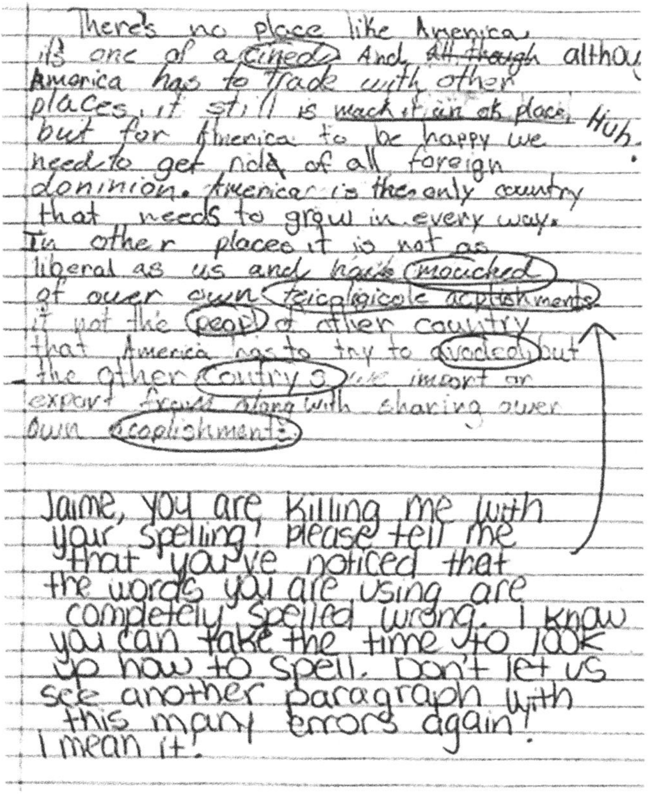

There's no place like America,
its one of a kind. And, although althou
America has to trade with other
places, it still is much it an ok place. Huh.
but for America to be happy we
need to get nold of all foreign
doninion. America is the only country
that needs to grow in every way.
In other places it is not as
liberal as us and have mouched
of ouer own reicologicole acptishments
if not the peopl of other country
that America nos to try to avodeol but
the other coutry 9 we import or
export frown along with sharing ouer
own acoplishments.

Jaime, you are killing me with
your spelling! Please tell me
that you've noticed that
the words you are using are
completely spelled wrong. I know
you can take the time to look
up how to spell. Don't let us
see another paragraph with
this many errors again!
I mean it.

Figure 8.7   Jaime's Paper

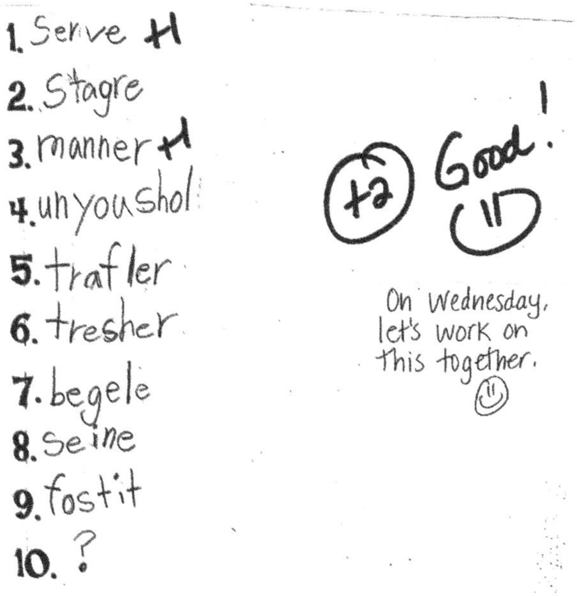

1. Serve +1
2. Stagre
3. manner +1
4. un you shol
5. trafler
6. tresher
7. begele
8. seine
9. fostit
10. ?

(+2) Good!
11

On Wednesday,
let's work on
this together.
☺

Figure 8.8   Melissa's Spelling Test

Accommodations in testing are provided so that students with dyslexia can demonstrate their knowledge of the content without the interference of their reading and spelling difficulties. Examples include extended time (the most common accommodation), untimed exams, and oral exams. One important determination is deciding how much extra time an individual needs on exams (e.g., .25, .50, or double time).

> **DON'T FORGET**
>
> The most common accommodation for individuals with dyslexia is extended time, typically 50%, although the student's performance should be monitored to ensure that this amount of time is enough or is not too much.

Dyslexia Interventions and Recommendations: A Companion Guide to the Tests of Dyslexia (TOD™) (Mather et al., 2024c), provides examples of accommodations that individuals with dyslexia often need.

In some cases, a teacher may feel that an accommodation is unfair or unnecessary. In such instances, teachers should carefully review the student's Individualized Education Program (IEP). As an example, Marcos, a fourth-grade student, has both dyslexia and dyscalculia. He has an IEP that states he can use a calculator for math. One day, given a math homework assignment, Marcos asked his teacher if he could use his calculator. The teacher replied, "Yes, if you show your work." One may wonder how it would be possible to show one's work when using a calculator, but the next day, Marcos handed in the picture in Figure 8.9 with his assignment. In presentations, Rick Lavoie (1989) would remind the audience that the word "fair" does not mean equal but that instead, everyone gets what they need.

Many students with dyslexia may benefit from the use of assistive technology. Rapid Reference 8.17, prepared by Emily Mather, provides examples of assistive technology that can benefit students with dyslexia.

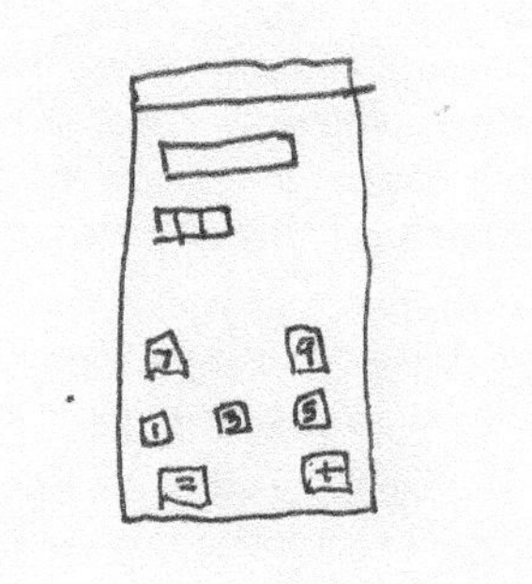

Figure 8.9   Marcos's Homework

≡ *Rapid Reference 8.17*

Examples of Assistive Technology

Audio Books Access

Learning Ally (previously named Recording for the Blind & Dyslexic): The Learning Ally Audiobook Solution® offers human-read audiobooks that provide struggling readers with access to the current school curriculum, helping them gain confidence, keep grade-level pace, and find success in the classroom. Learn more at www.learningally.org.

OverDrive Education: Overdrive Education provides a digital library of 5,000+ videos and audiobooks in addition to customized academic content to help schools support students and to support students in meeting their learning and reading goals. Learn more at www.overdrive.com.

Bookshare: Bookshare® offers ~1.2 million eBooks and audiobooks completely free of charge for schools and students in the United States with qualifying disabilities, including dyslexia. Learn more at www.bookshare.org.

Notetaking

Notability: The Notability app operates with iOS and macOS. Notability Starter offers free services for notetaking and audio recording. A subscription to Notability Plus provides users with automatic audio transcription capabilities. Learn more at www.notaility.com.

Evernote: The Evernote app operates with Microsoft Windows, macOS, Android, and iOS. It offers free, AI-powered audio transcription services. Several subscription plans are available that offer more features. Learn more at www.evernote.com.

Reading

C-Pen: C-Pen offers a lineup of scanning pens with real-time text-to-speech capabilities. The Reader 2, Exam Reader 2, and Reader 3 serve as excellent options to support reading at home and in the classroom, while the Secure Reader is an appropriate choice for workplace use. Learn more at www.cpen.com.

Read&Write: This subscription-based literacy support tool is offered by Everway (formerly Texthelp) and assists users with reading and writing tasks through features like text-to-speech, word prediction, dictionaries, proofreading and highlighting tools. It is compatible with nearly all web browsers and both Android and iPhone, and it can also be used as a browser extension for both Google Chrome and Microsoft Edge. Learn more at www.texthelp.com

Speechify: Speechify offers free text-to-speech services. A paid subscription gives users access to 200+ natural voices and 60+ different languages. Speechify is compatible with nearly all web browsers and both Android and iPhone. Learn more at www.speechify.com.

Voice Dream: This subscription-based text-to-speech service offers a wide range of features, including adjustable reading speeds, synchronized text highlighting, a personal pronunciation dictionary, and offline functionality. Learn more at www.voicedream.com.

Kurzweil 3000: Kurzweil 3000 provides text-to-speech functionality in addition to word prediction, highlighting, and audio notetaking. It is compatible with both Microsoft Windows and macOS, and browser extensions are also available for Firefox, Google Chrome, and Microsoft Edge. Learn more at www.kurzweil.edu.

NaturalReader: NaturalReader provides free text-to-speech services for both personal and commercial use. It is available as both a web-based application and desktop software, offering features like MP3 conversion, optical character recognition, and customizable reading speeds. Learn more at www.naturalreaders.com.

Writing

Grammarly: Grammarly offers free, AI-powered writing assistance that checks grammar, spelling, clarity, and punctuation across multiple platforms. Further, it provides suggestions for improving style, conciseness, and overall readability. Learn more at www.grammarly.com.

Ginger: Ginger provides access to a free AI writing assistant that checks texts for grammar, spelling, and style. Several subscriptions are available and include access to additional tools, such as a Microsoft Office add-in and text translation in 40+ languages. Learn more at www.gingersoftware.com.

Ghotit: Ghotit is a literacy software designed to support individuals with dyslexia and dysgraphia. It offers advanced spelling and grammar correction, word prediction, and text-to-speech to improve reading and writing skills. The software is compatible with Windows, Mac, iOS, and Android devices. Learn more at www.ghotit.com.

Speech-to-Text

Otter.ai: Otter.ai provides speech-to-text services in English, French, and Spanish. It offers basic (free) and paid subscriptions that meet a variety of personal and professional needs. Learn more at www.otter.ai.

Apple Dictation: Apple Dictation is a free, built-in feature available on Apple devices, including iPhone, iPad, Mac, and Apple Watch. It allows users to convert spoken words into text across various applications and in multiple languages.

Google Voice Typing: Google Voice Typing is a free speech-to-text tool built into Google Docs and Google Slides that allows users to dictate text and commands using their voice. It supports multiple languages.

Students with dyslexia do appreciate the help and support that they receive from their teachers. Peter, a sixth-grade student, wrote this apologetic note in Figure 8.10 to his teacher:

Translation: Miss O, I am sorry I called you an old goat today. You have really helped me with my writing this year.

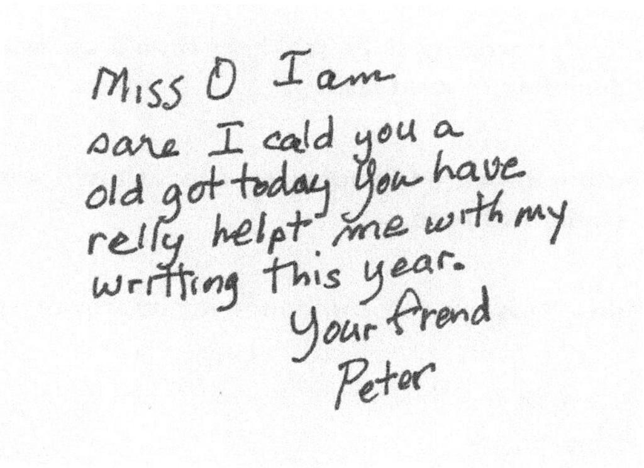

Figure 8.10   Peter's Note to his Teacher

✒ TEST YOURSELF ✒

1. **By the end of kindergarten, most students can segment words with three or four phonemes.**
   True or False?

2. **Orthographic mapping is the process by which readers acquire sight words.**
   True or False?

3. **How many phonemes do you hear in the word "fox"?**
   (a) 1
   (b) 2
   (c) 3
   (d) 4

4. **Connected phonation techniques present**
   (a) the sounds in a word with short pauses.
   (b) the sounds in a word in a continuous stream.
   (c) each sound in isolation.
   (d) the sounds with a one-second break.

5. **If a child cannot segment the phonemes in words, what is typically the easiest skill to master?**
   (a) Segmenting each sound in a multisyllabic word
   (b) Segmenting a two-syllable word into its two parts
   (c) Segmenting a compound word into its parts
   (d) Segmenting each sound in a one-syllable word

6. **When teaching children to blend sounds in words it is advisable to begin with words that have**
   (a) letters with continuant sounds.
   (b) letters with stop sounds.
   (c) short vowel sounds.
   (d) long vowel sounds.

7. **To improve student's decoding skills, teachers should ask students who are struggling with decoding to read fast.**
   True or False?

8. **When implementing Repeated Reading, teachers should select text that is difficult for the student to read.**
   True or False?

9. **Which of the following is not recommended for improving spelling?**
   (a) Have students copy their spelling words 5 times each.
   (b) Include spelling words that the student misspells when writing.
   (c) Use a spelling flow list.
   (d) Have students spell the words from memory.

10. The most common type of accommodation in testing for students with dyslexia is

(a) use of spell-check.

(b) use of audiobooks.

(c) provision of extended time.

(d) having test content read aloud.

Answers: 1. True; 2. True; 3. d; 4. b; 5. c; 6. a; 7. False; 8. False; 9. a; 10. c

REFERENCES

Archer, A. L., & Hughes, C. A. (2011). *Explicit instruction: Effective and efficient teaching.* Guilford.

Aspiranti, K. B., Reynolds, J. L., Henze, E. E., Grekov, P., & Martinez, J. C. (2024). An analysis of word/sound boxes and their effects on basic literacy skills. *Education and Treatment of Children, 47,* 271–283.

Blachman, B. A., Ball, E. W., Black, R., & Tangel, D. M. (2000). *Road to the code: A phonological awareness program for young children.* Brookes.

Catts, H. W., & Petscher, Y. A. (2022). Cumulative risk and resilience model of dyslexia. *Journal of Learning Disabilities, 55*(3), 171–184. https://doi.org/10.1177/00222194211037062

Cleary, B. (1979). *Ramona and her mother.* William Morrow.

Colenbrander, D., Kohnen, S., Beyersmann, E., Robidoux, S., Wegener, S., Arrow, T., Nation, K., & Castles, A. (2022). Teaching children to read irregular words: A comparison of three instructional methods. *Scientific Studies of Reading, 26*(6), 545–564. https://doi.org/10.1080/10888438.2022.2077653

Ehri, L. C. (1998). Grapheme-phoneme knowledge is essential for learning to read words in English. In J. L. Metsala & L. C. Ehri (Eds.), *Word recognition in beginning literacy* (pp. 3–40). Lawrence Erlbaum.

Ehri, L. C. (2000). Learning to read and learning to spell: Two sides of a coin. *Topics in Language Disorders, 20*(3), 19–36.

Ehri, L. (2022). Sight word learning supported by systematic phonics instruction. *Nomanis, 14,* 27–28.

Elkonin, D. B. (1973). U.S.S.R. In J. Downing (Ed.), *Comparative reading: Cross-national studies of behavior and processes in reading and writing* (pp. 551–579). Macmillan.

Erbeli, F., Rice, M., Xu, Y., Bishop, M. E., & Goodrich, J. M. (2024). A meta-analysis on the optimal cumulative dosage of early phonemic awareness instruction. *Scientific Studies of Reading, 28*(4), 345–370. https://doi.org/10.1080/10888438.2024.2309386

Gillingham, A., & Stillman, B. (1956). *Remedial training for children with specific disability in reading, spelling and penmanship* (5th ed.). Educators Publishing Service.

Gonzalez-Frey, S. M., & Ehri, L. C. (2021). Connected phonation is more effective than segmented phonation for teaching beginning readers to decode unfamiliar words. *Scientific Studies of Reading, 25*(3), 272–285. https://doi.org/10.1080/10888438.2020.1776290

Grace, K. (2022). *Phonics and spelling through phoneme–grapheme mapping.* Really Great Reading.

Hasbrouck, J., & Glaser, D. (2011). *Fluency: Understanding and teaching this complex skill: Training manual.* Gibson, Hasbrouck & Associates.

International Dyslexia Association. (2019). *Educator training initiatives brief.* Structured Literacy: An Introductory Guide. https://dyslexiaida.org/

Kemp, N., Parrila, R. K., & Kirby, J. R. (2009). Phonological and orthographic spelling in high-functioning adult dyslexics. *Dyslexia, 15*(2), 105–128. https://doi.org/10.1002/dys.364

Kilpatrick, D. A. (2015). *Essentials of assessing, preventing, and overcoming reading difficulties*. Wiley.

Kilpatrick, D. (2016). *Equipped for reading success: A comprehensive, step-by-step program for developing phonemic awareness and fluent word recognition*. Casey & Kirsch.

Lavoie, R. (1989). *The F.A.T. City Workshop: How difficult can this be?* PBS Video.

Lee, J., & Yoon Yoon, S. (2017). The effects of repeated reading on reading fluency for students with reading disabilities: A meta-analysis. *Journal of Learning Disabilities, 50*, 213–224. https://doi.org/10.1177/0022219415605194

Mather, N., & Wendling, B. J. (2024). *Essentials of dyslexia assessment and intervention* (2nd ed.). Wiley.

Mather, N., McCallum, R. S., Bell, S. M., & Wendling, B. J. (2024c). *Dyslexia interventions and recommendations: A companion guide to the Tests of Dyslexia (TOD™)*. Western Psychological Services.

Moats, L. (2019). Structured Literacy: Effective instruction for students with dyslexia and related reading difficulties. *Perspectives on Language and Literacy, 45*(2), 9–11.

Moats, L. C. (2020). *Speech to print: Language essentials for teachers* (3rd ed.). Brookes.

Odegard, T. N. (2020). Structured literacy is exemplified by an explicit approach to teaching. *Perspectives on Language and Literacy, 46*, 21–23.

Orton-Gillingham Academy. (2020). What is the Orton-Gillingham approach? https://www.ortonacademy.org/resources/what-is-the-orton-gillingham-approach/

Rehfeld, D. M., Kirkpatrick, M., O'Guinn, N., & Renbarger, R. (2022). A meta-analysis of phonemic awareness instruction provided to children suspected of having a reading disability. *Language, Speech, and Hearing Services in Schools, 53*(4), 1177–1201. https://doi.org/10.1044/2022_LSHSS-21-00160

Ring, J. J., Avrit, K. J., & Black, J. L. (2017). Take Flight: The evolution of an Orton Gillingham-based curriculum. *Annals of Dyslexia, 67*(3), 383–400. https://doi.org/10.1007/s11881-017-

Ross, K. M., & Joseph, L. M. (2019). Effects of word boxes on improving students' basic literacy skills: A literature review. *Preventing School Failure: Alternative Education for Children and Youth, 63*, 43–51.

Samuels, S. J. (1979). The method of repeated readings. *Reading Teacher, 32*, 403–408.

Skinner, C. H., McLaughlin, T. F., & Logan, P. (1997). Cover, copy, and compare: A self-managed academic intervention effective across skills, students, and settings. *Journal of Behavioral Education, 7*(3), 295–306. https://doi.org/10.1023/A:1022823522040

Snow, C. E., & Juel, C. (2005). Teaching children to read: What do we know about how to do it? In M. J. Snowling & C. Hulme (Eds.), *The science of reading: A handbook* (pp. 501–520). Blackwell. https://doi.org/10.1002/9780470757642.ch26

Stevens, E. A., Walker, M. A., & Vaughn, S. (2017). The effects of reading fluency interventions on the reading fluency and comprehension performance of elementary students with learning disabilities: A synthesis of the research from 2001 to 2014. *Journal of Learning Disabilities, 50*, 576–590. https://doi.org/10.1177/0022219416638028

Willows, D. M., & Terepocki, M. (1993). The relation of reversal errors to reading disabilities. In D. M. Willows, R. S. Kruk, & E. Corcos (Eds.), *Visual processes in reading and reading disabilities* (pp. 31–56). Lawrence Erlbaum.

Wong, B. Y. L. (1986). A cognitive approach to teaching spelling. *Exceptional Children, 53*(2), 169–173. https://doi.org/10.1177/001440298605300210

Nine

ILLUSTRATIVE CASE REPORTS FOR THE TOD-S AND TOD-E

The purpose of this chapter is to illustrate how three major components of the TOD can be helpful in determining risk and probability of dyslexia and the need for services to individuals who have limitations in reading, including: the direct assessments (i.e., TOD-S and TOD-E); the rating scales for Parents/Caregivers and Teachers, and the intervention guidebook. The TOD-S can be administered across the age span, from kindergarten to adulthood. The TOD-E can be administered to children in Grades K–2, whereas the TOD-C can be administered to children from Grades 1–12 and adults. The TOD-E Rating Scales are appropriate for individuals in Grades K–2, and the TOD-C Rating Scales are appropriate for individuals in Grades 1–12 and adults.

Although further documentation, such as classroom observations, other standardized tests, work samples, and rating scales, are often required to justify the implementation of accommodations or support eligibility decisions, the main purpose of these reports is to illustrate the type of information that can be obtained specifically from the TOD-S and TOD-E, supported by data from the TOD Rating Scales. Familiarity with the TOD test content and interpretive options (presented in Chapters 1 through 8 of this book) is required to fully understand the information presented here.

Each case typically includes the following indicators of performance: traditional standard scores with a population mean set to 100 with a standard deviation of 15, T-scores, percentiles, age- or grade-equivalents, the Dyslexia Risk Index (DRI) on the TOD-S, and, for the TOD-E, an additional global score—a probability index, the Early Dyslexia Diagnostic Index (EDDI). The types of scores emphasized for each report, however, differ slightly to illustrate the use of various types of scores. Chapter 5 provides detailed descriptions of how to interpret these scores. These five case reports are all actual cases, but the names, schools, and birthdates have been changed to protect confidentiality. The first three cases are based on a TOD-S administration and, due to the grade or age of the examinees, the TOD-C Rating Scales were administered. The last two cases are based on administration of the TOD-E, which includes the three TOD-S tests and the TOD-E Rating Scales.

DON'T FORGET

The TOD-S and the TOD Rating Scales can be used to screen for dyslexia, and when used with the TOD-E, increase the accuracy of the diagnosis. When administering the rating scales along with the TOD-S, select either the TOD-E or the TOD-C Rating Scale based on the examinee's age or grade. TOD-E Rating Scales are appropriate for Grades K–2, and the TOD-C Rating Scales are appropriate for Grades 1–12 and adults.

1. TOD-S and TOD-C Parent/Caregiver and Teacher Rating Scales: Aliza, a nine-year-old 3rd grade female student referred for dyslexia screening.
2. TOD-S and TOD-C Parent/Caregiver and Self-Rating Scales: Emma, a 10-year-old 5th grade female student with a family history of dyslexia and extensive tutoring.
3. TOD-S and TOD-C Self-Rating Scale: Drew, a 42-year-old male, self-referred for dyslexia screening because he has long suspected that he has dyslexia.
4. TOD-S, TOD-E, TOD-E Parent/Caregiver Rating Scale: Tessa, a six-year-old female kindergarten student referred by her parents for dyslexia assessment because of poor performance on her school's universal reading screeners.
5. TOD-S, TOD-E, TOD-E Parent/Caregiver Rating Scale: Jesse, a seven-year-old male first-grade student with ADHD referred by his mother due to extreme difficulty acquiring beginning reading skills.

CASE 1: CONFIDENTIAL PSYCHOEDUCATIONAL REPORT

Name: Aliza McGhee	School: Wildwood Elementary
Date of Birth: 03/03	
Sex: Female	Grade: 3
Date of Testing: 03/08	Age: 9 years, 0 months

REASON FOR REFERRAL AND BACKGROUND INFORMATION

Referral Question

Aliza was referred for a dyslexia screening by her father at the suggestion of her teacher. She attends a small independent school. Most of her instruction is provided by a single teacher, and her class size is small (eight students). Her teacher noted that Aliza's spelling is weak, which negatively affects her written expression.

Family and Social History

Aliza is an only child. Her parents divorced about two years ago; they are both healthcare professionals and amiably co-parent. Both were supportive of Aliza's being screened for dyslexia. There is no known family history of dyslexia, but there is a history of attention-deficit/hyperactivity disorder (ADHD) on both sides of the family. Aliza spends approximately equal time with both parents, who live within a couple of miles of each other. She has her own room in each home. Neither parent has remarried, and there are no other children in either home. Aliza is said to get along "pretty well" with her classmates, who are also her friends and playmates. She participates in Taekwondo, piano, and voice lessons outside of school. She enjoys reading graphic novels, drawing, and doing crafts.

Developmental and Medical History

Aliza is in good health, and her birth history was unremarkable. She reportedly met developmental milestones within typical age expectations. Her last physical exam was at the beginning of grade 2. Results were normal as were results of vision and hearing screenings done at that time. Aliza takes no medications, has had no major accidents or illnesses, nor has she ever been hospitalized.

Educational History

Aliza has been in her current school setting since she began preschool at the age of three. Her school does not give typical grades, but her parents receive monthly narrative reports that document Aliza's progress. Her progress reports have all indicated satisfactory performance, although her teacher noted recently that Aliza seems to struggle to remember how to spell words when she writes, and she sometimes cannot read back what she has written. The curriculum is heavily experience-based and includes both crafts and gardening, which Aliza enjoys.

ASSESSMENT PROCEDURES AND INSTRUMENTS

Tests of Dyslexia Screener (TOD-S) (Digital Form)*
TOD-C Parent/Caregiver Rating Scale; TOD-C Teacher Rating Scale
Interview

*Age-based norms were used to calculate Aliza's scores on the TOD-S.

Assessment Observations and Interview

Assessment was accomplished in one session, lasting about 30 minutes. Aliza separated readily from her father. She was friendly and appropriately talkative. Her vocabulary was appropriate for her age. She appeared to put forth good effort. She shared that she likes to read (mostly graphic novels) and to do math problems but likes the activities they do at school (i.e., crafts and gardening) more. Given adequate rapport, the results are considered to be accurate and valid.

Understanding Test Scores

To understand the scores in this report, the following definitions are provided. A common type of standard score (SS) has a population mean of 100 and standard deviation of 15; this type of standard score is used in the TOD. For this type of standard score, the broad range of average extends from 90 to 110. Percentile ranks are rank scores; a student who scores at the

75th percentile performed equal to or better than 75% of the norm group and equal to or below 25% of the norm group. The TOD also provides age and/or grade equivalent scores, depending on which norms are used to generate TOD scores. The TOD Rating Scales provide another type of standard score, the "T" score, which has a mean of 50 and standard deviation of 10.

TESTS OF DYSLEXIA-SCREENER (TOD-S)

The Tests of Dyslexia are a set of nationally normed tests designed to provide screening and comprehensive assessment of dyslexia. Aliza was administered the digital version of the TOD-S, which yields a Dyslexia Risk Index (DRI). Aliza achieved a DRI standard score of 100, 50th percentile, and is in the Possible Risk range for dyslexia. This score indicates average basic reading skills.

Aliza scored in the Average range on the two tests that comprise the DRI: Letter and Word Choice (standard score of 99, 47th percentile) and Question Reading Fluency (standard score of 102, 55th percentile). She performed in the high end of the Average range on the Picture Vocabulary test, a measure of receptive vocabulary (standard score of 109, 73rd percentile). Her Picture Vocabulary performance is not significantly higher than her performance on the DRI nor on either of the tests that make it up. Figure 9.1 illustrates her scores on the TOD-S.

		Raw score						
Test number	Test name	Raw score	Ability score	Standard score	Confidence interval: 90%	%ile rank	Equivalent: Child age	Descriptive range
1S	Picture Vocabulary	22	127	109	98 - 120	73	11:0 to 11:5	Average
2S	Letter and Word Choice	23	119	99	89 - 109	47	9:0 to 9:5	Average
3Sb	Question Reading Fluency	34		102	97 - 107	55	9:6 to 9:11	Average

Score Summary

Dyslexia Risk Index (DRI)

Sum of standard scores for DRI (Letter and Word Choice + Reading Fluency)	DRI standard score: Child age	Confidence interval: 90%	%ile rank	Risk of dyslexia based on DRI*
201	100	92 - 108	50	Possible Risk

* No to Low Risk (110 and above); Possible Risk (90-109); At-Risk (89 and below).

Standard Score Comparisons of TOD-S Tests and DRI

TOD-S scores compared	Difference in standard scores	Significant difference	Percentage of sample with this difference
Picture Vocabulary vs. Dyslexia Risk Index	9	No	

Comparison between DRI and PV, as well as any other significant differences are listed. Nonsignificant differences are not included in this table.

Figure 9.1   Aliza's Scores on the TOD-S

TOD-C RATING SCALES

The TOD Rating Scale scores are reported in T-scores, which have a mean of 50 and standard deviation of 10. Scores of 59 and below are considered low to moderate risk of dyslexia. Scores between 60 and 69 indicate high risk, and scores of 70 and above indicate very high risk. Aliza's father completed the TOD-C Parent/Caregiver Rating Scale, and her teacher completed the TOD-C Teacher Rating Scale. Both raters' responses yielded scores in the average range. Aliza's father's ratings yielded a T-score of 55, 69th percentile, indicating Low to Moderate risk for dyslexia. Her teacher's ratings yielded a T-score of 49, the 46th percentile, indicating Low to Moderate risk as well. Parent responses indicated "minor difficulty" in all areas assessed except for "some difficulty" with orthographic processing, basic reading skills, and motivation for reading. In an interview, her father shared that Aliza prefers graphic novels and that he is encouraging her to read traditional chapter books in addition to the graphic novels. Her teacher's ratings yielded "minor" difficulty with most areas assessed except no difficulties with general reasoning and "some" difficulties with attention, spelling and memory. Figures 9.2 and 9.3 display the results for the TOD-C Parent/Caregiver and Teacher Rating Scales.

SUMMARY AND RECOMMENDATIONS

Aliza is a nine-year-old third grader referred for dyslexia screening primarily because of some difficulty with spelling. She attends a nontraditional school with a heavily experience-based curriculum. Results of the TOD-S tests and TOD-C Rating Scales (completed by her father

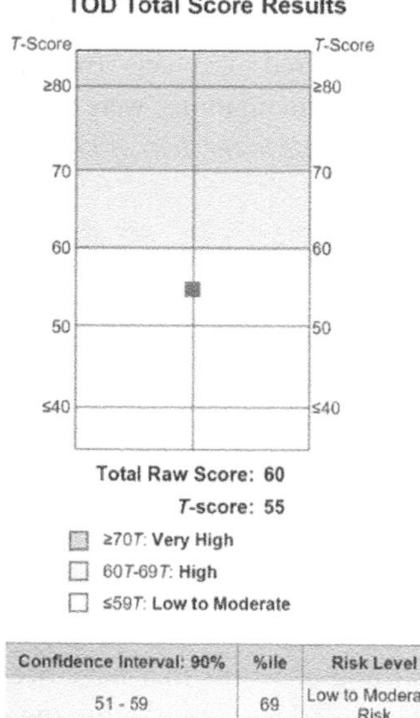

Confidence Interval: 90%	%ile	Risk Level
51 - 59	69	Low to Moderate Risk

Category	Degree of Difficulty			
Vocabulary and Reasoning	None	Minor	Some	Major
VC = Verbal Comprehension		X		
GR = General Reasoning		X		
Linguistic Risk Factors				
PP = Phonological Processing		X		
OP = Orthographic Processing			X	
RAN = Rapid Automatized Naming *				
ME = Memory		X		
Reading and Spelling				
BRS = Basic Reading Skills			X	
RF = Reading Fluency		X		
RC = Reading Comprehension		X		
SP = Spelling		X		
Contributing Factors				
MoR = Motivation (for Reading)			X	
A = Attention		X		

* **Note:** Category not measured on this form.

Figure 9.2 TOD-C Parent/Caregiver Rating Scale Results for Aliza

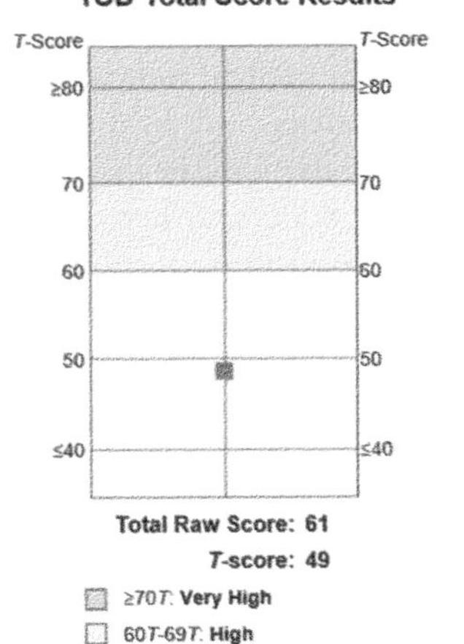

Confidence Interval: 90%	%ile	Risk Level
46 - 52	46	Low to Moderate Risk

Category	Degree of Difficulty			
Vocabulary and Reasoning	None	Minor	Some	Major
VC = Verbal Comprehension		X		
GR = General Reasoning	X			
Linguistic Risk Factors				
PP = Phonological Processing		X		
OP = Orthographic Processing		X		
RAN = Rapid Automatized Naming *				
ME = Memory			X	
Reading and Spelling				
BRS = Basic Reading Skills		X		
RF = Reading Fluency		X		
RC = Reading Comprehension	X			
SP = Spelling			X	
Contributing Factors				
MoR = Motivation (for Reading)		X		
A = Attention		X		

* **Note:** Category not measured on this form.

Figure 9.3   TOC-C Teacher Rating Scale Results for Aliza

and her teacher), when considered together, indicate low risk for dyslexia. It appears that Aliza may have some mild difficulties with spelling compared to same-age peers and grade expectations, but they do not rise to the level to be considered a Specific Learning Disorder. Still, Aliza may benefit from systematic and explicit instruction in spelling, consistent with the International Dyslexia Association's definition of Structured Literacy (https://dyslexiaida.org/what-is-structured-literacy/). The following recommendations were taken from *Dyslexia Interventions and Recommendations: A Companion Guide to the Tests of Dyslexia* (Mather et al., 2024c).

- Teach Aliza to read and spell the following 37 rimes, which can be used to make over 500 primary words (in a syllable, a rime is the ending part that begins with a vowel): *-ack, -ain, -ake, -ale, -all, -ame, -an, -ank, -ap, -ash, -at, -ate, -aw, -ay, -eat, -ell, -est, -ice, -ick, -ide, -ight, -ill, -in, -ine, -ing, -ink, -ip, -ir, -ock, -oke, -op, -or, -ore, -uck, -ug, -ump,* and *-unk.*
- Aliza may benefit from using a verbal mnemonic to master an unusual spelling pattern. For example, teach Aliza the *-ould* spelling pattern with the mnemonic "oh (*o*) you (*u*) little (*l*) dog (*d*)." For the *-ight* spelling pattern, teach her the mnemonic "I (*i*) go (*g*) home (*h*) tonight (*t*)."
- Use the Cover-Copy-Compare (CCC) strategy to help Aliza master the spelling of words. The CCC strategy can be used to reinforce learning of words that have been studied previously as well as with new words. (a) Select up to 10 words and write them in the left column of a piece of lined paper that has three columns. (b) Ask Aliza to study the first word, cover it, write it in the adjacent column, and then compare for accuracy. (c) If it is correct, move on to the next word. If it is not, repeat the first step, write the word in the third column, and check for accuracy again (Skinner et al., 1997).

DON'T FORGET

TOD Rating Scales can provide additional valuable information to help indicate whether there is a need for further, more comprehensive testing.

Finally, there is a reported history of ADHD in the family. Some indicators of memory difficulties and attention difficulties were noted in the rating scales. If limited attention becomes a more prominent concern, then further assessment for ADHD may be warranted, pending Aliza's school performance and progress. It was a pleasure to work with Aliza; I'm available for consultation, further assessment, and/or monitoring her progress as needed.

DON'T FORGET

Although the TOD-S is a screener, results can be linked to interventions and recommendations from the *Dyslexia Interventions and Recommendations: A Companion Guide to the Tests of Dyslexia*.

CASE 2: TOD-S EVALUATION

Name: Emma Boswell	
Date of Birth: 11/02	Grade: 5
Date of Testing: 08/28	Age: 10–10

Reason for Referral

Emma was referred by her parents to determine whether a comprehensive evaluation for dyslexia would be beneficial at this time. There is a strong family history of reading difficulties with her mother, father, brother, and grandfather all having had difficulty learning to read and spell.

Present Placement and Services

Currently, Emma is a 10-year-old student who will soon enter the fifth grade. She has been identified as a student with an Other Health Impairment due to a diagnosis of ADHD. She currently attends the Lincoln School, a private school that serves students with dyslexia, ADHD, and other learning disabilities. Her teachers report that Emma struggles with self-monitoring, impulsivity, word attack skills, reading comprehension strategies, multi-step computations, and focusing for long periods of time. In addition, her work pace is inconsistent. Emma now has a Service Plan through the public school system that is for students who qualify for an Individualized Education Program (IEP) but are attending a private school or are homeschooled.

Background Information

Emma was first evaluated at the age of three and met the eligibility criteria of IDEA for Speech or Language Impairment. She received one year of speech therapy. She was then re-evaluated at the age of four and was found ineligible under the Individuals with Disabilities Education Act (IDEA); therefore, her speech services were dropped. The speech-language pathologist informed her mother that Emma's difficulties were with language and not speech.

Prior to entering kindergarten in August, Emma was administered the Barton Student Screener. The results indicated that she needed specific instruction in phonological awareness and both letter names and sounds. Emma then participated in the Lincoln School's intensive *Ready to Read* program as a kindergartner. Although she attended school in her local school district for kindergarten, first, and second grade, in first grade she started receiving supplemental after-school tutoring at the Lincoln School. During these years, Emma had a comprehensive Section 504 plan that was developed for "suspected" dyslexia and included accommodations, such as allowing: (a) assignments/assessments to be answered orally, handwritten, or typed; (b) extended time as needed for all assignments as well as assessments; and (c) completion of work in a quiet area/alternate location.

In May, when Emma was in second grade, a comprehensive educational evaluation was completed at school. The results indicated average overall intelligence with low scores in phonological memory (primarily nonsense repetition), working memory, and a slow oral reading rate. Emma also had a speech and language evaluation that was requested by her local school district. The results indicated "probable" dyslexia. A strength was noted in vocabulary with weaknesses noted in working memory, hearing and repeating nonsense words, and phonological processing. The conclusion from this assessment was that Emma was ineligible under IDEA because she did not meet the criteria for special education that required a significant discrepancy (22 points) between her cognitive ability and academic achievement.

Because she was not going to receive additional support beyond her 504 plan in the public school, her parents moved Emma to Lincoln's separate day school. She has attended Lincoln for the past two years and has received one hour daily of one-to-one reading instruction using the Wilson Reading System˚. Her mother notes that fifth grade will be her final year at Lincoln because she is "doing outstanding."

Test and Procedures

Tests of Dyslexia-Screener (TOD-S)*
Record review
Parent interview
TOD-C Parent/Caregiver and TOD-C Self-Rating Scales
Analyses of writing samples

*The TOD-S was scored using grade norms.

Behavior During Testing

Emma was seen for one formal testing session (morning). She arrived early to the evaluation and was ready to work. She was attentive, responsive, and appeared to try her best. At the end of the session, Emma said to the evaluator, "I hope I don't have dyslexia. It would make it hard to read like it is for my brother." She also stated that she enjoyed the tasks and could see how they could help identify students with dyslexia. Considering that Emma was tested in a quiet, one-to-one environment and was attentive, these results are considered to be a valid assessment of her present level of skills.

TOD-C Parent/Caregiver and TOD-C Self-Rating Scales

Emma's mother completed the TOD-C Parent/Caregiver Rating Scale. She noted a significant family history of dyslexia (all family members) and reported that Emma reads slowly, lacks interest in reading, has trouble spelling words that are not spelled like they sound, and has trouble managing time and planning and completing tasks. The Rating Scale T-score of 71 indicates a Very High Risk for dyslexia with less than 2% of the population scoring in this range.

Emma also completed the TOD-C Self-Rating Scale. With the exception of no difficulty in Verbal Comprehension, she indicated some degree of difficulty in all of the other categories. The obtained T-score of 68 indicates a High Risk for dyslexia.

Tests of Dyslexia (TOD-S)

Emma was administered the three tests of the TOD-S designed to screen for dyslexia risk. Based on her overall performance, her Dyslexia Risk Index (DRI) fell in the "Possible Risk for dyslexia" range (DRI SS = 102; PR = 55th).

She performed in the Above Average range when asked to identify specific vocabulary words (Picture Vocabulary, 87th percentile). She was asked to look at four pictures and then circle the one that best depicted a word presented orally by the evaluator. Following the administration of Picture Vocabulary, she stated that her older brother would easily know the meanings of several words that she did not know.

When compared to her grade-peers, Emma performed in the Average range on a spelling task (Letter and Word Choice, 61st percentile). The evaluator orally presented a word, such as "table," and Emma was asked to circle the correct spelling from a choice of four similar options (e.g., *tabel, table, tabul, tabble*). She also performed in the Average range on a reading fluency task that was timed for three minutes (Question Reading Fluency, 50th percentile). Emma silently read questions and then circled a response from a row of four words.

Analysis of Classroom Writing Samples

Several present day and past writing samples were analyzed. A sample from third grade, before she started getting structured help, is appended to the end of this report (see Figure 9.4). Error analysis of this sample indicates a significant weakness in orthographic processing. Emma spelled words the way they sound (e.g., *sed, a nuther, bruthr, gril*). She had a few b-d reversals (*dake* for back, *dut* for but) and a backward *J*, and she misspelled several high-frequency words (e.g., they, were, said, does).

After two years of intensive intervention, her writing and spelling have significantly improved, although there are still some spelling errors typical of individuals with dyslexia. For example, in one sample, she wrote *well* for while, *butiful* for beautiful, and *hear* for

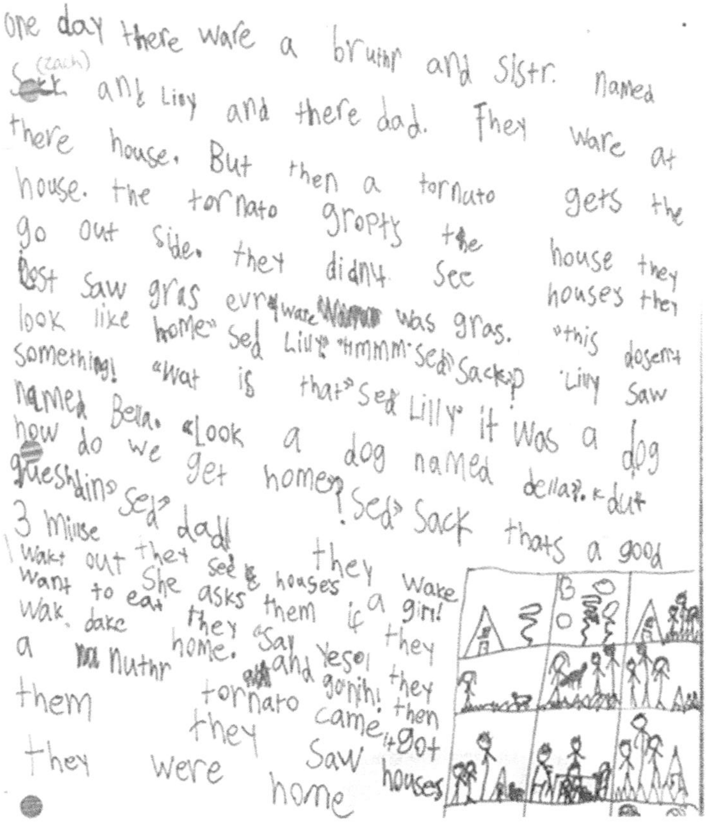

Figure 9.4 Emma's Story from Third Grade

here. In another sample, she spelled arguing as *arrging* and each other as one word: *echoter*. She wrote *park* for dark, confusing the letters *p* and *d*. Throughout these recent samples, she capitalized words that started with the letter D within sentences. This is a strategy students with dyslexia sometimes employ to help them distinguish between the letters *b* and *d*.

CONCLUSIONS

Although Emma achieved average scores on the two reading tests of the TOD-S, these findings do not rule out a diagnosis of dyslexia but instead demonstrate the positive effects of two years of systematic, intensive reading intervention. Based upon her family history, rating scale information, analysis of writing samples, results of past evaluations, and her history of intensive educational interventions, Emma does have dyslexia but is currently getting the type of help and support that she needs.

Recommendations

1. Because Emma will receive another year of intensive reading support, specific recommendations and a comprehensive evaluation are unnecessary at this point in time. At the end of this year, prior to returning to public school, it would be beneficial to provide a more comprehensive evaluation that includes the TOD-C measures of working memory, orthographic processing, nonsense and irregular word reading (untimed and timed), irregular word spelling, and reading rate.
2. If Emma returns to public school in the following school year, she will require an IEP that provides the accommodations and instructional supports that are included on her present Service Plan.

CASE 3: CONFIDENTIAL PSYCHOEDUCATIONAL REPORT

Name: Drew Childs	School: N/A
Date of Birth: 03/25	
Sex: Male	Grade: N/A
Date of Testing: 05/07	Age: 42 years

REASON FOR REFERRAL AND BACKGROUND INFORMATION

Referral Question

Mr. Childs was self-referred for a dyslexia screening. He reported that he has long suspected that he has dyslexia but has not been previously evaluated. Referral concerns included difficulty with spelling and slow reading speed. Mr. Childs reported that he dreaded reading aloud when in school and struggled to complete lengthy reading assignments.

Family History

Mr. Childs is married with no children. He is the oldest of three siblings; his parents divorced when he was about 10 years old. He is in contact with all his family. There is no known history of reading disorders in his family, but there is a family history of attention-deficit/hyperactivity disorder (ADHD). He is the first person in his immediate family to earn a college degree.

Developmental and Medical History

Mr. Childs reported typical development as a child. He currently is, reportedly, in good health. He has always been very physically active and takes no routine medications. For the past two years, he has been wearing glasses for reading. He reported no history of hearing problems. Mr. Childs is skilled at kayaking and biking and enjoys running, hiking, camping, and being outdoors generally. He has a workshop in his home and enjoys woodworking.

Educational and Employment History

Mr. Childs attended public schools for grades K–12. He reported attending summer school following second grade to improve his reading and writing skills. Nonetheless, he made adequate grades through grades K–12, and he completed a Bachelor of Arts (majoring in photography). After working as a guide on hiking and kayaking expeditions for a few years, Mr. Childs completed a Master of Science degree in sport management. He has been employed for over 10 years as director of an outdoor adventure and recreation program at a major university. Mr. Childs oversees about 20 staff/employees and a number of graduate students in this role and teaches classes in sport management and ecology. He has received awards from his field's state and national organizations and provides leadership in outdoor sports/recreation in the city where he lives.

Although Mr. Childs has had a successful career, he expressed concerns about his difficulties with reading and, particularly, spelling. He shared that when he drafts an email to send to colleagues, students, or staff, he rereads it multiple times, using the word processing features to correct spelling. Even so, he still finds that his emails contain spelling mistakes. He also noted that the difficulties with spelling made him unwilling to pursue a doctoral degree, although he was recruited to do so by his major professor. Despite these difficulties, Mr. Childs has authored travel commentaries that have been posted online and shared in magazines focused on outdoor sport and nature.

ASSESSMENT PROCEDURES AND INSTRUMENTS

Tests of Dyslexia-Screener (TOD-S) (Paper and Pencil Format)*
TOD-C Self-Rating Scale
Interview

*Age-based norms were used for the TOD-S.

Assessment Observations and Interview

Assessment was accomplished in one session, lasting about an hour. Mr. Childs was affable and appeared to put forth good effort. He was forthcoming about his difficulties with reading and spelling. Given adequate rapport, the results are considered to be accurate and valid.

Understanding Test Scores

To understand the scores in this report, the following definitions are provided. A common type of standard score (SS) has a population mean of 100 and standard deviation of 15; this type of standard score is used in the TOD. For this type of standard score, the broad range of average extends from 90 to 110. Percentile ranks are rank scores; an individual who scores at the 75th percentile performed equal to or better than 75% of the norm group and equal to or below 25% of the norm group. The TOD Rating Scales provide another type of standard score, the T-score, which has a mean of 50 and standard deviation of 10. The TOD does not provide grade and age equivalents for adults.

TESTS OF DYSLEXIA-SCREENER (TOD-S)

The Tests of Dyslexia (TOD) are a set of nationally normed tests designed to provide screening and comprehensive assessment of dyslexia. Mr. Childs was administered the paper and pencil version of the TOD-S, which yields a Dyslexia Risk Index (DRI).

Mr. Childs achieved a DRI standard score of 83, which is at the 13th percentile and in the At-Risk range for dyslexia. This score indicates limited basic reading skills and need for further assessment and gathering of additional data (e.g., educational and family history, rating scale data).

Mr. Childs scored in the Below Average range on the two tests that comprise the DRI: Letter and Word Choice, standard score of 86, 19th percentile, and Question Reading Fluency, standard score of 83, 13th percentile. In contrast, he performed in the Above Average range on the Picture Vocabulary test, a measure of receptive vocabulary. His Picture Vocabulary performance is significantly higher than his performance on the DRI and on the two tests that make it up. The difference between Mr. Childs' Picture Vocabulary and DRI scores is extremely uncommon, occurring in only 1%–5% of the standardization sample. Figure 9.5 illustrates his scores on the TOD-S.

The TOD-S Dyslexia Risk Index (DRI) estimates the risk for dyslexia. Mr. Childs' DRI fell in the Below Average range and indicates moderate to significant risk (At-Risk) for dyslexia. This low score suggests Mr. Childs has limited basic reading skills and will need further assessment. Other information, such as educational and family history and rating scale data, should also be considered.

Picture Vocabulary

Picture Vocabulary (1S), a measure of receptive vocabulary knowledge, requires selecting one out of four pictures that best illustrates words that the examiner says orally. Mr. Childs' standard score fell into the Above Average range, indicating advanced receptive vocabulary knowledge.

Letter and Word Choice

Letter and Word Choice (2S), a measure of orthographic knowledge, requires selecting the correct spelling of a word from four similar choices (e.g., *prak, park, karp, rakp*). Mr. Childs'

Score Summary								
Test number	Test name	Raw score		Standard score	Confidence interval: 90%	%ile rank	Equivalent: Adult age	Descriptive range
		Raw score	Ability score					
1S	Picture Vocabulary	28	157	112	101 - 123	79	N/A	Above Average
2S	Letter and Word Choice	22	133	87	78 - 96	19	N/A	Below Average
3Sb	Question Reading Fluency	39		82	77 - 87	12	N/A	Below Average

Dyslexia Risk Index (DRI)				
Sum of standard scores for DRI (Letter and Word Choice + Reading Fluency)	DRI standard score: Adult age	Confidence interval: 90%	%ile rank	Risk of dyslexia based on DRI*
169	83	76 - 90	13	At-Risk

* No to Low Risk (110 and above); Possible Risk (90-109); At-Risk (89 and below).

Figure 9.5   Mr. Childs' Scores on the TOD-S

standard score fell into the Below Average range, indicating weaknesses in spelling and recognizing orthographic patterns.

Question Reading Fluency

Question Reading Fluency (3Sb), a measure of reading rate and comprehension, requires reading questions silently and then selecting the correct response from among four choices. His standard score fell into the Below Average range, indicating difficulty reading and answering questions quickly.

Note. Descriptions of Mr. Child's performance on the DRI and the three tests from the TOD-S are taken directly from the TOD-S Score Report.

TOD-C SELF-RATING SCALE

TOD Rating Scale scores are reported in T-scores, which have a mean of 50 and standard deviation of 10. Scores of 59 and below are considered low to moderate risk of dyslexia. Scores between 60 and 69 indicate high risk, and scores of 70 and above indicate very high risk. Mr. Childs completed the TOD-C Self-Rating Scale. His ratings yielded a T-score of 72, 99th percentile, indicating Very High risk for dyslexia. He reported considerable difficulties in reading, spelling, and related skills.

SUMMARY AND RECOMMENDATIONS

Mr. Childs requested a screening to determine if he should pursue an evaluation for dyslexia. He is an active, healthy 42-year-old male who holds a master's degree in the area of sport management. He directs and teaches in an outdoor recreation program at a major university. Mr. Childs reported a history of struggling to learn to read, poor spelling, and slow reading. He received extra help in reading in the elementary grades. Mr. Childs' performance on the TOD-S indicates he is at-risk for dyslexia. His scores on two tests measuring word identification, spelling, orthography, and reading fluency are weak (below average), compared to above-average performance on a measure of receptive vocabulary. In addition, his responses to the TOD-C Self-Rating Scale indicated very high risk for dyslexia. These screening results indicate a high likelihood that Mr. Childs does have dyslexia, and further assessment (e.g., the TOD-Comprehensive) is recommended.

American Psychiatric Association Diagnostic and Statistical Manual, 5th edition, Text Revision (DSM-5-TR) Diagnostic Impressions:

F81.0 Specific Learning Disorder with impairment in reading (word reading accuracy, reading rate, or fluency) (provisional, pending further assessment)
F81.81 Specific Learning Disorder with impairment in written expression (spelling accuracy) (provisional, pending further assessment)

In many ways, Mr. Childs presents with a pronounced pattern of strengths and relative weaknesses often associated with average or high-ability individuals with dyslexia. Dr. Sally Shaywitz in *Overcoming Dyslexia* (S. Shaywitz & Shaywitz, 2020) aptly characterized dyslexia as a "weakness in a sea of strengths." The term dyslexia is simply an alternative way of referring to a specific learning disorder in basic reading skills or reading fluency.

As noted, screening data (TOD-S test and TOD-C Self-Rating Scale results) are consistent with Mr. Childs' reported history, indicating a strong likelihood of dyslexia, which can be further confirmed by a more comprehensive assessment. To address some on-the-job concerns related to difficulty with reading and spelling, Mr. Childs may benefit from using text to speech (e.g., audiobooks) as an alternate way to access reading material. For writing, he may benefit from ensuring he understands how to use all of the features of the word processing programs he uses (e.g., spell check, grammar check, word prediction, thesaurus). He may also benefit from using assistive technology, such as smart pens, for reading and notetaking. Further, he may consider using speech to text (dictation) software for drafting his writing. It has been a pleasure to work with Mr. Childs. I am available for consultation and/or further assessment as needed.

> **DON'T FORGET**
>
> Dyslexia occurs across the age span. The TOD-S results combined with TOD-C Self-Rating Scale data can provide evidence that a comprehensive evaluation is needed. Figure 9.6 provides a Dyslexia Risk Checklist that evaluators can use to summarize information from the TOD-S and the TOD Rating Scales to help inform decisions about the need for further assessment.

	Yes	No
1. The Dyslexia Risk Index (DRI) standard score is below 90.	☐	☐
2. The DRI score is significantly lower than the Picture Vocabulary (1S) test score.	☐	☐
3. A family history of reading difficulty exists (parent or sibling).	☐	☐
4. A family history of spelling difficulty exists (parent or sibling).	☐	☐
5. A history of early speech/language impairments exists.	☐	☐
6. A history of attentional difficulties exists.	☐	☐
7. Reading and/or spelling difficulties are reported on the Teacher Rating Scale.	☐	☐
8. The examinee has received reading interventions or accommodations in the past.	☐	☐

*High comorbidity with syslexis.

Figure 9.6   Dyslexia Risk Checklist

CASE 4: CONFIDENTIAL PSYCHOEDUCATIONAL REPORT

Name: Tessa McCall	School: Sweetgrass Elementary
Date of Birth: 07/28	
Sex: Female	Grade: Kindergarten
Dates of Testing: 04/25, 4/28	Age: 6 years, 9 months

REASON FOR REFERRAL AND BACKGROUND INFORMATION

Referral Question

Tessa was referred by her parents for a reading evaluation. Referral concerns included difficulty mastering letter sounds and sight words and trouble blending sounds into words. Her parents report that she has consistently obtained low scores on her school's universal reading screening despite receiving extra reading instruction at school.

Family History

Tessa is an only child who lives with her biological parents. Her father is an attorney, and her mother is a part-time paralegal and part-time stay-at-home mother. Both parents report that they are in good health. There is a family history of reading difficulties (paternal siblings) and attention-deficit/hyperactivity disorder (ADHD) on both sides of the family.

Developmental and Medical History

Tessa was born the result of a normal pregnancy, though labor was induced about a week early due to concerns about intrauterine development. Regardless, Tessa appeared to be healthy at birth with average length and weight. Parents described Tessa as a highly alert baby and toddler, although she walked independently somewhat late (14–15 months) and toilet trained late (3.5 years of age). Parents report she has always been sensitive to loud sounds. Tessa spoke early, though her speech was difficult to understand. She displayed mild speech articulation errors. She was observed informally by a speech-language pathologist the summer before beginning kindergarten. The speech-language pathologist indicated that her articulation errors were likely developmental in nature and did not recommend speech services at the time. At age six, Tessa is reported to have a sophisticated vocabulary but makes unusual speech errors (e.g., she says "lellow" for "yellow" and "remember" for "remember"). She sometimes omits the beginning sound in a word or transposes it with a sound later in the word. Tessa's last physical examination was during the summer before beginning kindergarten. She was reportedly in good health and passed vision and hearing screenings.

Social and Family History

Tessa has friends of similar age both at home and school and is described as kind and helpful. She likes drawing in her playroom at home. She plays well with others and on her own. She is involved in ballet and tap dancing and has taken swimming lessons and played soccer. She is in the Brownie Girl Scouts. Tessa has a large and supportive extended family that she sees regularly. Nonetheless, at home, Tessa can be resistant to change and becomes emotional easily at times when asked to do something she doesn't want to do (e.g., clean her room, practice with letters or words). She also tends to be reserved when she initially meets someone new. Despite resisting practice with letters and words, Tessa loves being read to; parents read to her nightly before bed. She has bookshelves full of books in her room and enjoys looking at them and talking about the pictures and characters.

Educational History

Tessa attended preschool at an area church with a large and established preschool program. Due to some concerns about developmental maturity, her parents made the decision to keep her with the younger children at age four so that she was in the pre-K class at age five. Tessa seemed to enjoy preschool, and no behavior problems were noted. She was, however, somewhat resistant to learning the "sight words" sent home as after-school work from her pre-K class. Tessa began kindergarten at her zoned public school at age six and is currently in the spring semester of her kindergarten year. Tessa has been receiving extra support in reading through her school's response to intervention program. The support provided focuses primarily on acquiring letter-sound knowledge. Although Tessa has made progress, reportedly, her rate of progress is not as expected for students in kindergarten. Tessa's kindergarten teacher described Tessa as kind, well-behaved, and always eager to help. She indicated that Tessa is no more active or fidgety than her peers in class, although she has to be prompted to persevere with reading-related tasks. Tessa reportedly seems to grasp mathematical concepts with relative ease.

Assessment Procedures and Instruments

Tests of Dyslexia Screener (TOD-S)* (paper and pencil format)
Tests of Dyslexia-Early (TOD-E)*
TOD-E Parent/Caregiver Rating Scale
Interviews

*Because Tessa began kindergarten at age six, meaning she is a little older than most of her kindergarten peers, grade-based norms were used to calculate her standard scores on the TOD-S and TOD-E.

Note: To illustrate the content, parts of this report, as noted, provide direct excerpts from the TOD-S and TOD-E score reports.

Assessment Observations and Interview

Assessment was accomplished in two sessions, the first one lasting about 30 minutes and the second one lasting about an hour. Tessa was dressed casually in a colorful shirt and leggings on both days of assessment. She carried a stuffed animal with her each time. She has dark wavy hair and brown eyes. Tessa was accompanied by her mother for the assessment sessions and separated readily, though she seemed shy at first. With praise and encouragement, she seemed to put forth good effort. Tessa stood while completing some of the tasks and was fidgety at times. Given adequate rapport, results are considered accurate and valid.

Understanding Test Scores

The TOD uses a common type of standard score (SS), which has a population mean of 100 and standard deviation of 15; this type of standard score is used in the TOD. The broad range of average extends from 90 to 110. Percentiles are rank scores; a student who scores at the 75th percentile performed equal to or better than 75% of the norm group and equal to or below 25% of the norm group. The TOD also provides age and grade equivalents, depending on which norms are used to generate scores. The TOD Rating Scales provide another type of standard score, the T-score, which has a mean of 50 and standard deviation of 10.

TESTS OF DYSLEXIA-SCREENER (TOD-S)

The TOD is a comprehensive battery that includes a set of nationally normed tests designed to provide both screening and a comprehensive assessment of dyslexia. Tessa was administered the paper and pencil version of the TOD-S, which yields a Dyslexia Risk Index (DRI).

Tessa achieved a DRI standard score of 86, which is at the 18th percentile and in the At-Risk range for dyslexia. This score indicates limited basic reading skills and need for further assessment and additional information (e.g., educational and family history, rating scale data). Figure 9.7 illustrates her scores on the TOD-S.

On the two tests that comprise the DRI, Tessa scored in the Average range (lower end) on Letter and Word Choice (standard score of 91, 27th percentile) and in the Below Average range on Word Reading Fluency (standard score of 88, 21st percentile). In contrast, she performed in the Well Above Average range on the Picture Vocabulary test, standard score of 120, 91st percentile, a measure of receptive vocabulary. Her Picture Vocabulary performance is significantly higher than her performance on the DRI and on each of tests that make it up; differences this large occur in only 1%–5% of the TOD-S standardization sample.

The DRI operationalizes an estimate of risk of dyslexia. Tessa's DRI score is in the Below Average range and indicates that she is At-Risk for dyslexia. Her score on the Picture Vocabulary test indicates advanced to very advanced receptive vocabulary.

Tessa scored in the lower end of the Average range on Letter and Word Choice, a measure of orthographic knowledge. This test requires selecting the correct letter or correct spelling of a word from four choices (e.g., *prak, park, karp, rakp*), indicating difficulty spelling and recognizing orthographic patterns. Tessa's score on the Word Reading Fluency test, a

		Score Summary						

Test number	Test name	Raw score		Standard score	Confidence interval: 90%	%ile rank	Equivalent: Child grade	Descriptive range
		Raw score	Ability score					
1S	Picture Vocabulary	25	119	120	110 - 130	91	2 - Spring	Well Above Average
2S	Letter and Word Choice	13	88	91	83 - 99	27	K - Fall	Average
3Sa	Word Reading Fluency	10		88	82 - 94	21	K - Fall	Below Average

Dyslexia Risk Index (DRI)				

Sum of standard scores for DRI (Letter and Word Choice + Reading Fluency)	DRI standard score: Child grade	Confidence interval: 90%	%ile rank	Risk of dyslexia based on DRI*
179	86	76 - 96	18	At-Risk

* No to Low Risk (110 and above); Possible Risk (90-109); At-Risk (89 and below).

Figure 9.7 Tessa's TOD-S Scores

measure of word reading rate, was Below Average, indicating a slow reading rate when reading single words.

TOD-E RATING SCALES

TOD-E Rating Scales standard scores are reported as T-scores, which have a mean of 50 and standard deviation of 10. Scores of 59 and below are considered low to moderate risk. Scores between 60 and 69 indicate high risk for dyslexia and scores of 70 and above indicate very high risk. Tessa's father and mother independently completed the TOD-E Parent/Caregiver Rating Scale. Mr. McCall's ratings yielded a T-score of 60, 84th percentile, indicating a High risk for dyslexia. Similarly, Ms. McCall's ratings yielded a T-score of 61, 86th percentile, indicating a High risk for dyslexia. Their ratings indicate Tessa is experiencing considerable difficulties in both reading and spelling. Tessa's performance on the TOD-S, along with results from TOD-E Parent/Caregiver Rating Scale, indicate the need for more comprehensive assessment.

TESTS OF DYSLEXIA-EARLY (TOD-E)

Because the results of the TOD-S and the TOD-E Parent/Caregiver Rating Scale both indicated Tessa is experiencing difficulties in reading and spelling and related skills and is at-risk for dyslexia, the TOD-E was administered. The TOD-E yields an Early Dyslexia Diagnostic Index (EDDI) that indicates the probability of dyslexia as well as several other composites and individual scores on key measures of linguistic processing skills that underlie acquisition of reading and spelling and on key reading and spelling measures.

TOD-E Indexes

Tessa's EDDI standard score was 80, 9th percentile, in the Below Average range (lower end), indicating a High Probability of dyslexia. Figure 9.8 presents Tessa's scores on the indexes followed by descriptions of each index and information about Tessa's performance.

Early Dyslexia Diagnostic Index (EDDI), Early Reading and Spelling Index (ERSI), and Early Linguistic Processing Index (ELPI) Standard Scores					
TOD Index	**Sum of standard scores**	**Index standard score: Child grade**	**Confidence interval: 90%**	**%ile rank**	**Descriptive range**
Early Dyslexia Diagnostic Index	697	80	77 - 83	9	Below Average
Early Reading and Spelling Index	434	82	77 - 87	12	Below Average
Early Linguistic Processing Index	263	83	79 - 87	13	Below Average

Descriptive ranges (based on standard scores): Significantly Below Average (69 and below); Well Below Average (70-79); Below Average (80-89); Average (90-109); Above Average (110-119); Well Above Average (120 and above).

Probability of dyslexia based on EDDI standard score *	High Probability of Dyslexia

*Extremely Low (120 and above), Very Low (110-119), Low to Moderate (90-109), High (80-89), Very High (70-79), Extremely High (69 and below)

Figure 9.8   Tessa's TOD-E Index Scores

Note. The descriptions of the EDDI, TOD-E Index scores, composite scores, and TOD-E test scores and information related to Tessa's performance are taken directly from the TOD-E score report.

Early Dyslexia Diagnostic Index

The TOD-E Early Dyslexia Diagnostic Index (EDDI), derived from eight tests, provides a standard score that defines the probability of dyslexia. The EDDI standard score fell into the Below Average range and indicates that the probability of dyslexia is high. This score indicates limited performance on tests of linguistic processing and early reading and spelling skills.

Early Reading and Spelling Index

The TOD-E Early Reading and Spelling Index (ERSI) is derived from five tests that measure different aspects of beginning reading and spelling, such as letter and word recognition, word or sentence reading fluency, knowledge of phonics, letter and sight word recognition, and identification of sounds within words. These five factors assess basic foundational reading skills. The ERSI is part of the Early Dyslexia Diagnostic Index (EDDI) and can also be interpreted independently when an index of reading and spelling ability is needed. The ERSI standard score fell into the Below Average range and indicates limited performance on tests of beginning reading/spelling.

Early Linguistic Processing Index

The TOD-E Early Linguistic Processing Index (ELPI) is derived from three tests that measure different aspects of basic linguistic processing skills, such as rhyming, early rapid letter naming, and segmenting skills. These three factors assess foundational linguistic processing abilities that underlie beginning reading. The ELPI is part of the EDDI and can also be interpreted independently when an index of linguistic processing risk factors is needed. The ELPI standard score fell into the Below Average range and indicates limited performance on tests of basic linguistic processing abilities.

TOD-E Composites

Figure 9.9 presents Tessa's scores on the composites from the TOD-E, followed by descriptions of each test and information about Tessa's performance.

Early Sight Word Acquisition

The Early Sight Word Acquisition composite, a measure of phoneme, grapheme, and orthographic knowledge, includes Letter and Word Choice (2S) and Letter and Sight Word Recognition (7E). The tasks in this composite require selecting the correct spelling of a word from four choices, naming specific letters, and reading high-frequency words. The standard score obtained on this composite fell into the Below Average range. This score range indicates limited orthographic knowledge.

Score Summary of TOD-E Composites					
TOD-E composite	Sum of standard scores	Composite standard score: Child grade	Confidence interval: 90%	%ile rank	Descriptive range
Early Sight Word Acquisition	178	86	79 - 93	18	Below Average
Early Phonics Knowledge	168	82	76 - 88	12	Below Average
Early Basic Reading Skills	176	86	82 - 90	18	Below Average
Early Phonological Awareness	180	87	81 - 93	19	Below Average

Descriptive ranges (based on standard scores): Significantly Below Average (69 and below); Well Below Average (70-79); Below Average (80-89); Average (90-109); Above Average (110-119); Well Above Average (120 and above).

Figure 9.9   Tessa's TOD-E Composite Scores

Early Phonics Knowledge

The Early Phonics Knowledge composite, a measure of knowledge of beginning phonics concepts, includes Sounds and Pseudowords (4E) and Letter and Sound Knowledge (9E). The tasks in this composite require naming the sounds of letters, reading phonically regular nonsense words, and identifying first, last, and middle sounds in words that are presented orally. The standard score obtained on this composite fell into the Below Average range. This score range indicates limited phoneme-grapheme knowledge.

Figure 9.10 presents Tessa's scores on the individual tests of the TOD-E, followed by descriptions of each and information about Tessa's performance.

Score Summary								
Test number	Test name	Raw score	Ability score	Standard score	Confidence interval: 90%	%ile rank	Equivalent: Child grade	Descriptive range
1S	Picture Vocabulary	25	119	120	110 - 130	91	2 - Spring	Well Above Average
2S	Letter and Word Choice	13	88	91	83 - 99	27	K - Fall	Average
3Sa	Word Reading Fluency	10		88	82 - 94	21	K - Fall	Below Average
4E	Sounds and Pseudowords	6		79	73 - 85	8	< Start grade	Well Below Average
5E	Rhyming	8		91	85 - 97	27	K - Fall	Average
6E	Early Rapid Number and Letter Naming	30		83	74 - 92	13	< Start grade	Below Average
7E	Letter and Sight Word Recognition	12		87	83 - 91	19	K - Fall	Below Average
8E	Early Segmenting	9		89	84 - 94	23	K - Fall	Below Average
9E	Letter and Sound Knowledge	15		89	84 - 94	23	K - Fall	Below Average

Descriptive ranges (based on standard scores): Significantly Below Average (69 and below); Well Below Average (70-79); Below Average (80-89); Average (90-109); Above Average (110-119); Well Above Average (120 and above).

Figure 9.10   Tessa's TOD-E Test Scores

Sounds and Pseudowords

Sounds and Pseudowords (4E), a measure of phonics knowledge, requires naming the sounds of letters and then reading phonically regular nonsense words. The standard score obtained on this test fell into the Well Below Average range. This score range indicates very limited knowledge of sound-letter (phoneme-grapheme) correspondences.

Rhyming

Rhyming (5E), a measure of phonological awareness, requires pointing to a picture that rhymes with a word and then producing a word that rhymes. The standard score obtained on this test fell into the Average range. This score range indicates average rhyming skills, an important phonological awareness ability.

Early Rapid Number and Letter Naming

Early Rapid Number and Letter Naming (6E), a measure of rapid automatized naming (RAN), requires rapidly retrieving and naming a random sequence of three numbers (*1, 2, 3*) and three letters (*A, B, C*) within one minute. The standard score obtained on this test fell into the Below Average range. This score range indicates limited rapid automatized naming ability.

Letter and Sight Word Recognition

Letter and Sight Word Acquisition (7E), a measure of early basic reading skills, requires naming specific letters and reading basic sight words. The standard score obtained on this test fell into the Below Average range. This score range indicates limited letter knowledge and early reading skills.

Early Segmenting

Early Segmenting (8E), a measure of phonological awareness, requires breaking apart compound words, syllables, and phonemes. The standard score obtained on this test fell into the Below Average range. This score range indicates limited segmenting ability, an essential skill for spelling.

SUMMARY AND RECOMMENDATIONS

Tessa's performance on the TOD-E exemplifies both the "unexpected" and "expected" aspects of dyslexia. Her receptive vocabulary (as measured by the TOD-S Picture Vocabulary test) is significantly higher than her EDDI; the difference between these scores occurred in less than 1% of the TOD-E standardization sample. Similarly, her Picture Vocabulary score is significantly higher than all of her TOD-E composite scores, with the differences occurring in less than 5% of the TOD-E sample. These differences indicate that, although Tessa has a well-developed vocabulary, her reading, spelling, and linguistic processing abilities are much weaker, as is often common in individuals with dyslexia. In contrast, Tessa's scores on the two composites that comprise the EDDI (ERSI and ELPI) are not significantly different, consistent with the notion that individuals with weaknesses in certain linguistic processing abilities are at risk for difficulties in acquiring reading and spelling skills.

American Psychiatric Association Diagnostic and Statistical Manual, 5th edition, Text Revision (DSM-5-TR) Diagnostic Impression:

F81.0 Specific Learning Disorder with impairment in reading (word reading accuracy)

Tessa presents with a pronounced pattern of strengths and relative weaknesses often associated with average or high-ability individuals with dyslexia. Assessment data (TOD-S, TOD-E Rating Scales, and TOD-E) indicate a high probability of dyslexia. Further, family history, history of speech irregularities, and need for extra support in reading are additional risk factors that support a diagnosis of dyslexia. Results should be reviewed by Tessa's teachers and the school staff to inform her educational programming. She is in need of intensive, explicit, and systematic instruction in reading and spelling, consistent with the Structured Literacy approach as described by the International Dyslexia Association: https://dyslexiaida.org/what-is-structured-literacy/. Although Tessa has made some progress in tiered intervention, results of assessment suggest she is in need of more intensive instruction.

Based on Tessa's performance on the TOD-S and TOD-E, the following instructional recommendations were selected from the *Tests of Dyslexia Interventions and Recommendations: A Companion Guide to the Tests of Dyslexia.*

1. Begin with spelling consonant-vowel-consonant (CVC) words. Have Tessa practice spelling words by first changing the beginning sound (e.g., hat, bat, sat) and then changing the ending sound (e.g., bat, bag, ban). Eventually, progress to changing the medial vowel sound (e.g., hit, hot, hut, hat).

2. Do not have Tessa attempt to learn sight words (regular or irregular words that a reader recognizes immediately without needing to use decoding strategies) through visual rote memorization. Instead, teach Tessa how to acquire sight words through the process of orthographic mapping (the process of assigning individual speech sounds [phonemes] to the letters that represent those sounds [graphemes]). Teach Tessa how to make connections between the phonemes in words and the related graphemes. Even after many exposures, Tessa may continue to use a blending strategy (i.e., merging together sounds or parts of words to create spoken words) to pronounce even simple words. Provide sufficient practice so that words can eventually be retrieved as sight words from memory.

3. Each day, introduce three or four words with regular sound–symbol correspondence. Provide daily practice until Tessa masters these words. Have Tessa write the words in isolation and in sentences. Ask if the words are similar to any other words Tessa has already learned. Discuss and practice other words that share the same phonograms (letters or letter combinations that represent a speech sound).

4. Help Tessa increase the number of words recognized by sight. Have Tessa note the associations between the most salient sounds in a word and the representative letters. Ask Tessa to sound out a word letter by letter and then to say it. After Tessa has sounded out a given word several times, the word's letter sequence will become bonded with the phonemes (individual speech sounds) in the spoken word, and its meaning becomes stored in memory. As Tessa masters an increasing number of orthographic patterns, her sight vocabulary will grow.

5. Teach Tessa phonemes (individual speech sounds) and then demonstrate how these sounds are represented by written letters. Have Tessa say the phonemes in a word and then map those sounds to their corresponding letters (graphemes, i.e., the letter or letter combination that represents a single speech sound) to spell words. Begin instruction with simple consonant-vowel-consonant (CVC) words and then progress to one-syllable words that contain consonant blends (two or three consonants that keep their identities, e.g., *st, br*).

6. Tessa will benefit from practice in orthographic mapping (the process of assigning individual speech sounds to the letters that represent those sounds). For example, say: "*Map*" and then segment (break apart) the word into its three sounds. Print the word *map* and point to each letter as you say each sound. Spend 5–10 minutes each day practicing orthographic mapping. Begin the instruction with words that have regular phoneme–grapheme correspondence.

DON'T FORGET

When an examinee is relatively older or younger than most peers in their assigned grade, use grade-based norms to generate standard scores on the TOD direct assessments. This is especially true for children in the lowest grades when literacy development is rapid.

CASE 5: PSYCHOEDUCATIONAL EVALUATION

Student: Jesse Graham	School: Sundale Elementary School
Birthdate: 09/07	Grade: 1.7
Age: 7–6	Test dates: February 15, 16
Parents: Sophia and Anthony Graham	Evaluator: Lynne E. Jaffe, Ph.D.

REASON FOR REFERRAL

Jesse was referred by his mother due to his extreme difficulty learning basic reading and spelling skills, despite obvious strengths in world knowledge and oral language. She wanted information regarding the reasons for his difficulties in addition to recommendations for effective instruction.

BACKGROUND

Developmental and Family History

Jesse was born at 38 weeks gestation, weighing 6 lb. 0 oz. His mother stated that he met all of his childhood developmental milestones, including language, on time. He's a physically active child, small for his age, and looks younger. Mr. and Mrs. Graham also have a two-year-old son, Thomas. English is the only language spoken in the home.

Due to severe behavioral difficulties and frequent emotional outbursts throughout kindergarten and first grade, Jesse was evaluated last summer by Dr. Robin Solnick, M.D., pediatric psychiatrist, and diagnosed with ADHD-Combined Presentation. After a trial of Focalin, which made Jesse highly anxious, she prescribed a low dose of Vyvanse, to which Jesse has acclimated well. Jesse attends a Taekwondo class twice a week and recently received a stripe on his belt for attention and effort. Mrs. Graham was diagnosed with ADHD as a freshman in college; Mr. Graham is not aware of any diagnosed disabilities in his family.

Educational History

Jesse attended preschool at Happy Valley Daycare and entered kindergarten at Tyndall Academy, a charter school, on his fifth birthday. He was the youngest child in his class. He had difficulty participating in group activities and tended to wander off. When presented with a task that was difficult for him, he cried, refused to attempt it, and often ran to the back of the classroom. Attentional and behavioral difficulties continued in first grade to the extent that Jesse frequently had to be removed from the classroom due to extended emotional outbursts. Because he benefitted so little from the academic instruction in first grade and appeared socially immature as well, his parents, with the approval of the school staff, decided to have him repeat first grade. To avoid the social stigma of retention, the Grahams enrolled Jesse in Sundale Elementary, their district public school.

Subsequent to his diagnosis of ADHD, with the Vyvanse and in his new school, Jesse's participation in academic work has improved. He is willing, albeit with considerable support, to tackle academic tasks even when he finds them difficult. He has made friends in his classroom and is socially appropriate on the playground during recess. Ms. Santiago, his teacher, reported that he is "wicked smart," has a surprisingly good vocabulary for a seven-year-old, and acquires mathematical concepts easily. He is fairly automatic with addition and subtraction facts and can add and subtract with multiple-digit numbers without regrouping. For reading and spelling, the class has been using the Wilson Fundations® program. The instruction has been focused on phonological awareness skills, the primary sounds of letters, and sounding out simple, phonically regular closed-syllable words. Ms. Santiago noted that Jesse is still unable to say the entire alphabet and, despite making an effort, he struggles to sound out simple words and does not remember any sight words. Sometimes, when particularly frustrated, Jesse begins to cry and is then embarrassed in front of his classmates. He no longer has temper tantrums, however, and has a place in the back of the classroom that he can go to when he feels overwhelmed.

BEHAVIORAL OBSERVATIONS

Jesse said that he likes school; his favorite part is recess and playing games with his friends. He commented that he likes his teacher and described Ms. Santiago as "super easy-going." Jesse was tested over two sessions for approximately two hours each, in a quiet room, with frequent breaks. He had taken Vyvanse about an hour and a half before each session. As an incentive for focused attention and effort, he earned play money after each test with which he could buy Pokémon cards during breaks. He had no trouble keeping track of how many more dollars he needed to buy his next card.

TESTS ADMINISTERED

Tests of Dyslexia-Early (TOD-E) (Grade norms)
TOD-E Parent/Caregiver Rating Scale

Woodcock-Johnson V (WJ V) (Grade norms)
   Oral Language Samples
   Oral Comprehension
   Picture Vocabulary
   Story Comprehension

EXPLANATION OF SCORES AND SCORE RANGES

Jesse's scores on the tests administered are reported as standard score ranges (SS) and percentile ranks (PR). The Appendix contains a score table for all of the tests administered. First-grade norms were used rather than age norms for several reasons. Jesse started kindergarten on the day he turned five. His immaturity and difficulty with attention were such that he did not benefit from the reading or writing instruction offered in kindergarten or in the previous first-grade classroom. As he is repeating first grade, it seems appropriate to monitor his progress against the children with whom he is being educated rather than those a grade ahead of him. Table 9.1 shows descriptors for the standard score and percentile rank ranges.

Note: Some of the examples of test items in this report are similar to the actual items but are fabricated to maintain confidentiality of the items.

TEST RESULTS

Oral Language

On the TOD-E, Jesse's vocabulary performance was in the Average range (Picture Vocabulary: SS 99, PR 47). His score might have been higher, but, in his haste, he missed a defining detail in an item he likely knew. One indication of his more advanced vocabulary was his use of self-talk (e.g., "carnivore means predator") before circling the appropriate picture. In order to establish a more comprehensive baseline of Jesse's oral language, and to rule out the possibility of a developmental language disorder, tests from the WJ V Oral Language cluster were administered. These tests required Jesse to name pictures, to use one sentence to describe given pictures, and to retell the details and answer questions about stories told orally. His Oral Language cluster score (SS 102, PR 55) and all four tests were well within the average range for his grade (Oral Language Samples: SS 109, PR 73; Oral Comprehension: SS 101, PR 53; Picture Vocabulary: 95, PR 37; Story Comprehension: PR 104, PR 61).

Table 9.1 Descriptors of Standard Scores and Percentile Rank Ranges

Standard Scores	Percentile Ranks	Descriptors
120 and above	>90	Well Above Average
110–119	75–90	Above Average
90–109	25–73	Average
80–89	9–23	Below Average
70–79	2–8	Well Below Average
69 and below	<2	Significantly Below Average

Phonological/Phonemic Awareness

Phonological awareness is the understanding that a stream of speech can be broken down into smaller units such as words, syllables, and sounds. These abilities include rhyming, blending sounds into words, and segmenting words into their component sounds. These skills are critical in learning to sound out words for reading and spelling and, thus, create the foundation for developing the large bank of sight words necessary for fluent reading and comprehension. On the composites, although still a weakness, Jesse's performance was the highest on the TOD-E Early Phonological Awareness, scoring in the Below Average range (SS 88, PR 21). His performance on Rhyming was in the Average range (SS 94, PR 34). He clearly understands the concept of rhyming; his errors were often due to providing nonsense words, despite reminders to use real words. Other error responses had the correct vowel sound but an incorrect final consonant, especially on final plosive sounds. For example, when asked to choose from four pictures the one that rhymed with "mop," he chose "knob" rather than "stop" and pronounced it as "nog."

Jesse's performance in segmenting was in the Below Average range (Early Segmenting: SS 88, PR 21). He segmented two- and three-syllable words into single syllables and segmented two-sound words correctly, but he broke three-sound words into onset and rime. On later informal testing, he was able to blend two sounds into a word (vowel + consonant) but could not blend three sounds (consonant, vowel, consonant) into a familiar word.

In addition to requiring knowledge of the sounds of certain letters, the Letter and Sound Knowledge test requires the examinee to recognize the location of a sound in a word (e.g., Which letter makes the first sound in the word *bank*?). Jesse demonstrated considerable difficulty with this. His performance, bordering the Well Below Average and Significantly Below Average ranges, was the same as or higher than only 2% of his grade-peers (SS 70, PR 2). He identified letters that made the initial sound in a word but could not identify any digraphs (two letters that represent one sound) or blends (a combination of two or more letters that retain individual sounds). He demonstrated considerable difficulty with final sounds and reached a ceiling before the test moved to medial sounds.

Early Phonics Skills

All three composites indicating early reading skills scores bordered the Well Below Average and Significantly Below Average range (Early Phonics Knowledge: SS 70, PR 2; Early Basic Reading Skills: SS 69, PR 2; Early Sight Word Acquisition: SS 71, PR 3), indicating notably low skills in letter-sound correspondence, word attack, and word recognition. In comparison to other students his age, only 2%–3% scored as low as or lower than Jesse in these beginning skills. Over the course of testing, when attempting to read real words, Jesse was motivated to make a serious attempt. His attempts in sounding out familiar, phonically regular two- and three-letter words were occasionally successful (e.g., it, mat), but, sometimes, he said the sounds and then blended them out of order.

On the Sounds and Pseudowords test (SS 73, PR 4), Jesse's performance was as low or lower than 96% of his grade-peers. He misidentified the location of sounds in words, including the first sound. For example, when asked which word began with the /r/ sound, he chose "car." Jesse could not read any of the pseudowords but tried to sound out each letter, consistently confusing *b/d* and sounding out the letter *g* as /n/.

In later informal testing, Jesse was not able to recite the alphabet in order but named random letters, sometimes repeating. When asked to sing (rather than say) the alphabet song, he did so up to G, then couldn't go any further. Given lowercase letter tiles, he confused b/d and misnamed j, g, p, z, l, v. He gave the correct primary sounds of most of the letters except for e, f, g, j, u, v, w. Within the tests, he frequently said "E" for upper- and lower-case C, even when asked to identify C and E and testing the limits on a repeated test. He did not correctly pronounce any consonant digraphs or blends.

Early Sight Word Acquisition

Jesse did not demonstrate any sight recognition of common words. Jesse's score on the Letter and Word Choice test is highly inflated (SS 81, PR 10). Given a letter name and a choice of four letters, Jesse identified all of the letters correctly. Asked to identify the correct spelling of a word given orally, he identified none of the "simpler" words but guessed correctly on five words that were far above his grade level and his reading ability.

On the Letter and Sight Word Recognition test (SS 73, PR 4), Jesse misnamed several letters, sounded out only two two-letter words, and recognized none as whole words. On the Word Reading Fluency test (SS 63, PR 1), when asked to choose which of four words matched a given picture, he recognized none of the words on sight. Rather, in the time allowed, he sounded out five of six three-letter words correctly. After that, he guessed.

Rapid Automatized Naming (RAN)

RAN assesses the ability to rapidly recognize and name a visual symbol. Jesse performed in the Low Average range on the test of Early Rapid Number and Letter Naming (SS 84, PR 14). When asked to name repeating series of the most common three letters and numbers, his responses were both slow and inaccurate, indicating that Jesse does not have the names of letters memorized to an automatic level and/or has difficulty with speed of retrieval. He made no errors on numbers.

Orthographic Processing

Longstanding research in reading disabilities indicates that RAN is correlated with orthographic processing. Orthographic processing is the ability to rapidly and accurately form visual images of individual letters, letter combinations, and spelling patterns in memory. When reading, a person who has these patterns set in memory recognizes words and letter patterns automatically, triggering the associated sound and facilitating the acquisition of sight words. In turn, this facilitates fluent reading and, consequently, comprehension.

The foundation for orthographic processing is phonics knowledge and the ability to blend sounds into words and segment words into sounds. After sounding out a word several times, the letter pattern is embedded in memory, forming an orthographic image. Subsequently, the word is recognized "on sight" and triggers its sound. Orthographic processing is also necessary for recognition of irregular words, i.e., words that do not follow the phonics patterns of our language, such as "the" and "some," and so cannot be sounded out.

Jesse has not developed sufficient phonics skills on which to layer orthographic processing and did not demonstrate automatic recognition of any words during the reading tests. He did

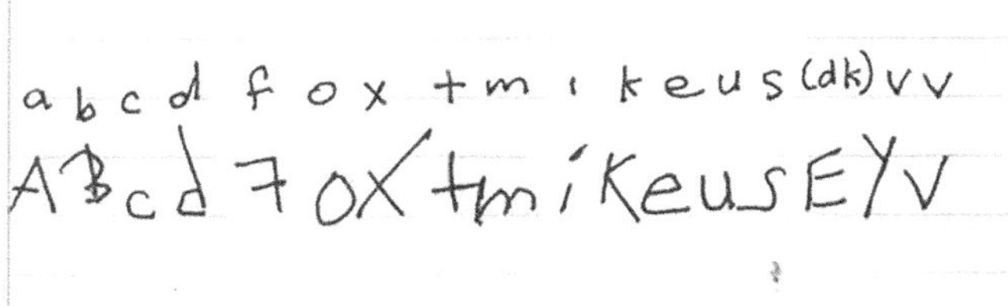

Figure 9.11   Jesse's Writing of the Alphabet

attempt to sound out words but was generally unsuccessful. To become a competent and fluent reader, Jesse must first have the names and sounds of letters embedded in memory and available for retrieval, along with the ability to blend and segment sounds.

Writing

Because Jesse was unable to say the entire alphabet and did not know the names of all of the letters, it was important to see which letters he could write. Jesse was given a choice of several types of writing paper with different types of guidelines, but he chose regular notebook paper. A graphic of his alphabet writing with the name of the letter he indicated he had written inserted above it by the evaluator, as shown in Figure 9.11. He wrote a backward F. He named each letter but called the Y "V" and did not know the name of the uppercase E. Jesse writes some of his letters and numbers from the bottom up, usually facing the correct direction.

Jesse's handwriting shows no evidence of formal instruction in any style. His pencil grasp looks functional, but most of the movement when he is writing comes from his wrist. He was not able to tap each finger to his thumb in sequence, indicating difficulty with fine-motor planning and integration.

INDEXES

The TOD-E provides indexes that represent critical constructs related to dyslexia: Early Linguistic Processing (phonological/phonemic processing and rapid automatized naming) and Early Reading and Spelling (phonics knowledge and word identification). In contrast to Jesse's age-appropriate oral language abilities, his Early Linguistic Processing Index is in the Below Average range, indicating difficulty with phonological and phonemic abilities (SS 85, PR 16) despite considerable instructional time spent on these skills in the classroom. This index score appears high considering the difficulties that Jesse demonstrated on segmenting and rapid letter naming but is elevated by his higher score on the Rhyming test. More telling is Jesse's Early Reading and Spelling Index, which is Significantly Below Average (SS 55, PR 0.1), as low or lower than 999 of 1,000 of his grade-peers, despite the inclusion of the inflated Letter and Word Choice score. As an indication of how disparate Jesse's early reading skills are from his phonological skills (low as they are), less than 1% of Jesse's grade-peers will have such an extreme difference between the Early Linguistic Processing Index and the Early Reading and Spelling Index. The Early Dyslexia Diagnostic Index (EDDI) indicates a person's likelihood of having dyslexia. His EDDI score fell in the Significantly Below Average range, indicating an Extremely High Probability of dyslexia. Only 2% of the population has scores within this range.

TOD-E PARENT/CAREGIVER RATING SCALE

Jesse's mother completed the TOD-E Parent/Caregiver Rating Scale. Her responses yielded a T-score of 66, at the 95th percentile, indicating High Risk of dyslexia. Her responses indicate Jesse has no difficulty with general reasoning, minor difficulty with verbal comprehension; some difficulty with phonological processing, orthographic processing, rapid automatized naming, memory, and basic reading skills and spelling; and major difficulty with motivation for reading. Figure 9.12 presents the results.

SUMMARY

On the TOD-E, Jesse demonstrated average vocabulary knowledge in comparison with his grade-peers. On the oral language tests of the WJ V, he demonstrated average oral language abilities in comparison with his grade-peers. In contrast, his phonological and phonemic awareness abilities were in the Below Average range. Jesse is very significantly delayed in his development of early phonics skills, including his knowledge of letter names and sounds,

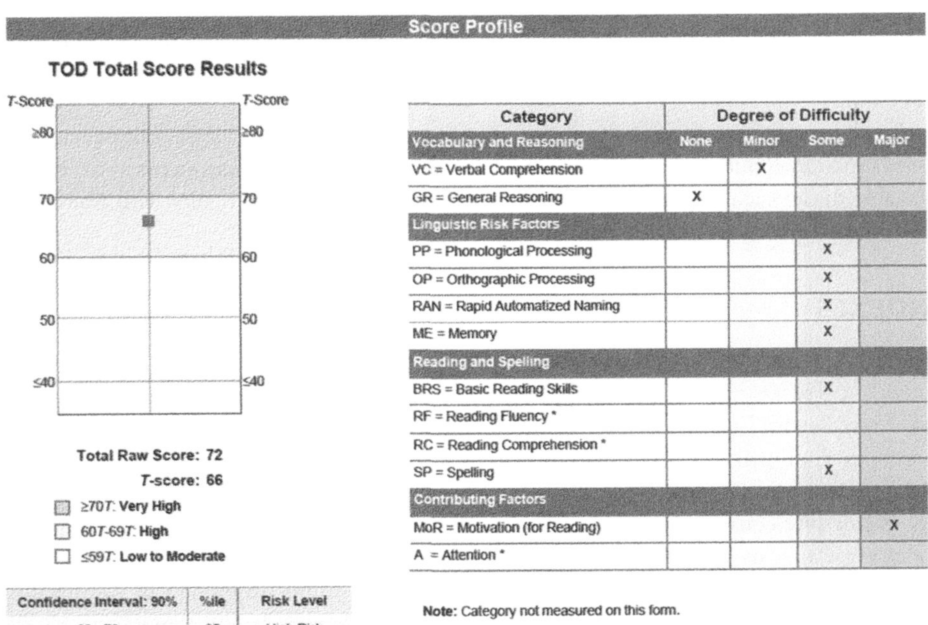

Category	Degree of Difficulty			
Vocabulary and Reasoning	None	Minor	Some	Major
VC = Verbal Comprehension		X		
GR = General Reasoning	X			
Linguistic Risk Factors				
PP = Phonological Processing			X	
OP = Orthographic Processing			X	
RAN = Rapid Automatized Naming			X	
ME = Memory			X	
Reading and Spelling				
BRS = Basic Reading Skills			X	
RF = Reading Fluency *				
RC = Reading Comprehension *				
SP = Spelling			X	
Contributing Factors				
MoR = Motivation (for Reading)				X
A = Attention *				

Note: Category not measured on this form.

The Rating Scale T-score indicates a High Risk for dyslexia. Considerable specific difficulties in reading, spelling, and related skill areas are likely present. Item-level responses, as well as additional data from TOD tests, will be helpful in understanding the specific areas of difficulty.

Figure 9.12   TOD-E Parent/Caregiver Rating Scale Results for Jesse

ability to blend sounds into words, and recognition of basic sight words, especially given the reading instruction program used in his classroom.

DIAGNOSTIC IMPRESSIONS

The current test results strongly indicate that Jesse has dyslexia. Dyslexia is a specific learning disability that impairs the acquisition of basic reading and spelling skills. In turn, these deficits cause difficulties with reading fluency, reading comprehension, and written expression. According to research, the major cognitive correlates of dyslexia include weaknesses in one or more of the following abilities: phonological awareness, orthographic awareness, memory, rapid naming, and processing speed. Other abilities that do not require reading, such as general intelligence, oral language, mathematics, and general knowledge, are often unimpaired, as is true in Jesse's case. A more comprehensive assessment of Jesse's cognitive and academic abilities is recommended to determine areas of cognitive, linguistic, and academic strength that should be supported and challenged as well as other areas of difficulty, such as handwriting, that may require intervention.

RECOMMENDATIONS

Use of Wilson Fundations®

Jesse's school is using the Wilson Fundations® program, a structured literacy program, to teach beginning reading and spelling skills. This is an appropriate program for Jesse's needs; thus, a detailed set of reading and spelling recommendations is not included in this report. If used as intended by someone well trained in the program, Fundations® incorporates the skills that Jesse needs in the correct sequence. The important principle is that *every skill* introduced is practiced until it is mastered before moving onto the next skill. Then, while practicing the new skill, the previous skill(s) is incorporated and reinforced until it becomes automatic.

Fundations® has multiple tiers in how it is presented.

Jesse requires Tier 2 intervention.

- Tier 1: Prevention: Intended for general instruction: Participation in whole-class Fundations® standard lesson—30 minutes daily
- Tier 2: Early Intervention: Intended for at-risk students needing strategic intervention. Targeted individual or small group intervention lessons focused on specific areas of difficulty as well as those needing more practice—30 minutes three to five times a week

If at all possible, to avoid possible refusal to engage due to embarrassment, intervention-level instruction would best be provided in a private area where Jesse's difficulties will not be obvious to other children. Wilson provides teacher support through videos and an online Fundations® Learning Community. Jesse should start at the kindergarten level.

Activities to Use Simultaneously or as Reinforcement of Fundations®

The following activities may prove useful in the classroom and/or at home.

Alphabet and Letter Names

1. To help Jesse learn the alphabet and the names of the letters, teach him to sing the alphabet song, incorporating letter tiles. Break up the song into the melodic parts so that he only has to memorize one part at a time. (e.g., a b c d e f g—h i j k l m n o p—q r s—t u v—w x y [and] z). Practice each part multiple times, pointing to the letter as he sings its name. Be careful that the letters "l m n o" do not become one word, "elemenno," which is common for young children. Do this with both upper- and lowercase letters separately.

2. After practicing each part of the alphabet, mix up letter tiles for only those letters practiced. Have Jesse put them in order, name them, mix them up again, and repeat. Practice each set as it is learned and then incorporate previous letters until he can name every letter, on command, out of order.

3. As Jesse is unclear as to the difference between upper- and lowercase letters, provide matching and sorting activities. At first, provide upper- and lowercase alphabet strips to use as a reference, and then have him work from memory. Some activities include:

   a. Using letter tiles, mix up upper- and lowercase letters and have Jesse practice matching upper- to lowercase letters. At this point, the letters need not be in alphabetical order.

   b. Have Jesse sort the letters into two piles—uppercase and lowercase—and put them into alphabetical order.

   c. Move to more advanced activities, such as having Jesse circle and name all of the uppercase letters on a page of text. On another sheet, have him circle and name only the lowercase letters.

Blending and Segmenting

1. Jesse understands the concept of blending and segmenting sounds but needs practice and reinforcement. A helpful activity uses interlocking cubes that each represent a sound. Interlock the cubes and tell Jesse the word they represent (e.g., sun). Then break the cubes apart, explaining that you are breaking the word into its sounds. Space the cubes a few inches apart, and point to each cube, saying its sound, with a pause in between each sound. Gradually move the cubes closer together, saying the sounds with shorter pauses. Continue until you have pushed together and locked the cubes, say the whole word, and lift the interlocked cubes as a unit to show that you now have a whole word.

2. When teaching segmentation of words into individual sounds, start with two-phoneme words composed of a consonant and a long vowel sound, such as ape, eat, knee, and toe. Long vowel sounds are easier to perceive than short vowel sounds. For words with initial consonants, use those with "stretchy sounds," such as /m/ and /s/, as these are easier to articulate in isolation. Progress to three-sound words with a consonant-vowel team-consonant pattern, such as soap and rain. Be careful not to use final consonant sounds, such as /l/ or /r/, that change the sound of the preceding long vowel.

Basic Reading Skills Reinforcement Activities

Due to Jesse's attention problems, especially when his medication effects may be waning, incorporate fun activities into reading.

1. When Jesse has learned to sound out phonically regular words, alter simple board games to include a reading or spelling step. For example, make small cards with one word (or, later, one sentence) on each card and pile them face down on the board. Player 1 reads the word/sentence then takes his turn. Provide whatever reading support Jesse needs so that the game remains fun. Consistent difficulty indicates the need for additional instruction; the skill level required by the game is too advanced. Games that lend themselves to this type of activity include Chutes and Ladders and Uncle Wiggly. These game alterations can be used to reinforce many skills:
   a. Phoneme-grapheme relationships: use individual letters and ask for the sounds.
   b. Phonics study: use nonsense words that are structured like real words.
   c. Irregular word recognition: Use irregular words.
2. Once Jesse has learned to sound out three-sound words and knows some basic sight words (e.g., the, is, says), a good source of decodable books, in addition to Fundations® and Wilson Reading, is DOG ON A LOG Books by Pamela Brookes. The words in the stories in these books progress in accordance with the Wilson Reading System. They are available at Amazon.com.

Handwriting

1. Teach Jesse handwriting using the Fundations® handwriting style and program. For most lowercase letters, once a student has put his pencil down on the paper, he can complete the letter without picking it up again. The Fundations® paper uses names for the lines (plane, grass, worm) so that the teacher can use a verbal cue as to how to draw the letter. Do not use a stick-and-ball handwriting style as it increases the burden on visual-fine motor coordination.
2. As Jesse frequently confuses b and d, use a strategy to help him remember which is which. Several strategies are included in the Strategy section of this report.
3. To increase interest in practicing letter formation, provide different surfaces (e.g., shaving cream, whiteboard, wet sand, chocolate pudding on a cookie sheet) and different writing implements (e.g., colored markers, glitter pens).
4. If Jesse continues to have significant difficulty with letter formation after focused intervention using the Fundations® handwriting instruction, then seek the consultation of an occupational therapist to help him develop the dexterity needed specifically for that task.

Oral Language

If Jesse continues to have difficulty recognizing intermediate or final plosive sounds within words, then refer him to a licensed speech-language pathologist for an evaluation.

DON'T FORGET

When deciding whether to administer the TOD-E or TOD-C for students in Grades 1 and 2, consider the present reading development of the examinee. For children who are not yet reading connected text, administer the TOD-E, as it is more appropriate for prereaders and emerging readers.

TEST YOURSELF

1. **The TOD-S can be administered either digitally or in paper and pencil format.**
   True or False?

2. **The TOD-S can do all but which of the following?**
   (a) Provide an estimate of risk of dyslexia
   (b) Provide diagnosis of dyslexia
   (c) Help determine the need for further assessment
   (d) Be linked to instructional recommendations

3. **Both the TOD-E and the TOD-C Rating Scales can be used to screen for dyslexia.**
   True or False?

4. **For examinees in grades 1 and 2, when deciding whether to administer the TOD-E or TOD-C, evaluators should consider whether the examinee**
   (a) has been retained.
   (b) can read connected text.
   (c) has received reading intervention.
   (d) has a family history of reading difficulties.

5. **It is advisable to use grade-based norms to generate TOD-E results when a student**
   (a) has been retained a grade.
   (b) is very mature for their grade.
   (c) is very immature for their grade.
   (d) none of the above.

6. **The "unexpected" aspect of dyslexia refers to stronger performance on Picture Vocabulary as compared to the EDDI.**
   True or False?

7. **The TOD Rating Scales can provide**
   (a) a dyslexia diagnosis.
   (b) an estimate of risk for dyslexia.
   (c) samples of student work.
   (d) a direct assessment of examinee performance.

8. **When deciding whether to administer the TOD-E or TOD-C for students in Grades 1 and 2, either option is equally appropriate.**
   True or False?

9. **The ELPI on the TOD-E includes measures of**
   (a) receptive vocabulary.
   (b) early letter and word reading skills.
   (c) foundational linguistic processing skills.
   (d) early spelling skills.

10. **Higher standard scores on the TOD-E EDDI indicate greater risk for dyslexia.**
    True or False?

Answers: 1. True; 2. b; 3. True; 4. b; 5. a; 6. True; 7. b; 8. False; 9. c; 10. False

REFERENCES

Mather, N., McCallum, R. S., Bell, S. M., & Wendling, B. J. (2024c). *Dyslexia interventions and recommendations: A companion guide to the Tests of Dyslexia (TOD)*. Western Psychological Services.

Shaywitz, S., & Shaywitz, J. (2020). *Overcoming dyslexia* (2nd ed.). Knopf.

Skinner, C. H., McLaughlin, T. F., & Logan, P. (1997). Cover, copy, and compare: A self-managed academic intervention effective across skills, students, and settings. *Journal of Behavioral Education, 7*(3), 295–306. https://doi.org/10.1023/A:1022823522040

Ten

ILLUSTRATIVE CASE REPORTS FOR THE TOD-C

The purpose of this chapter is to illustrate how three major components of the Tests of Dyslexia (TOD) can be helpful in determining and providing services to individuals who have limitations in reading, including the direct assessment elements (i.e., TOD-C); the rating scales (for parents/caregivers, teachers, and examinees); and the intervention guidebook, *TOD Intervention and Recommendations: A Companion Guidebook to the Tests of Dyslexia* (Mather et al., 2024c). Although further documentation, such as classroom observations, other standardized tests, and work samples, may be required to justify the implementation of accommodations or support eligibility decisions, the main purpose of these reports is to illustrate the type of information that can be obtained specifically from the TOD-C. Familiarity with the TOD-C test content, administration/scoring, and interpretive options (presented in Chapters 1 through 8 of this book) is required to fully understand the information presented here.

Each case typically includes the following indicators of performance: standard scores (SS), percentiles (PR), age- or grade-equivalents, risk indexes, and probability indexes; however, the types of scores emphasized for each report differ slightly to illustrate the use of these scores. Chapter 5 provides detailed descriptions of how to interpret these scores. These are all actual case reports, but the names, schools, and birthdates have been changed to protect confidentiality. The following cases are presented:

1. Tests of Dyslexia-Screener (TOD-S), Tests of Dyslexia-Comprehensive (TOD-C), and TOD-C Parent/Caregiver and Self-Rating Scales: Illustrates use of the Dyslexia Diagnostic Index (DDI), along with the rating scales, to indicate probability of dyslexia. Javier is a 15-year-old male who was referred by his school counselor due to low grades in English class and difficulty with reading assignments.

2. TOD-S, TOD-C, and TOD-C Parent/Caregiver and Teacher Rating Scales: Illustrates use of selected TOD-S and TOD-C tests and rating scales to identify a specific learning disability/disorder in reading and to generate educational recommendations. June is an 11-year-old female, 6th grade student, who was referred by her mother and reading teacher to determine reading strengths and weaknesses.

3. TOD-S, TOD-C, and TOD-C Parent/Caregiver and Self-Rating Scales: Illustrates the use of the TOD-C battery to indicate probability of dyslexia, identify a specific learning disability, and generate educational recommendations. Gillian is a nine-year-old, 3rd grade student, who was referred by her parents for a dyslexia assessment because of a lack of progress in reading despite a history of school-based intervention.

All components of the TOD (TOD direct assessments and the TOD Rating Scales) can be scored electronically to generate score reports. Except for the adult sample, which can only be scored with age norms, the TOD direct assessment results can be scored using either age-based or grade-based norms. These reports can be downloaded in Microsoft Word and in PDF format, allowing the evaluator flexibility in integrating TOD results into their own evaluation reports. In some of the cases in this Chapter, sections of the TOD score reports have been cut and pasted into the reports. In addition to score reports, instructional recommendations from the *TOD Dyslexia Interventions and Recommendations* guidebook are included in the reports and can be generated electronically by the "Create Intervention Report" function on the TOD scoring platform. The evaluator selects appropriate instructional recommendations based on the examinee's performance on the TOD tests. Appendix B includes examples of TOD score reports with questions that provide practice in interpreting the TOD scores.

> # DON'T FORGET
>
> **Key Information Typically Included in a Case Report**
>
> Identifying information
>
> Reason for referral
>
> Background information
>
> Tests administered
>
> Behavioral observations
>
> Interpretation of test results and the rating scales
>
> Conclusions and recommendations

CASE 1: CONFIDENTIAL PSYCHOEDUCATIONAL REPORT

Name: Javier Williams	School: Westley School
Date of Birth: 10/26	
Sex: Male	Grade: 9
Dates of Testing: 05/30	Age: 15 years, 7 months

REASON FOR REFERRAL AND BACKGROUND INFORMATION

Reason for Referral

Javier was referred for a psychoeducational evaluation by his school counselor due to concerns about weak performance and low grades in his freshman English class. Javier has had difficulties in understanding and completing assigned reading and related assignments. His parents provided background information.

Family History

Javier's parents are both engineers and business owners. He has a younger sister who excels academically. There is no known family history of learning or attentional difficulties. English is the first language of Javier, his sibling, and his parents.

Family and Social Interaction

Javier's relationship with his parents and siblings is described as "good, very close." His parents reported that the family enjoys doing things together and that Javier rarely needs discipline. Javier helps out with routine family chores. His sleep habits are normal. Javier enjoys good peer relationships which mostly center around sports activities. He is an outstanding basketball player and started on his school's varsity team as a freshman. In part, he transferred to Wesley in order to play on the basketball team. Javier also enjoys golf and has become quite an accomplished golfer. He plays recreationally and on his school team.

Developmental History

Javier was born five weeks premature and remained in neonatal care for several weeks prior to coming home. Despite this, he has always been tall for his age. Javier walked at 12 months and began talking at about 2.5 years. He began speaking and learning to read later than his sibling.

Medical History

Javier has no history of major illnesses. He did, however, have tubes inserted in his ears as a toddler due to chronic ear infections. He takes no routine medications and has not been hospitalized. Javier passed vision and hearing screenings at the time of his last physical examination about a year ago.

Educational History

Javier attended grades K–8 in a public school district; he enrolled in Wesley, an independent school, as a freshman. His parents reported that his academic grades in K–8 were mostly As and Bs but that he has always struggled with reading. He participated in extracurricular tutoring in reading during kindergarten through the second grade but did not receive extra help in school. His parents reported that Javier comprehends well when he can listen to text but not when he has to read it himself. He is enrolled in college preparatory level classes at his current school. His grades last year were As and Bs in all subjects except English (D). Mathematics is reportedly a strength, and his grades in Algebra this year for both semesters were As.

According to the school counselor, earlier this school year, Javier was screened for attention-deficit hyperactivity disorder (ADHD), and the results were negative. He was given the Wechsler Intelligence Scale for Children-V, an individually administered cognitive abilities test as part of his school's standardized testing program. The results indicated strengths in visual spatial and fluid reasoning abilities. Javier has not previously participated in any other psychoeducational testing.

Assessment Procedures and Instruments

Tests of Dyslexia (TOD): TOD-Screener (TOD-S); TOD-Comprehensive (TOD-C)*
TOD Rating Scales: Parent/Caregiver; Self-Report
Interviews
Record Review

*Age-based norms were used to calculate Javier's SS on the TOD-S and TOD-C.

Assessment Observations and Interview

The assessment was accomplished in one session lasting about 1.5 hours with a short break. Javier was accompanied by his mother. He was polite and friendly and put forth good effort. Javier presented as a tall adolescent male with an athletic build. He used his right hand for writing tasks. He wrote in print rather than cursive, his handwriting was legible, and the letters and words in his writing were appropriately spaced. Given adequate rapport, the results of this evaluation are considered accurate and valid.

Understanding Test Scores

The TOD-S and TOD-C provide standard scores (SS) that have a population mean of 100 and standard deviation of 15 with the broad range of average extending from 90 to 110. Percentiles are rank scores; a student who scores at the 75th percentile performed equal to or better than 75% and equal to or below 25% of the norm group. The TOD provides grade or age equivalent scores, depending on which norm sample is used to generate the examinee's scores. The TOD-C Rating Scales provide another type of SS, the "T-score," which has a mean of 50 and standard deviation of 10.

TESTS OF DYSLEXIA-SCREENER (TOD-S) AND COMPREHENSIVE (TOD-C)

The TOD are a set of nationally normed tests designed to provide screening and comprehensive assessment of dyslexia. Together, the TOD-S and TOD-C provide direct measures of linguistic processing, reading and spelling skills, vocabulary, and general reasoning. Javier was administered the TOD-S, which yields a Dyslexia Risk Index (DRI), and tests from the TOD-C which yield a Linguistic Processing Index (LPI), a Reading and Spelling Index (RSI), a Dyslexia Diagnostic Index (DDI), and a Vocabulary and Reasoning Composite (VR2) derived from a number of individually administered tests as shown in Figure 10.1. Javier was administered the three tests of the TOD-S and the first seven tests of the TOD-C.

On the TOD-S, Javier achieved a DRI SS of 78, which is at the 7th percentile and in the at-risk range for dyslexia. Javier's SS on the two TOD-S tests that make up the DRI were Letter and Word Choice, 88, 21st percentile, Below Average range; and Question Reading Fluency, 74, 7th percentile, Well Below Average range. In contrast, his SS on the Picture Vocabulary test was in the Average range, 100, 50th percentile. Javier's Picture Vocabulary score was significantly higher than his DRI score; a difference this large occurred only in 10–15% of the TOD standardization sample.

Score Summary								
Test number	Test name	Raw score Raw score	Raw score Ability score	Standard score	Confidence interval: 90%	%ile rank	Equivalent: Child age	Descriptive range
1S	Picture Vocabulary	20	134	100	89 - 111	50	15:0 to 16:11	Average
2S	Letter and Word Choice	17	123	88	79 - 97	21	10:0 to 10:5	Below Average
3Sb	Question Reading Fluency	29		74	69 - 79	4	8:6 to 8:11	Well Below Average
4C	Phonological Manipulation	41		95	89 - 101	37	13.0 - 13.11	Average
5C	Irregular Word Spelling	27		84	81 - 87	14	11.6 - 11.11	Below Average
6C	Rapid Letter Naming	87		89	79 - 99	23	12.0 - 12.5	Below Average
7C	Pseudoword Reading	36		86	82 - 90	18	9.6 - 9.11	Below Average
8C	Word Pattern Choice	27		89	79 - 99	23	11.0 - 11.5	Below Average
9C	Word Memory	8		102	92 - 112	55	17.0 - 18.11	Average
10C	Picture Analogies	34		124	116 - 130	95	> Stop age	Well Above Average

Figure 10.1   Javier's Scores on the TOD-S and TOD-C Tests

Javier's TOD-C index scores were DDI, SS of 83, 13th percentile (Below Average range, High Probability of Dyslexia); RSI, SS of 79, 8th percentile (Well Below Average range); and LPI, SS of 91, 27th percentile (Average range, lower end). Figure 10.1 presents Javier's scores on the TOD-S and the first seven TOD-C tests.

The DDI is comprised of eight tests (i.e., two sets of four tests that make up the LPI and RSI). On the four tests that comprise the LPI, Javier's performance ranged from average (Phonological Manipulation, a measure of advanced phonological skills, and Word Memory, a measure of verbal working memory) to below average (Rapid Letter Naming, a measure of rapid automatized naming or RAN, and Word Pattern Choice, a measure of orthographic knowledge of English spelling), yielding an overall score in the low end of the average range. Individuals with dyslexia typically exhibit a weakness in one or more of the linguistic processing tests that make up the LPI. In Javier's case, his scores were below average on the TOD-C measures of RAN and orthographic processing. Because his scores on Phonological Manipulation and Word Memory were average, his overall LPI was in the lower end of the average range. It is likely that the early intervention he received helped boost his phonological skills. He did, however, have weaknesses in two key areas of linguistic processing: RAN and orthography.

On the four tests that comprise the RSI, Javier's performance ranged from well below average (Question Reading Fluency, a measure of silent reading

DON'T FORGET

The DDI provides an indicator of the probability of dyslexia based on the examinee's performance on measures of key linguistic processing and reading and spelling skills. An examinee may earn scores in the average range on some of these skills and still have a high probability of dyslexia, especially if they have received intervention.

fluency) to below average (Letter and Word Choice, a measure of ability to recognize/ identify letters and correctly spelled words; Irregular Word Spelling, a measure of ability to spell words that have an irregular element; and Pseudoword Reading, a measure of basic reading skills that requires the ability to apply both phonological and orthographic knowledge).

Javier was also administered the Picture Analogies test, a measure of nonverbal, fluid reasoning. He achieved an SS of 124, 95th percentile in the Well Above average range. Scores from the Picture Analogies test and the Picture Vocabulary test from the TOD-S, which measures receptive vocabulary, comprise the VR2 Composite an estimate of overall cognitive ability. Javier's VR2 SS was 115, 84th percentile in the Above Average range. His VR2 score can be contrasted with various scores from the TOD-S and TOD-C. Javier's VR2 was significantly higher than his DDI score; a difference this large occurred only in 1–5% of the TOD standardization sample. Javier's pattern of performance on the TOD exemplifies the "unexpected" aspect that many experts consider characteristic of dyslexia.

TESTS OF DYSLEXIA RATING SCALES

Rating Scale scores are reported in T-scores, which have a mean of 50 and standard deviation of 10. Unlike the SS on the direct assessment components of the TOD, high T-scores on the rating scales are indicative of poor performance. For example, scores of 59 and below are considered low to moderate risk, scores between 60 and 69 indicate high risk for dyslexia, and scores of 70 and above indicate very high risk. Javier's mother completed the Parent/ Caregiver Form; her ratings yielded a T-score of 61, 86th percentile, which is in High Risk range. Her ratings indicated Javier has significant difficulty with reading motivation and some difficulty with basic reading skills, reading fluency, reading comprehension, and phonological skills. Javier completed the Self-Rating Form; his ratings yielded a T-score of 70, 98th percentile, and is in the Very High Risk range. His ratings indicated significant difficulties with reading motivation, reading fluency, and phonological skills and some difficulty with reading comprehension, basic reading skills, and memory.

SUMMARY AND RECOMMENDATIONS

Javier was referred for an assessment due to persistent difficulties with reading and poor performance in his freshman English class, despite several years of early intervention. Javier's performance on the TOD-S indicated that he is at high risk for dyslexia, and results from the TOD-C indicated a high probability of dyslexia. Parent/caregiver and teacher rating scales also indicated that he is at risk for dyslexia. Javier performed in the average range on vocabulary tasks. In contrast, he scored in the well above average range on a nonverbal, fluid reasoning task. It is somewhat surprising that Javier's vocabulary skills are not more in line with his reasoning abilities, but unfortunately, over time, the vocabulary skills of individuals who read infrequently tend to lag behind peers who do spend time reading (Stanovich, 1986).

Diagnostic Impressions

F81.0 Specific Learning Disorder with impairment in reading (word reading accuracy; reading rate or fluency)

Javier's pattern of performance is consistent with criteria for identification of a specific learning disorder in reading, based on the American Psychiatric Association's Diagnostic and Statistical Manual, 5th edition, Text Revision (DSM-5-TR™). In many ways, Javier presents with a pronounced pattern of strengths and relative weaknesses often associated with average or high-ability individuals with dyslexia. Results should be reviewed and used to aid in educational planning for Javier by a school-based team. Javier appears to be experiencing significant difficulties in major life skills (i.e., reading) and as such, accommodations under Section 504/ADA are recommended. Given the pattern of scores, he may also be eligible for special education services, a decision to be made by the school-based team.

Recommended Accommodations

Extended time (1.5 time) for tests and assignments that involve reading

Text instructions read aloud

Use of text-to-speech technology for reading assignments (Learning Ally is a potential resource)

Use of spell check

Do not penalize spelling in routine assignments

Instructional Recommendations

Javier needs explicit, systematic instruction such as is recommended by the International Dyslexia Association (i.e., Structured Literacy). Because he has a busy schedule of school, homework, sports, and sports practice and conditioning, he may benefit from participating in on-line tutoring that is systematic, explicit, and interactive, such as MindPlay Education. Individual subscriptions are available from https://parents.mindplay.com/account/plans. Frequent (e.g., 30 minutes five times per week) participation in such a program can strengthen his reading skills in a manner that is user friendly and that fits into his schedule.

Javier has significant strengths in his nonverbal, visual–spatial, and fluid reasoning abilities. These strengths can be used to help him with reading comprehension and written expression (e.g., use of graphic organizers, charts, maps, and graphs).

Further assessment (e.g., additional tests from the TOD-C and a measure of written expression) may be helpful in determining specific instructional recommendations for Javier.

It has been a pleasure to work with Javier. I am available for consultation regarding his progress as needed. Selected cognitive and academic skills should be re-evaluated within three years, but some may warrant earlier re-evaluation to determine progress.

CASE 2: PSYCHOEDUCATIONAL EVALUATION

Name: June Roberts	
Date of Birth: June 19	Dates of Evaluation: February 20 & 21
Grade: 6th	Sex: Female
Evaluator: Janice Sammons, Ph.D.	Age: 11 years, 8 months

REASON FOR REFERRAL

June was referred for an evaluation by her mother with the goal of determining her strengths and needs in reading and spelling. June's reading teacher, Dr. Amanda Turner, recommended that reading testing should be administered to help determine if June has dyslexia.

BACKGROUND INFORMATION

June is an 11-year-old girl in the sixth grade. She lives in Colorado with her parents and younger brother, Matthew (age seven). June's parents are both dentists. There is no family history of ADHD, dyslexia, or any other condition.

Developmental History

June is the product of an uneventful pregnancy and healthy birth, born at 40.5 weeks gestation with a weight of 8 pounds, 13 ounces. Developmental milestones were reportedly reached within typical limits, including speech. At the age of seven, June received speech therapy for articulation errors, primarily difficulty pronouncing the /r/ and /s/ sounds. She was treated for occasional ear infections as a child by her pediatrician. In the second grade, June had a neuropsychological evaluation which was recommended by her teacher after she noticed that June was experiencing difficulty with reading. A copy of that report was not available.

Currently, the family lives in a rural area. June enjoys drawing and painting, photography, studying birds, and hiking. She also loves playing with her brother and visiting her grandparents. When asked about friendships, her mother reported that June is somewhat indifferent to people that she does not know or does not know well. She has one good friend who is her age with whom she shares a love of drawing and birds and cats. No behavior problems were endorsed. Her mother also noted that June has a large vocabulary.

June attended kindergarten starting at age four. She did not learn any letters while attending kindergarten, nor did she show any desire to learn them. From first through 6th grade, she has attended Mansfield School, an independent private K–8 school with high academic standards. Both June's mother and her reading teacher reported that reading progress is "slow going."

OBSERVATIONS

June was seen for two formal testing sessions. Throughout both evaluation sessions, she demonstrated adequate comprehension and appeared to do her best. She often persisted on tasks that were challenging.

TESTS ADMINISTERED

Tests of Dyslexia-Comprehensive (TOD-C)*
TOD-C Rating Scales
Parent Interview
Review of Records

*Age-based norms were used to calculate June's SS on the TOD-C.

Note: Figure 10.3 provides the individual test scores and Figure 10.5 the composite scores.

Vocabulary

June was administered the two TOD vocabulary tests (TOD-S Picture Vocabulary and TOD-C Listening Vocabulary). For the TOD-S Picture Vocabulary test, June was asked to look at four pictures and circle the one that best depicts a word presented orally by the evaluator. On this test, she demonstrated Above Average receptive vocabulary knowledge (TOD-S Picture Vocabulary, 88th percentile).

She also performed in the Well Above Average range on the Listening Vocabulary test (Listening Vocabulary, 98th percentile). Listening Vocabulary is a measure of listening comprehension and receptive vocabulary knowledge. June was asked to listen to a question and four choices and then choose a response. Overall, June performed in the Well Above Average range on receptive vocabulary tasks (TOD-C Vocabulary Composite, 96th percentile).

Linguistic Processing Index (LPI)

June was administered a set of tests from the TOD-C designed to measure several underlying skills that are predictive of reading and spelling difficulties. Performance on these linguistic processes can indicate risk of dyslexia. On the LPI, her scores on the Phonological Manipulation and Working Memory tests were in the Average range. In contrast, her scores on the Rapid Letter Naming test fell in the Well Below Average range (SS = 78), and her score on Word Pattern Choice test was in the Below Average range (SS = 84).

Phonological Awareness

The Phonological Awareness composite is a measure of four different phonological awareness abilities: blending, segmenting, substitution, and deletion. June performed in the Average range on a measure of phonological awareness and working memory which requires substituting sounds and deleting sounds in words (TOD-C Phonological Manipulation, 68th percentile). She performed in the Average range when asked to combine phonemes and then pronounce a whole word (Blending, 55th percentile). Furthermore, she performed in the Well Above Average range when asked to segment words into their phonemes (individual speech sounds) (Segmenting, 93rd percentile). Overall, June demonstrated above average phonological awareness abilities, important skills that support learning to read and spell.

Rapid Automatized Naming (RAN)

In contrast, June performed in the Well Below Average range on a rapid letter naming task (TOD-C Rapid Letter Naming, 7th percentile). Rapid Letter Naming is a measure of RAN which requires quickly retrieving and naming a random sequence of six confusable letters (*b, d, p, q, n, u*) within one minute. June also performed in the Below Average range when asked to rapidly retrieve and name a random sequence of three numbers (*3, 6, 9*) and three letters (*E, F, L*) (Rapid Number and Letter Naming, 21st percentile). Overall, June's RAN performance was below average.

Auditory Working Memory

June demonstrated Above Average auditory working memory ability (TOD-C Auditory Working Memory, 79th percentile). Auditory working memory is a measure of the ability to hold information in immediate memory and then manipulate it. Specifically, when asked to listen to a series of words and then repeat them in reverse order, June performed in the

Average range (Word Memory, 70th percentile). In addition, June performed in the Above Average range when asked to listen to a series of letters and then repeat the letters in reverse order (Letter Memory, 81st percentile).

Orthographic Processing

June exhibited significant difficulties on orthographic processing tasks. The TOD-C Orthographic Processing composite is a measure of the ability to quickly

> **DON'T FORGET**
>
> Individuals with dyslexia may not exhibit difficulties in all areas of linguistic processing as assessed by the TOD. As individuals age, they often exhibit an uneven pattern of scores with difficulties in reading fluency, spelling, and orthographic processing. If they have received systematic instruction, they will most likely not have weaknesses in phonological awareness and phonics.

recognize common English spelling patterns. For example, when asked to select the correct spelling of a word from four choices (e.g., *prak, park, karp, rakp*), June performed in the Well Below Average range (Letter and Word Choice, 5th percentile). In addition, when asked to look at a row of four-letter groups and then choose the one that looks most like a real English word within a two-minute time limit, June performed in the Below Average range (Word Pattern Choice, 14th percentile). Overall, June's orthographic knowledge was well below average.

Reading and Spelling

June was first administered the TOD-S Screener (comprised of three tests) in order to determine a Dyslexia Risk Index (DRI), which helped to determine whether a more in-depth assessment was needed. June's performance on the DRI (See Figure 10.2) indicated that she is At-Risk for dyslexia (TOD-S DRI, 4th percentile). Based on this information, June was administered additional measures to assess her reading and spelling skills. Based on tests 2 and 3 from the TOD-S and 4–9 from the TOD-C, her Dyslexia Diagnostic Index (DDI) suggested a High Probability of dyslexia (See Figure 10.4). The following descriptions provide more details regarding June's performance in specific areas related to reading and spelling.

Basic Reading Skills

June performed in the Below Average range on a set of basic reading tasks (TOD-C Basic Reading Skills, 19th percentile). Specifically, June performed in the Average range when asked to read aloud phonically regular nonsense words (Pseudoword Reading, 53rd percentile). She successfully decoded two- and three-syllable pseudowords but occasionally mixed up *bs* and *ds* when pronouncing the pseudowords. She performed in the Well Below Average range on a measure of exception word reading that requires reading aloud words that contain an irregular element that cannot be pronounced through the application of phonics alone (Irregular Word Reading, 6th percentile). June has not yet developed automatic word identification skills. Although she identified several words accurately, as compared to most peers, she required increased time and greater attention to the phonological and orthographical aspects of each word in order to pronounce the word correctly.

Sight Word Acquisition

June performed in the Well Below Average range on word recognition tasks (TOD-C Sight Word Acquisition Composite, 6th percentile). The tests in this composite require recognizing and reading aloud words that have an irregular element under untimed and timed conditions. Orthographic knowledge also plays a role in word recognition and spelling. As previously reported, June performed poorly on the Irregular Word Reading test. Similarly, she performed in the below average range when asked to quickly read words aloud that contain an irregular element within a one-minute limit.

Phonics Knowledge

June exhibited a relative strength when asked to demonstrate her knowledge of phonics (TOD-C Phonics Knowledge Composite, 39th percentile). As previously reported, June performed in the Average range when asked to read aloud phonically regular nonsense words (Pseudoword Reading, 53rd percentile). Similarly, June performed in the Average range when asked to read aloud phonically regular nonsense words as quickly as possible within a one-minute limit (Rapid Pseudoword Reading, 34th percentile).

Decoding Efficiency

The Decoding Efficiency Composite, a measure of automaticity with basic reading skills, includes two timed tests. As previously reported, June performed in the Average range when asked to read aloud phonically regular nonsense words as quickly as possible within a one-minute limit (Rapid Pseudoword Reading, 34th percentile). In contrast, June performed in the Below Average range for exception word reading, which requires quickly reading aloud words that contain an irregular element within a one-minute time limit (Rapid Irregular Word Reading, 10th percentile). Reading words with irregular elements quickly and efficiently is very difficult for June.

Spelling

The TOD-C Spelling Composite includes two tests, a measure of orthographic knowledge, that require spelling words with an irregular element and a measure of words that follow the spelling rules of English. June performed in the Below Average Range on the irregular spelling test (Irregular Word Spelling, 16th percentile). In contrast, she performed in the Average range with words that are phonically regular (Regular Word Spelling, 27th percentile). Letter reversals (b/d) were observed; however, June self-corrected as needed. In general, June's spelling ability and orthographic knowledge fell in the Below Average range (Spelling, 21st percentile).

Reading Fluency

Several reading fluency and comprehension tests from the TOD-C were administered. June performed in the Well Below Average range on a set of reading fluency tasks (Reading Fluency Composite, 7th percentile). When asked to silently read a question and circle the correct answer within time limits, June's score fell in the Well Below Average range (Question Reading Fluency, 7th percentile). She read and answered only 25 questions but had 100% accuracy. In addition, when asked to read aloud a grade-level (grade 6) passage for one minute, June performed in the Well Below Average range (Oral Reading Efficiency, 4th percentile). She struggled to read words accurately and automatically. June also performed in the Below Average range on a timed test when asked to read paragraphs and answer questions (Silent Reading Efficiency, 19th percentile). June's difficulty reading words automatically is interfering with her reading comprehension. Her performance on timed reading comprehension tasks also placed her in the Below Average range compared to her age peers (Reading Comprehension Efficiency, 10th percentile).

TOD-C RATING SCALES

June's mother and reading teacher completed the TOD-C Rating scales, designed for parents/caregivers and teachers (separate forms). Her mother's ratings (See Figure 10.6) indicated a Moderate risk level for dyslexia while her teacher's ratings (See Figure 10.7) indicated a Very High risk level. Specifically, areas of "some" or "major" difficulty identified by both raters included orthographic processing, memory, basic reading skills, reading fluency, and spelling. Her mother and teacher both identified attention as "some degree of difficulty."

CONCLUSIONS

June is an 11-year-old girl with vocabulary knowledge in the Well Above Average range (TOD-C Vocabulary Composite, SS = 126). In contrast, she demonstrated Below Average performance in basic reading skills (TOD-C Basic Reading Skills, SS = 87), Well Below Average performance on reading fluency tasks (TOD-C Reading Fluency, SS = 78), and Below Average performance on reading comprehension tasks (TOD-C Reading Comprehension Efficiency, SS = 81). These findings are consistent with a diagnosis of a Specific Learning Disorder (also known as Specific Learning Disability [SLD] under IDEA) in the area of basic reading skills (also known as dyslexia).

RECOMMENDATIONS

Given June's diagnosis of an SLD in the area of reading, she should qualify for special education services. She will benefit from individualized, highly structured reading and spelling intervention from a reading specialist to help improve her sight-word reading, spelling, and reading rate.

Instruction and Interventions for Reading

As noted in the report, based on her advanced vocabulary, June demonstrates unexpected underachievement in both reading and spelling. The following recommendations are provided for June, her parents, and her teachers.

Basic Reading Skills

1. June needs an instructional program in basic reading and spelling skills that is systematic in introduction, practice, and reinforcement of phoneme-grapheme relationships, sight words, syllabication rules, structural analysis, and spelling rules. In a systematic program, skills are presented in graduated steps, from simple to complex, with students achieving mastery before the next skill is introduced. Practice assignments on the current skill incorporate previously learned skills, providing opportunities for June to develop automaticity.

2. Teach June how to use structural analysis to decode multisyllabic words. Ensure that she "over learns" these skills so that she can see unfamiliar words as a sequence of recognizable word parts. Teach her to identify both meaning parts (prefixes, suffixes, and root words) and pronunciation parts (common clusters and syllables). Teach June the six most common syllable types. Explain to her how recognizing the syllable structure will aid with word pronunciation and, importantly, help her know how to pronounce the vowel sounds in words. An excellent program supporting such instruction is *REWARDS (Secondary) Reading Excellence: Word Attack and Rate Development Strategies* (A. L. Archer, M. M. Gleason, V. Vachon). Available from Amazon.

Sight Word Acquisition

June would benefit from instruction in morphology. Recommendations can then focus upon mastery of base words and affixes. Notably, only 18 prefixes (e.g., *un-, re-, in-, pre-*) are used in 95% of all words with prefixes. Practice in reading and spelling these prefixes can help June pronounce multisyllabic words. In general, instruction designed to help June master sight words should draw attention to why words are spelled the way they are and the relationships among the word's spelling, meaning, and word origin.

1. Help June build an efficient sight vocabulary. Provide instruction that will help June develop a connection between a word's pronunciation and its printed form. Discuss the patterns in the word and provide repeated exposures. June will benefit from multiple exposures in order to recognize a word quickly.
2. Introduce the concept that there are three types of words: (a) words that are regular and are spelled exactly as they sound; (b) words that are not regular but have frequent spelling pattern that must be memorized; and (c) words that are irregular and include a part that must be memorized.

Reading Fluency

To help increase her reading rate, use the Great Leaps Reading Program. Through work in Phonics, Phrases, and Stories, June will improve her reading fluency and reading comprehension. Online tutoring is also available. Website: https://greatleaps.com/

Irregular Word Spelling

1. When June is learning the spelling of an irregular word, have her look at the word, cover it, and then write it from memory, saying the word while writing it. Ask June to underline the tricky part of the word and then enter the word alphabetically into a word box. Review the word as needed.
2. One program that would be beneficial is *Spellography*. This program will teach her common spelling rules and explain why words are spelled the way they are.
3. As June moves ahead in grade levels and writing expectations increase, she may benefit from voice recognition software to alleviate spelling and handwriting difficulties. Teach June how to use voice-activated word processing programs or voice recognition software. June would speak into a microphone, and the text is then translated into a word processing format on the computer. Although this procedure is not error free, it will significantly reduce the demands on spelling, allowing June to concentrate more fully on expressing and organizing her ideas. One example of voice recognition software

is Dragon NaturallySpeaking (dragondictations.org). June may also have success with a computer's "built in" dictation processor.

Accommodations

1. Copying: Limit near- or far-point copying activities. When copying is necessary, do not require speed or accuracy.
2. Alternative testing location: Due to June's specific reading disability, she may benefit from a quiet, distraction-free environment to complete tests.
3. Note-taking support: June may experience difficulties keeping up with writing due to spelling difficulties. When following lectures, taking notes, and writing down assignments, June may benefit from the use of a notetaker. A copy of the teacher's notes may also be a reliable source for content that June will be responsible to learn.
4. Since June has significant needs in basic academic skills (e.g., basic reading skills, spelling, and reading rate), it may be difficult for her to keep up with her grade peers without accommodations and supports. June will need assistance in accessing the curriculum when reading is required. June is able to learn concepts when academic accommodations and modifications are made. For example, in a social studies class, June can understand the content but needs a way to access the information. If extensive reading is required, then this information may be presented in another way (e.g., use of audio books).

Note: Several of these recommendations were taken directly from: Mather et al. (2024c). *Dyslexia interventions and recommendations: A companion guide to the Tests of Dyslexia (TOD).* Western Psychological Services.

Additional Resources

Websites

- International Dyslexia Association. Website: http://eida.org/
- Learning Disabilities Association of America (LDA) Website: http://www.ldanatl.org/
- Information and inspiration for parents and teachers of children with learning disabilities (Rick Lavoie, M.A., M.Ed.) Website: http://www.ricklavoie.com
- Website on learning disabilities and ADHD. Website: ldonline.org

Recommended Books

Mather, N., & Wendling, B. J. (2024). *Essentials of dyslexia: Assessment and intervention* (2nd ed.). Wiley.
Shaywitz, S., & Shaywitz, J. (2020). *Overcoming dyslexia: A new and complete science-based program for reading problems at any level* (2nd ed.). Knopf.

I enjoyed working with June and her family. If you have any questions about these findings or this report, please do not hesitate to contact me.

TOD TEST RESULTS

Figures 10.2–10.7 present June's Score Report for the TOD-C and the rating scales. Figure 10.2 displays the results of the TOD-S tests and the DRI. Figure 10.3 shows the TOD-C individual test scores. Figure 10.4 shows the DDI SS Profile. Figure 10.5 presents the TOD-C Composite scores. Figures 10.6 and 10.7 show the results of the Parent/Caregiver Rating Scale and the Teacher Rating Scale.

| | | Raw score | | | | | | |
Test number	Test name	Raw score	Ability score	Standard score	Confidence interval: 95%	%ile rank	Equivalent: Child age	Descriptive range
					Score Summary			
1S	Picture Vocabulary	22	138	118	105 - 130	88	17:0 to 18:11	Above Average
2S	Letter and Word Choice	9	108	76	65 - 87	5	7:4 to 7:7	Well Below Average
3Sb	Question Reading Fluency	25		78	72 - 84	7	7:8 to 7:11	Well Below Average

Dyslexia Risk Index (DRI)

Sum of standard scores for DRI (Letter and Word Choice + Reading Fluency)	DRI standard score: Child age	Confidence interval: 95%	%ile rank	Risk of dyslexia based on DRI*
154	74	65 - 83	4	At-Risk

* No to Low Risk (110 and above); Possible Risk (90-109); At-Risk (89 and below).

Figure 10.2   June's Score Report for the TOD-S tests and DRI

Test number	Test name	Raw score	Ability score	Standard score	Confidence interval: 95%	%ile rank	Equivalent: Child age	Descriptive range
1S	Picture Vocabulary	22	138	118	105 - 130	88	17:0 to 18:11	Above Average
2S	Letter and Word Choice	9	108	76	65 - 87	5	7:4 to 7:7	Well Below Average
3Sb	Question Reading Fluency	25		78	72 - 84	7	7:8 to 7:11	Well Below Average
4C	Phonological Manipulation	42		107	100 - 114	68	15.0 - 16.11	Average
5C	Irregular Word Spelling	20		85	81 - 89	16	9.0 - 9.5	Below Average
6C	Rapid Letter Naming	53		78	66 - 90	7	7.8 - 7.11	Well Below Average
7C	Pseudoword Reading	40		101	96 - 106	53	12.0 - 12.5	Average
8C	Word Pattern Choice	15		84	71 - 97	14	7.8 - 7.11	Below Average
9C	Word Memory	8		108	96 - 120	70	17.0 - 18.11	Average
10C	Picture Analogies							
11C	Irregular Word Reading	28		77	71 - 83	6	7.8 - 7.11	Well Below Average
12C	Oral Reading Efficiency**	43		74	64 - 84	4	1 - Fall	Well Below Average
13C	Blending	20		102	94 - 110	55	12.6 - 12.11	Average
14C	Segmenting	26		122	113 - 130	93	> Stop age	Well Above Average
15C	Regular Word Spelling	23		91	86 - 96	27	10.0 - 10.5	Average
16C	Silent Reading Efficiency	16		87	76 - 98	19	< Start age	Below Average
17C	Rapid Number and Letter Naming	82		88	76 - 100	21	9.0 - 9.5	Below Average
18C	Letter Memory	9		113	101 - 125	81	> Stop age	Above Average
19C	Rapid Pseudoword Reading	29		94	81 - 107	34	9.6 - 9.11	Average
20C	Rapid Irregular Word Reading	54		81	69 - 93	10	8.0 - 8.5	Below Average
21C	Symbol to Sound Learning							
22C	Listening Vocabulary	32		130	123 - 130	98	> Stop age	Well Above Average
23C	Geometric Analogies							

Descriptive ranges (based on standard scores): Significantly Below Average (69 and below); Well Below Average (70-79); Below Average (80-89); Average (90-109); Above Average (110-119); Well Above Average (120 and above).

**Child Oral Reading Efficiency scores are available in grade-based norms only.

Figure 10.3   June's Test Scores for TOD-C (includes TOD-S)

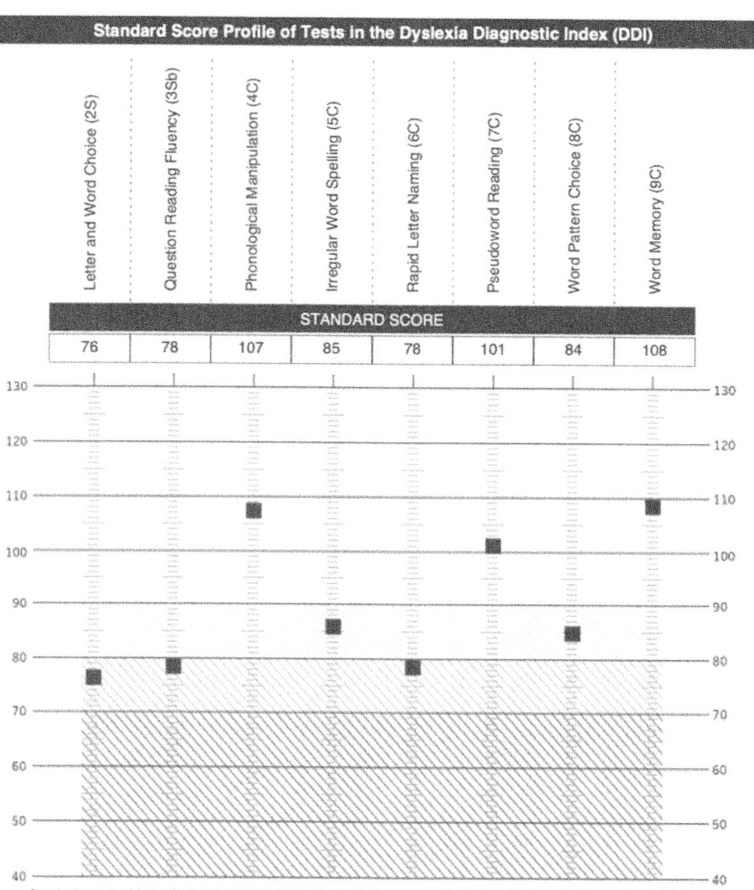

Figure 10.4   June's DDI Standard Score Profile

TOD-C composite	Sum of standard scores	Composite standard score: Child age	Confidence interval: 95%	%ile rank	Descriptive range
Sight Word Acquisition	158	77	70 - 84	6	Well Below Average
Phonics Knowledge	195	96	91 - 101	39	Average
Basic Reading Skills	178	87	80 - 94	19	Below Average
Decoding Efficiency	175	86	82 - 90	18	Below Average
Spelling	176	88	81 - 95	21	Below Average
Reading Fluency	152	78	70 - 86	7	Well Below Average
Reading Comprehension Efficiency	165	81	78 - 84	10	Below Average
Phonological Awareness	331	113	106 - 120	81	Above Average
Rapid Automatized Naming	166	81	78 - 84	10	Below Average
Auditory Working Memory	221	112	103 - 121	79	Above Average
Orthographic Processing	160	74	63 - 85	4	Well Below Average
Vocabulary	248	126	115 - 130	96	Well Above Average

Descriptive ranges (based on standard scores): Significantly Below Average (69 and below); Well Below Average (70-79); Below Average (80-89); Average (90-109); Above Average (110-119); Well Above Average (120 and above).

Figure 10.5   June's TOD-C Composite Scores

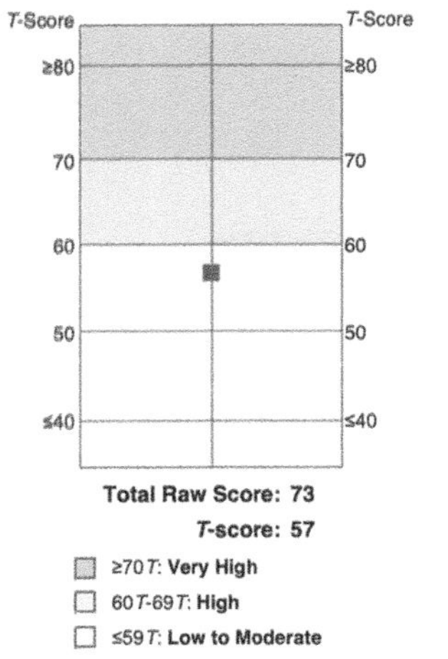

Confidence Interval: 95%	%ile	Risk Level
53 - 61	76	Low to Moderate Risk

Category	Degree of Difficulty			
Vocabulary and Reasoning	None	Minor	Some	Major
VC = Verbal Comprehension		X		
GR = General Reasoning		X		
Linguistic Risk Factors				
PP = Phonological Processing		X		
OP = Orthographic Processing			X	
RAN = Rapid Automatized Naming *				
ME = Memory			X	
Reading and Spelling				
BRS = Basic Reading Skills			X	
RF = Reading Fluency			X	
RC = Reading Comprehension		X		
SP = Spelling			X	
Contributing Factors				
MoR = Motivation (for Reading)		X		
A = Attention			X	

* **Note:** Category not measured on this form.

Figure 10.6 Parent/Caregiver Rating Scale Completed by June's Mother

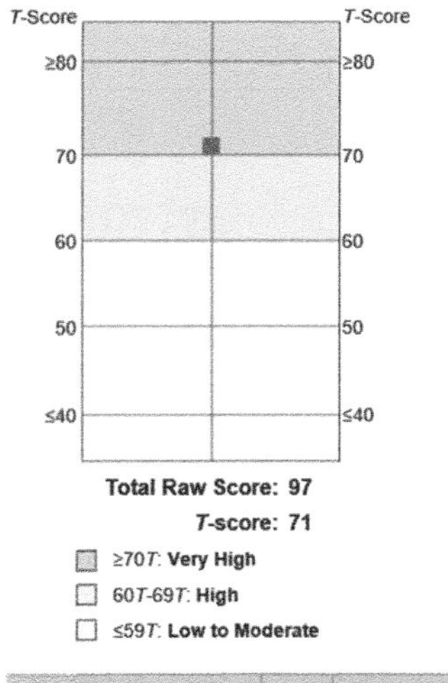

Confidence Interval: 90%	%ile	Risk Level
68 - 74	98	Very High Risk

Category	Degree of Difficulty			
Vocabulary and Reasoning	None	Minor	Some	Major
VC = Verbal Comprehension		X		
GR = General Reasoning		X		
Linguistic Risk Factors				
PP = Phonological Processing			X	
OP = Orthographic Processing				X
RAN = Rapid Automatized Naming *				
ME = Memory				X
Reading and Spelling				
BRS = Basic Reading Skills			X	
RF = Reading Fluency				X
RC = Reading Comprehension			X	
SP = Spelling				X
Contributing Factors				
MoR = Motivation (for Reading)				X
A = Attention		X		

* **Note:** Category not measured on this form.

Figure 10.7 Teacher Rating Scale Completed by June's Teacher

CASE 3: CONFIDENTIAL PSYCHOEDUCATIONAL REPORT

Name: Gillian Kelly	School: Sweetgrass Elementary
Date of Birth: 11/16	
Sex: Female	Grade: 3
Date of Testing: 03/24	Age: 9 years, 4 months

REASON FOR REFERRAL AND BACKGROUND INFORMATION

Referral Question

Gillian was referred for a psychoeducational assessment by her parents to determine if she has a specific learning disorder, specifically dyslexia. Her parents were seeking information about the nature of Gillian's reading and related difficulties and hoped to get information useful for educational planning. Background information was provided by Gillian's parents who also provided copies of school records and previous evaluations. Gillian participated in speech therapy as a preschooler through the state's early intervention program. At her school, Gillian has participated in tiered instruction in reading and currently is receiving special education services as a student with a specific learning disability (SLD) in reading (in the area of reading fluency). She is currently completing 3rd grade at a local public elementary school where she has been enrolled since kindergarten.

Gillian's parents described her as friendly with a sense of humor. She can be a leader in some situations but is also aware that her reading and related performance is not commensurate with most of her same-grade peers. She appears eager to go to school and is generally described as happy.

Family History

Gillian's parents are both employed in professional positions. She has a younger brother who "breezes" through school. Her parents noted some history of attention difficulties (her father) and possible dyslexia (paternal grandmother).

Family and Social Interaction

Gillian enjoys a close relationship with both parents and with her brother, although she and her brother sometimes bicker. Gillian rarely needs discipline. When she does, her parents remove privileges. Gillian is assigned routine chores, such as cleaning her room. She gets along very well with peers, and not only enjoys outdoor activities but also enjoys doing crafts and playing with her dolls. She participates in dance and seems to have a natural talent for it.

Developmental History

No birth problems were reported by Gillian's parents. She met most developmental milestones within typical time limits, except for speech. She participated in speech therapy for speech sound articulation at age three.

Medical History

Gillian is reportedly healthy and has had no hospitalizations or serious illnesses. Gillian takes no routine medications. Her last complete physical exam was at the beginning of this school year; results including vision and hearing exam results were normal. No signs of attentional difficulties have been noted by parents or by Gillian's teachers.

Educational History

Gillian attended preschool before beginning kindergarten at a local public school where she is now in 3rd grade. She is said to like school and have good attendance. In grade 1, Gillian began receiving tiered instruction in reading through the state/district's response to intervention (RTI) program. Due to a lack of adequate progress, she was assessed and deemed eligible for special education services toward the end of last school year (end of her 2nd grade year). Unfortunately, according to the results of the universal screener used in the district, Gillian showed regression in her reading skills.

Results of recent school-based individual standardized achievement testing indicated that Gillian's reading scores are generally below average, whereas mathematics and written expression (not including spelling) are generally average.

Assessment Procedures and Instruments

Tests of Dyslexia (TOD): TOD-Comprehensive (TOD-C)*
TOD Rating Scales: Parent/Caregiver; Self-Report
Record Review
Interviews

*Age-based norms were used to calculate Gillian's scores on the TOD-C.

Assessment Observations and Interview

Assessment was accomplished in one session that lasted about two hours with a break. Gillian presented as an engaging, friendly, energetic, and polite nine-year-old. Her mother accompanied her for the assessment session, and Gillian separated easily from her. During assessment, Gillian attempted all tasks asked of her and did not exhibit atypical fidgetiness, anxiety, or difficulty attending. Her conversation skills seemed advanced. She wrote with her left hand, curving her hand slightly but not excessively as she wrote. Her pencil grip appeared to be typical.

Understanding Test Scores

To understand the scores in this report, the following definitions are provided. The TOD uses standard score (SS) with a population mean of 100 and standard deviation of 15. The average range extends from 90 to 110. Percentile ranks (PR) indicate the percentage of scores in a distribution that a score surpasses. An individual who scores at the 75th percentile performed equal to or better than 75% of the norm group and equal to or below 25% of the norm group. The TOD also provides age or grade equivalent scores, depending on which norms are used to generate scores. The TOD Rating Scales provide another type of SS, the T-score, which has a mean of 50 and standard deviation of 10. Unlike SS and PR, higher T-scores indicate greater difficulty.

TESTS OF DYSLEXIA-SCREENER

The TOD are a set of nationally normed tests designed to provide screening and comprehensive assessment of dyslexia. Gillian was administered the TOD-S, which yields a Dyslexia Risk Index (DRI), and the TOD-C, which yields a Linguistic Processing Index (LPI), a Reading and Spelling Index (RSI), and a Dyslexia Diagnostic Index (DDI). On the TOD-S, Gillian achieved a DRI SS of 77, which is at the 6th percentile and in the At-Risk range for dyslexia. Figure 10.8 illustrates Gillian's performance on the TOD-S.

On the two tests that comprise the DRI, Gillian scored in the Below Average range on Letter and Word Choice (SS of 83, 13th percentile) and in the Well Below Average range on Word Reading Fluency (SS of 76, 5th percentile). In contrast, on the Picture Vocabulary test, a measure of receptive vocabulary, she performed in the Average range (SS of 105, 63rd percentile). Her Picture Vocabulary performance is significantly higher than her performance on the DRI. Differences this large occurred in only 5% of the TOD-S standardization sample.

Below are descriptions of the TOD-S tests and information related to Gillian's performance. (Note: These descriptions are provided verbatim to illustrate information that is presented on the TOD-S Score Report).

Dyslexia Risk Index

The TOD-S Dyslexia Risk Index (DRI) provides a standard score that estimates the risk for dyslexia. The obtained DRI is in the Below Average range. This score indicates below average performance and moderate to significant risk (at-risk) for dyslexia. It indicates limited basic

Score Summary								
Test number	Test name	Raw score		Standard score	Confidence interval: 90%	%ile rank	Equivalent: Child age	Descriptive range
		Raw score	Ability score					
1S	Picture Vocabulary	21	125	105	94 - 116	63	10:0 to 10:5	Average
2S	Letter and Word Choice	15	105	83	73 - 93	13	6:8 to 6:11	Below Average
3Sb	Question Reading Fluency	16		76	71 - 81	5	< Start age	Well Below Average

Dyslexia Risk Index (DRI)				
Sum of standard scores for DRI (Letter and Word Choice + Reading Fluency)	DRI standard score: Child age	Confidence interval: 90%	%ile rank	Risk of dyslexia based on DRI*
159	77	69 - 85	6	At-Risk

* No to Low Risk (110 and above); Possible Risk (90-109); At-Risk (89 and below).

Figure 10.8   Gillian's Scores on the TOD-S

reading skills and the need for further assessment. Additional information should be considered, such as educational and family history, writing samples from the classroom, and rating scale data.

Picture Vocabulary

Picture Vocabulary (1S), a measure of receptive vocabulary knowledge, requires selecting one of four pictures that best depicts a word that the examiner presents orally. The standard score obtained on this test fell into the Average range. This score range indicates average receptive vocabulary knowledge.

Letter and Word Choice

Letter and Word Choice (2S), a measure of orthographic knowledge, requires selecting the correct letter or correct spelling of a word from four choices (e.g., *prak, park, karp, rakp*). The standard score obtained on this test fell into the Below Average range. This score range indicates limited spelling skills and ability to recognize orthographic patterns.

Question Reading Fluency

Question Reading Fluency (3Sb), a measure of reading rate and comprehension, requires reading questions silently and selecting the correct response from among four choices as quickly as possible. The standard score obtained on this test fell into the Well Below Average range. This score range indicates very limited ability to read and answer questions quickly.

TESTS OF DYSLEXIA-COMPREHENSIVE

Because Gillian's TOD-S scores indicate at-risk status for dyslexia, the TOD-C was administered. Gillian's TOD-C index scores were DDI, SS 76, 5th percentile (Very High probability of dyslexia/well below average); RSI, SS 78, 7th percentile (Well Below Average range); and LPI, SS 79, 8th percentile (Well Below Average range). Figure 10.9 presents Gillian's TOD-C Index scores.

Dyslexia Diagnostic Index (DDI), Reading and Spelling Index (RSI), and Linguistic Processing Index (LPI) Standard Scores					
TOD Index	**Sum of standard scores**	**Index standard score: Child age**	**Confidence interval: 90%**	**%ile rank**	**Descriptive range**
Dyslexia Diagnostic Index	673	76	72 - 80	5	Well Below Average
Reading and Spelling Index	329	78	71 - 85	7	Well Below Average
Linguistic Processing Index	344	79	73 - 85	8	Well Below Average

Descriptive ranges (based on standard scores): Significantly Below Average (69 and below); Well Below Average (70-79); Below Average (80-89); Average (90-109); Above Average (110-119); Well Above Average (120 and above).

Probability of dyslexia based on DDI standard score *	Very High Probability of Dyslexia

*Extremely Low (120 and above); Very Low (110-119); Low to Moderate (90-109); High (80-89); Very High (70-79); Extremely High (69 and below).

Figure 10.9   Gillian's TOD-C Index Scores

The DDI is made up of eight test scores, four of which comprise the RSI, and four of which comprise the LPI. On the four tests that comprise the RSI, Gillian performed as follows: Question Reading Fluency (well below average); Irregular Word Spelling (well below average); Pseudoword Reading (low end of average); and Word Pattern Choice (low end of average). On the four tests that comprise the LPI, Gillian scored as follows: Letter and Word Choice (below average); Phonological Manipulation (average); Rapid Letter Naming (significantly below average); and Word Memory (below average). She struggled most on Rapid Letter Naming, which is measure of rapid automatized naming, using confusable letters. Gillian made several errors discriminating between *b* versus *d* in particular. Below are descriptions of the TOD-C indexes and information about Gillian's performance on each. [The following descriptions are excerpted from the TOD™-C Score Report.]

Dyslexia Diagnostic Index

The TOD-C Dyslexia Diagnostic Index (DDI), derived from eight tests, provides a standard score that defines the probability of dyslexia. This is the most robust indication of whether or not dyslexia is present. The DDI standard score fell into the Well Below Average range and indicates that the probability of dyslexia is Very High. This score indicates very limited performance on tests of linguistic processing and reading and spelling skills.

Reading and Spelling Index

The TOD-C Reading and Spelling Index (RSI) is derived from four tests that measure different aspects of foundational reading skills, such as letter/word knowledge, reading fluency, irregular word spelling, and nonsense word reading. The RSI is part of the Dyslexia Diagnostic Index (DDI) and can also be interpreted independently when an index of reading and spelling ability is needed. The RSI standard score fell into the Well Below Average range and indicates very limited performance on tests of basic reading/spelling.

Linguistic Processing Index

The TOD-C Linguistic Processing Index (LPI) is derived from four tests that measure different aspects of linguistic processing, such as phonemic awareness, rapid automatized naming, orthographic knowledge, and working memory. These four factors are foundational for acquiring basic reading skills. The LPI is part of the Dyslexia Diagnostic Index (DDI) and can also be interpreted independently when an index of linguistic processing risk factors is needed. The LPI standard score fell into the Well Below Average range and indicates very limited performance on tests of linguistic processing.

Figure 10.10 presents Gillian's TOD-C Composite scores. Gillian performed in the average range on the TOD-C phonological tests, likely related to the intensive instruction she has received; however, her performance on the other key linguistic areas often implicated in dyslexia is weak and helps explain Gillian's weak reading and spelling scores. That is, she performed as follows on RAN (well below average); Auditory Working Memory (below average), and Orthographic Processing (below average).

	Score Summary of TOD-C Composites				
TOD-C composite	Sum of standard scores	Composite standard score: Child age	Confidence interval: 90%	%ile rank	Descriptive range
Basic Reading Skills	173	84	78 - 90	14	Below Average
Spelling	158	78	72 - 84	7	Well Below Average
Reading Fluency	152	78	71 - 85	7	Well Below Average
Reading Comprehension Efficiency	163	80	75 - 85	9	Below Average
Phonological Awareness	303	101	95 - 107	53	Average
Rapid Automatized Naming	153	74	72 - 76	4	Well Below Average
Auditory Working Memory	169	81	73 - 89	10	Below Average
Orthographic Processing	173	83	73 - 93	13	Below Average
Vocabulary and Reasoning 2	216	109	102 - 116	73	Average

Descriptive ranges (based on standard scores): Significantly Below Average (69 and below); Well Below Average (70-79); Below Average (80-89); Average (90-109); Above Average (110-119); Well Above Average (120 and above).

Figure 10.10   Gillian's TOD-C Composite Scores

Descriptions of the TOD-C composite scores and information about Gillian's performance on each test is presented below. (Note: These descriptions are provided verbatim to illustrate information that is presented in the TOD-C score report).

Basic Reading Skills

The Basic Reading Skills composite, a measure of two aspects of word reading (applying phonics and reading words with an irregular element), includes Pseudoword Reading (7C) and Irregular Word Reading (11C). The tasks in this composite require reading aloud pseudowords that are phonically regular and reading aloud words that have an irregular element. The standard score obtained on this composite fell into the Below Average range. This score range indicates limited basic reading skills.

Spelling

The Spelling composite, a measure of orthographic knowledge, includes Irregular Word Spelling (5C) and Regular Word Spelling (15C). The tasks in this composite require spelling words that have an irregular element and words that follow the spelling rules of English. The standard score obtained on this composite fell into the Well Below Average range. This score range indicates both very limited spelling ability and very limited orthographic knowledge.

Reading Fluency

The Reading Fluency composite, a measure of reading accuracy and rate, includes Question Reading Fluency (3Sb) and Oral Reading Efficiency (12C). The tasks in this composite, both timed, require reading and answering questions silently and reading a grade-level passage orally. The standard score obtained on this composite fell into the Well Below Average range. This score range indicates very limited reading accuracy and rate.

Reading Comprehension Efficiency

The Reading Comprehension Efficiency composite, a measure of rate and reading comprehension, includes Question Reading Fluency (3Sb) and Silent Reading Efficiency (16C). The tasks in this composite, both timed, require reading and answering questions silently, reading passages of increasing difficulty, and answering comprehension questions. The standard score obtained on this composite fell into the Below Average range. This score range indicates limited reading rate and comprehension.

Phonological Awareness

The Phonological Awareness composite, a measure of four different phonological awareness abilities (blending, segmenting, substitution, and deletion), includes Phonological Manipulation (4C), Blending (13C), and Segmenting (14C). The standard score obtained on this composite fell into the Average range. This score range indicates average phonological awareness abilities.

Rapid Automatized Naming

The Rapid Automatized Naming composite, a measure of naming speed, includes Rapid Letter Naming (6C) and Rapid Number and Letter Naming (17C). The tasks in this composite, both timed, require rapidly retrieving and naming confusable letters and a random mix of three numbers and three letters. The standard score obtained on this composite fell into the Well Below Average range. This score range indicates very limited rapid automatized naming (RAN) ability.

Auditory Working Memory

The Auditory Working Memory composite, a measure of the ability to hold information in immediate memory and then manipulate it, includes Word Memory (9C) and Letter Memory (18C). The tasks in this composite require listening to a series of words or letters and then repeating them in reverse order. The standard score obtained on this composite fell into the Below Average range. This score range indicates limited working memory.

Figure 10.11 presents Gillian's scores on the individual tests from the TOD-C, followed by descriptions of each test and information about Gillian's performance.

Phonological Manipulation

Phonological Manipulation (4C), a measure of phonological awareness and working memory, requires substituting sounds and deleting sounds in words. The standard score obtained on this test fell into the Average range. This score range indicates average phonological manipulation abilities.

Test number	Test name	Raw score		Standard score	Confidence interval: 90%	%ile rank	Equivalent: Child age	Descriptive range
		Raw score	Ability score					
4C	Phonological Manipulation	33		97	91 - 103	42	8.6 - 8.11	Average
5C	Irregular Word Spelling	7		77	74 - 80	6	6.4 - 6.7	Well Below Average
6C	Rapid Letter Naming	27		68	58 - 78	2	< Start age	Significantly Below Average
7C	Pseudoword Reading	29		93	89 - 97	32	7.8 - 7.11	Average
8C	Word Pattern Choice	13		90	80 - 100	25	7.0 - 7.3	Average
9C	Word Memory	4		89	79 - 99	23	6.0 - 6.3	Below Average
10C	Picture Analogies	26		111	103 - 119	77	17.0 - 18.11	Above Average
11C	Irregular Word Reading	24		80	75 - 85	9	7.0 - 7.3	Below Average
12C	Oral Reading Efficiency**	25		76	68 - 84	5	< Start grade	Well Below Average
13C	Blending	16		92	85 - 99	30	6.4 - 6.7	Average
14C	Segmenting	23		114	107 - 121	82	17.0 - 18.11	Above Average
15C	Regular Word Spelling	10		81	77 - 85	10	7.0 - 7.3	Below Average
16C	Silent Reading Efficiency	14		87	80 - 94	19	7.8 - 7.11	Below Average
17C	Rapid Number and Letter Naming	60		85	75 - 95	16	6.8 - 6.11	Below Average
18C	Letter Memory	3		80	70 - 90	9	6.0 - 6.3	Below Average
19C	Rapid Pseudoword Reading							
20C	Rapid Irregular Word Reading							
21C	Symbol to Sound Learning	18		106	102 - 110	66	17.0 - 18.11	Average
22C	Listening Vocabulary							
23C	Geometric Analogies							

Descriptive ranges (based on standard scores): Significantly Below Average (69 and below); Well Below Average (70-79); Below Average (80-89); Average (90-109); Above Average (110-119); Well Above Average (120 and above).

**Child Oral Reading Efficiency scores are available in grade-based norms only.

Figure 10.11   Gillian's Test Scores on the TOD-C

Irregular Word Spelling

Irregular Word Spelling (5C), a measure of exception word spelling, requires spelling words that contain at least one irregular element that is not spelled the way it sounds. The standard score obtained on this test fell into the Well Below Average range. This score range indicates very limited spelling ability, including the ability to recall irregular spelling patterns within words.

Rapid Letter Naming

Rapid Letter Naming (6C), a measure of rapid automatized naming (RAN), requires rapidly retrieving and naming a random sequence of six confusable letters (*b, d, p, q, n, u*) within one minute. The standard score obtained on this test fell into the Significantly Below Average range. This score range indicates extremely limited rapid automatized naming ability.

Pseudoword Reading

Pseudoword Reading (7C), a measure of phonics skills, requires reading aloud phonically regular nonsense words. The standard score obtained on this test fell into the Average range. This score range indicates average knowledge of phonics and ability to blend phonemes.

Word Pattern Choice

Word Pattern Choice (8C), a measure of orthographic knowledge, requires quickly looking at a row of four letter groups and then choosing the one that looks most like a real English word within a two-minute time limit. The standard score obtained on this test fell into the Average range. This score range indicates average orthographic knowledge of English letter patterns.

Word Memory

Word Memory (9C), a measure of verbal working memory, requires listening to a series of words and then repeating the words in reverse order. The standard score obtained on this test fell into the Below Average range. This score range indicates limited verbal working memory on this task.

Picture Analogies

Picture Analogies (10C), a measure of reasoning ability, requires understanding the relationship between pictures in order to solve an analogy. The standard score obtained on this test fell into the Above Average range. This score range indicates advanced reasoning ability on this task.

Irregular Word Reading

Irregular Word Reading (11C), a measure of exception word reading, requires reading aloud words that contain an irregular element that cannot be pronounced through the application of phonics alone. The standard score obtained on this test fell into the Below Average range. This score range indicates limited ability to recognize and read aloud words with irregular letter patterns.

Oral Reading Efficiency

Oral Reading Efficiency (12C), a measure of oral reading accuracy and efficiency, requires reading aloud a grade-level passage for one minute. The standard score obtained on this test fell into the Well Below Average range. This score range indicates very limited ability to decode words automatically and maintain an appropriate reading rate.

Blending

Blending (13C), a measure of phonological awareness, requires putting together compound words, syllables, and phonemes and then pronouncing the whole word. The standard score obtained on this test fell into the Average range. This score range indicates average ability to blend word parts and phonemes to pronounce regular, but unfamiliar, words.

Segmenting

Segmenting (14C), a measure of phonological awareness, requires breaking apart compound words, syllables, and phonemes. The standard score obtained on this test fell into the Above Average range. This score range indicates advanced ability to segment words into their parts and phonemes, abilities critical for spelling.

Regular Word Spelling

Regular Word Spelling (15C), a measure of written spelling, requires spelling words that are phonically regular and mostly spelled the way they sound. The standard score obtained on this test fell into the Below Average range. This score range indicates limited ability to spell words correctly, which requires segmenting the sounds in order and mapping each sound to the correct grapheme.

Silent Reading Efficiency

Silent Reading Efficiency (16C), a measure of reading rate and comprehension, requires reading passages of increasing difficulty and answering questions within a time limit. The standard score obtained on this test fell into the Below Average range. This score range indicates limited ability to read and comprehend connected text relatively quickly.

Rapid Number and Letter Naming

Rapid Number and Letter Naming (17C), a measure of rapid automatized naming (RAN), requires rapidly retrieving and naming a random sequence of three numbers (3, 6, 9) and three letters (E, F, L) within one minute. The standard score obtained on this test fell into the Below Average range. This score range indicates limited rapid automatized naming ability.

Letter Memory

Letter Memory (18C), a measure of working memory, requires listening to a series of letters and then repeating the letters in reverse order. The standard score obtained on this test fell into the Below Average range. This score range indicates limited working memory ability on this task.

Figure 10.12 illustrates a few of her spellings on Test 5C, Irregular Word Spelling. Gillian can segment individual sounds in words quite well (although slowly), but she does not yet consistently apply her phoneme-grapheme knowledge to sounding out words when reading or spelling. She reverses letters and numbers and has difficulty with sequencing of letters in words. She is just beginning to master understanding of spelling patterns but applies these patterns very inconsistently. Although she still has skills to master in phonological awareness and phonics, her greatest difficulties were on the composites of Orthographic Processing, Spelling, and Reading Fluency (all well below average). Basic Reading Skills and Reading Comprehension Efficiency were also weak (low average).

Gillian's pattern of performance on the TOD exemplifies the "unexpected" aspect that many experts (e.g., Catts & Petscher, 2022; S. Shaywitz & Shaywitz, 2020) consider to be characteristic

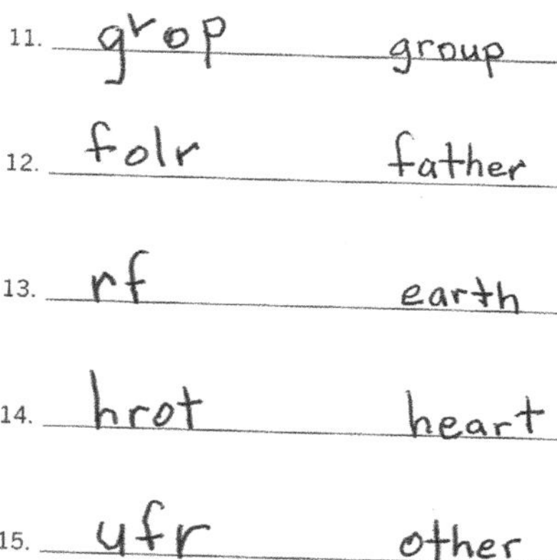

Figure 10.12   Gillian's Spellings on Test 5C, Irregular Word Spelling

of dyslexia. She achieved a Vocabulary and Reasoning-2 (VR2) composite SS of 109 (73rd percentile), in the high end of average range. This score can be contrasted with her DRI, which is statistically significantly weaker, occurring in only 1–5% of the TOD-C standardization sample. In addition, Gillian's pattern exemplifies the "expected" aspect of dyslexia described by the TOD authors; her LPI and her RSI are both well below average and weaker than her VR2.

TESTS OF DYSLEXIA RATING SCALES

TOD Rating Scale scores are reported in T-scores, which have a mean of 50 and standard deviation of 10. Scores of 59 and below are considered low to moderate risk. Scores between 60 and 69 indicate high risk for dyslexia, and scores of 70 and above indicate very high risk. Gillian's mother completed the Parent/Caregiver Form; her ratings yielded a T-score of 61, 86th percentile, which is in the High Risk range. Gillian completed the Self-Rating Form during the assessment session. Her ratings yielded a T-score of 60, 84th percentile, also in the High Risk range.

CAUTION

Not all individuals with dyslexia exhibit a clear-cut pattern of strengths in vocabulary and reasoning as compared to their linguistic and reading and spelling skills. Some have comorbid language difficulties which also negatively impact vocabulary acquisition. In addition, dyslexia occurs across the range of cognitive abilities. Especially for individuals with dyslexia who have participated in intensive instruction/intervention, all areas of linguistic processing may not be weak.

DON'T FORGET

Individuals with dyslexia typically have difficulty with reading **and** spelling, and, in some cases, their difficulties are most apparent in spelling, especially when they have received intensive instruction in basic reading skills. These individuals need continued intensive instruction to develop encoding (i.e., spelling) skills and to recognize and decode words.

SUMMARY AND RECOMMENDATIONS

The assessment results are consistent with a diagnosis of dyslexia with no indicators of attentional difficulties. Her reading and spelling skills are much weaker than her vocabulary and reasoning abilities. Although she has shown progress in developing phonological skills, her reading and spelling skills are hampered by reversals, difficulty with sequencing, and lack of automaticity and fluency. Her most significant areas of difficulty are in the areas of orthographic processing, spelling, and reading fluency. Her basic reading skills are still weak. Recent school-based assessment indicates Gillian's mathematical reasoning is average, but her math facts fluency is low average, in part because she sometimes misreads the math operation signs. Gillian's writing fluency is also slow, likely related to her lack of automaticity with spelling and letter formation.

Gillian has many strengths, including an engaging personality, strong vocabulary and listening comprehension, and a positive attitude. She is social and participates well in several sports. Thus far, she likes school and sees herself as a reader. Her parents are concerned, however, that she will lose confidence if she does not begin to make greater progress in reading, spelling, and writing.

Diagnostic Impressions from the American Psychiatric Association Diagnostic and Statistical Manual, 5th edition (DSM-5-TR):

F81.0 Specific learning disorder with impairment in reading (word reading accuracy, reading rate, or fluency)

F81.81 Specific learning disorder with impairment in written expression (spelling accuracy, grammar, and punctuation accuracy)

Gillian's pattern of performance meets criteria for the identification of a specific learning disorder in reading, based on the American Psychiatric Association's Diagnostic and Statistical Manual, 5th edition, Text Revision (DSM-5-TR). Findings are also consistent with the State Department of Education eligibility criteria for SLD in reading (basic reading skills, reading fluency) and in written expression.

In many ways, Gillian presents with a pronounced pattern of strengths and relative weaknesses often associated with average or high ability individuals with dyslexia. S. Shaywitz and Shaywitz (2020) aptly characterized dyslexia as a "weakness in a sea of strengths." The term *dyslexia* is simply an alternative way of referring to a specific learning disorder or disability in basic reading skills and/or reading fluency.

A school-based team should review these results to aid in educational planning for Gillian. She is in need of continued dyslexia-specific instruction consistent with Structured Literacy as described by the International Dyslexia Association (https://dyslexiaida.org/what-is-structured-literacy/). As noted, she has made progress in developing phonological skills, but instruction should continue in this area. She exhibited some subtle speech irregularities, such as mispronouncing common words (e.g., *degree* for *agree*). Further assessment in the area of speech production of multiple syllable words is recommended.

In general, Gillian should continue to benefit from explicit, systematic instruction to build phonology, phonics, and basic reading skills. She needs practice applying her skills by reading decodable books and explicit instruction in orthographic mapping, which will strengthen word recognition and spelling skills. Note: Specific instructional recommendations taken from the *TOD Intervention and Recommendations* guidebook and based on Gillian's performance on the TOD-C are provided below.

- Each day, introduce three or four words with regular sound–symbol (phoneme-grapheme) correspondence. Provide daily practice until Gillian masters these words. Have the student write the words in isolation and in sentences. Ask if the words are similar to any other words she has already learned. Discuss and practice other words that share the same phonograms. (A phonogram is a letter or letter combination that represents a speech sound).
- Explain to Gillian that there are three types of words: (a) words that are regular and are spelled exactly as they sound (sound words such as *cat* and *swim*); (b) words that are not regular but have a frequent spelling pattern that must be memorized (e.g., words such as *would* and *night*); and (c) words that are irregular and include a part of the word that must be memorized (e.g., words such as *said* and *they*). Explain to her that irregular words are often the most difficult to read and spell and that these words will require extra practice to master.
- Increase understanding of how the pronunciation of letters and words is related to their orthographic representations. Have Gillian process the sounds of each letter in a word to help recall the specific letter sequences and to establish familiarity with common letter patterns. For example, using word families with the same rime (e.g., -at, -an, -ig, -ight, -ound, -ack) have her add different onsets to the rime to build new words. (In a syllable, an onset is the initial consonant or group of consonants that precede the vowel; a rime is the ending part that begins with a vowel). These onsets can be consonants, including blends (two or three consonants that keep their identities) and digraphs (two letters that represent a single speech sound).
- Play a game in which you write a word, and Gillian can change only one letter to make a new word (e.g., sip, sin, tin, tip, tap, sap, map, mat). Pass the paper back and forth until one player cannot think of a new word.
- Gillian will benefit from practice in orthographic mapping (the process of assigning individual speech sounds to the letters that represent those sounds). For example, say: "map" and then segment (break apart) the word into its three sounds (/m/, /a/, /p/). Print the word "map" and point to each letter as you say each sound. Spend 5–10 minutes each day practicing orthographic mapping. Begin the instruction with words that have regular phoneme–grapheme correspondence. (A phoneme is an individual speech sound, and a grapheme is the letter or letter combination that represents a single speech sound).
- Use a speech-to-print approach to practice real words as Gillian sounds out words and then writes them. This activity requires Gillian to both segment (break apart) and blend (merge together) sounds. Start the instruction with only a few sounds and letters and have her sound out and spell consonant-vowel-consonant (CVC) words. Help her understand that

spoken words are composed of strings of sounds and that the letters we use stand for those sounds. Gradually introduce additional spelling patterns.

- Practice instant recognition of high-frequency words using a rapid word-recognition chart. Make a chart with five rows of six irregular or high-frequency words. Before timing Gillian, point to 8–10 words randomly as a warm-up. Time her for one minute, which may involve reading through the chart more than once; then, record the number of words read correctly in the minute. You can also make a chart that includes words with a common orthographic pattern (e.g., -tch) or a chart that contains decodable words.

- Use partner reading to provide practice in reading decodable text (reading material that includes words with regular sound–symbol correspondences and that is used to practice the application of common phonic elements). Pair Gillian (the reader) with another individual (the partner) who has a slightly higher reading level. Have the partner read a page aloud and then have Gillian reread the same page. Have the partners take turns reading aloud to each other. If the reader makes a mistake on a word, the partner should say, "Stop" and then have the reader look closely at the word and attempt to read it again. If the word is still incorrect, the partner should read the word. On another day, repeat this procedure, but pair Gillian with someone who has a slightly lower reading level. In this case, Gillian would be the partner, i.e., the first reader.

CLASSROOM AND STANDARDIZED TESTING ACCOMMODATION RECOMMENDATIONS

- Extended time (time and a half) on tests and assignments
- Note-taking assistance and/or access to instruct notes
- Use of text-to-speech software for reading assignments (Learning Ally can be a resource (https://learningally.org/).
- No penalty for spelling errors on routine assignments
- Minimize copying
- Provide strategies for correctly reading math signs (e.g., color code)

DON'T FORGET

Younger children with dyslexia often meet state criteria for a SLD in Basic Reading Skills. As they get older, they may also meet the criteria for SLD in Reading Fluency. Other reading-related skills (e.g., Reading Comprehension and Spelling) may also be weak.

It has been a pleasure to work with Gillian. I am available for consultation regarding her progress as needed. Selected cognitive and academic skills should be re-evaluated within three years, but some may warrant earlier re-evaluation to determine her progress.

✍ TEST YOURSELF ✍

1. **An examinee must score in the below average range on all four areas of linguistic processing assessed by the TOD-C in order to have a high probability of dyslexia.**
   True or False?

2. **Which of the following provides a probability that the examinee has a diagnosis of dyslexia?**
   (a) DRI
   (b) DDI
   (c) RSI
   (d) LPI

3. **The TOD-C direct assessment yields all but which of the following types of scores?**
   (a) Standard scores
   (b) Percentiles
   (c) Age-equivalents
   (d) T-scores

4. **Which of the following is not true of individuals with dyslexia?**
   (a) They typically have reading and spelling difficulties.
   (b) They tend to have most difficulty with reading comprehension.
   (c) They exhibit dyslexia characteristics across the age span.
   (d) Intensive instruction may improve their phonological skills.

5. **The unexpected "aspect" of dyslexia as measured by the TOD-C refers to significant differences between an examinee's**
   (a) reading and spelling skills.
   (b) linguistic processing abilities and reading and spelling skills.
   (c) vocabulary and reasoning abilities and reading and spelling skills.
   (d) vocabulary and reasoning abilities.

6. **The "expected" aspect of dyslexia refers to similar performance on an examinee's**
   (a) Linguistic Processing Index and Reading and Spelling Index.
   (b) Linguistic Processing Index and Vocabulary and Reasoning Composite.
   (c) Reading and Spelling Index and Vocabulary and Reasoning Composite.
   (d) Dyslexia Risk Index and Dyslexia Diagnostic Index.

7. **In addition to results of direct assessment, psychoeducational reports should include**
   (a) the reason for referral.
   (b) an interpretation of the results.
   (c) a summary of behavioral observations.
   (d) all of the above.

8. **The TOD software allows evaluators to select specific interventions based on an examinee's test performance.**
   True or False?

9. **Young students with dyslexia often meet state criteria for a Specific Learning Disability in which area?**
   (a) Basic Reading Skills
   (b) Oral Expression
   (c) Reading Comprehension
   (d) Written Expression

10. **Not all individuals with dyslexia exhibit a clear-cut pattern of strengths in vocabulary and reasoning as compared to their linguistic processing abilities and reading and spelling skills.**
    True or False?

Answers: 1. False; 2. b; 3. d; 4. b; 5. c; 6. a; 7. d; 8. True; 9. a; 10. True

REFERENCES

Catts, H. W., & Petscher, Y. (2022). A cumulative risk and resilience model of dyslexia. *Journal of Learning Disabilities, 55*(3), 171–184. https://doi.org/10.1177/00222194211037062

Mather, N., McCallum, R. S., Bell, S. M., & Wendling, B. J. (2024c). *Dyslexia interventions and recommendations: A companion guide to the Tests of Dyslexia (TOD)*. Western Psychological Services.

Shaywitz, S., & Shaywitz, J. (2020). *Overcoming dyslexia* (2nd ed.). Knopf.

Stanovich, K. E. (1986). Matthew effects in reading: Some consequences of individual differences in the acquisition of literacy. *Reading Research Quarterly, 22*, 360–407.

Appendix A

COMMONLY ASKED QUESTIONS

Who can use or purchase the TOD?

The components of the TOD can be used by a variety of personnel. For example, a classroom teacher may administer the TOD-Screener and complete the Teacher Rating Scale. Reading specialists, educational diagnosticians, psychologists, and speech-language pathologists are best suited to administer and interpret the TOD-Early or the TOD-Comprehensive due to their advanced coursework and experience with standardized tests. Teachers who are trained to administer the test and are supervised by professionals who have advanced training with standardized assessments may also administer the TOD-E or TOD-C. Administering a test requires one level of skill, whereas interpreting the results requires a higher level of skill. Therefore, a broader range of individuals can administer the test than can interpret the test. Interpretation requires a professional who is knowledgeable about dyslexia and has had formal training in test administration and scoring. Test publishers provide qualification guidelines to help determine who may purchase their tests. Western Psychological Services (WPS) has the following guidelines:

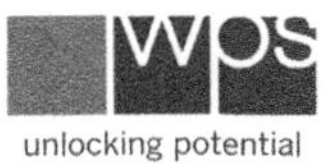

Qualification Guidelines

Letter code	Degree	Additional training	Products qualified to purchase
N	**Doctorate** A doctoral degree (e.g., PhD, PsyD, MD) in psychology or a related field (e.g., occupational therapy, speech–language pathology, special education)	None	All products
	Master's (plus additional training) A master's degree (e.g., MA, MS, MSW, CAGS) in psychology or a related field (e.g., occupational therapy, speech–language pathology, special education), plus additional training	Experience or training in neuropsychological assessment	
C	**Master's** A master's degree (e.g., MA, MS, MSW, CAGS) in psychology or a related field (e.g., occupational therapy, speech–language pathology, special education)	None	All products except advanced neuropsychological instruments
	Bachelor's (plus additional training) A bachelor's degree (e.g., BA, BS) in psychology or a related field (e.g., occupational therapy, speech–language pathology, special education), plus additional training	A license or certification from an agency/organization that requires training and experience in assessment	
B	**Bachelor's** A bachelor's degree (e.g., BA, BS) in psychology or a related field (e.g., occupational therapy, speech–language pathology, special education)	None	General screening materials, counseling materials, instructional materials, achievement tests
A	No degree requirement	None	Books and instructional materials only

WPS's qualification guidelines are for the purchase of materials through WPS. Additional training and experience may be required for the proper use of specific instruments.

WPS is a publisher and distributor of products that are used worldwide. We understand that many professionals with varying degrees and licensures use our products. The qualification guidelines described here are broad and do not provide an exhaustive list of which professionals may purchase our products.

Who can diagnose dyslexia?

There is no single job title that defines a person who can diagnose dyslexia. Originally, it was believed that dyslexia was a medical diagnosis. Today, it is viewed as an educational diagnosis. Dyslexia is recognized as a specific learning disability under the Individuals with Disabilities Education Act; it is also included in the Diagnostic and Statistical Manual of the American Psychiatric Association (DSM-5-TR) as a specific learning disorder in reading. Within a school setting, typically professionals within school-based teams who are well-versed in the characteristics of dyslexia and understand standardized assessments are best suited for making this diagnosis. The team could include reading specialists, school psychologists, educational diagnosticians, speech and language pathologists, and learning disability specialists. Within a private setting, this diagnosis would most commonly be made by a school psychologist, clinical psychologist, educational psychologist, neuropsychologist, dyslexia specialist, or speech-language pathologist.

What sets the TOD apart from other reading assessments?

Several factors set the TOD apart from other reading assessments. First, the TOD covers a wide age range and includes the major components that are needed for a comprehensive dyslexia assessment. One of the components is the TOD-Screener which is available in a print version and a digital version. Further assessment can be completed with the TOD-Early and the TOD-Comprehensive. There is no need to cobble together results from different tests with different norm groups. Second, the TOD differs from other reading assessments as it includes the reading and linguistic abilities that are most relevant to the diagnosis of dyslexia. The TOD includes measures of word recognition (untimed and timed), phonics knowledge, reading fluency, and comprehension efficiency (the ability to comprehend text under time pressure). The TOD also includes linguistic risk factors (e.g., phonological awareness, rapid automatized naming) that can help the examiner determine the factors that are affecting reading development. Third, the TOD includes measures of vocabulary and reasoning to help determine if the reading problem is specific and/or unexpected in relation to these abilities that do not require reading. Fourth, the TOD includes rating scales to help standardize the process of collecting information from parents, teachers, or individuals being assessed. Fifth, the TOD includes a guide to interventions to help facilitate the development of an instructional plan. Sixth, online scoring, reports, and intervention reports are available at no additional charge.

I am confused by the interpretive ranges for the DDI/EDDI. An average score of 90–109 doesn't seem to "fit" with the TOD DDI/EDDI Diagnostic Index Probability classification of "Low to Moderate Probability." Why isn't an average score just "low probability", not a range up to moderate probability?

The reason for moderate possibility is to be sure that high-ability examinees with dyslexia would not be missed by just using 'low' to describe this range. Students with a lot of intervention also could be missed if the range was just 'low'. Best practice suggests that a confidence band (+/−1 or more SEMs) should be considered when interpreting the obtained SS. A broader range of probability for the Dyslexia Diagnostic Index (DDI) or Early Dyslexia Diagnostic Index (EDDI) score in the 90–109 range provides more confidence in the classification. Other data such as rating scale information, Vocabulary and Reasoning scores, family history, and instructional history have to be considered as well. See page 80 of the Manual under Cautions for Interpreting the DDI for more explanations/rationales for the "Low to Moderate" range description.

Our school district won't let us use the term dyslexia or make a diagnosis of dyslexia. What should we do?

Some states or school districts may not want evaluators to use the word "dyslexia" as a diagnosis. In some cases, an evaluator may say: "exhibits characteristics of dyslexia." In other cases, the diagnosis may be a specific learning disability in basic reading skills or reading fluency (also known as dyslexia). The U.S. Department of Education (2015) released a Dear Colleague letter, stating that it was appropriate for school districts to use the terms, dyslexia, dyscalculia, and dysgraphia, in both evaluations and Individualized Education Programs (IEPs).

Why doesn't the TOD test for reading comprehension and written expression?

The TOD was designed to measure the abilities that are most relevant to the diagnosis of dyslexia: basic reading skills, reading fluency, and spelling. A few of the tests, however, do measure aspects of reading comprehension (e.g., TOD-3S: Question Reading Fluency and TOD-16C Silent Reading Efficiency). Poor reading comprehension and written expression are affected by dyslexia, but they are secondary consequences. Poor word reading or slow reading affects reading comprehension, and poor spelling affects written expression.

How early can a student be diagnosed with dyslexia?

Early warning signs for dyslexia can be identified in Pre-K–1. Although prior to formal reading instruction, it is difficult to make a definitive diagnosis of dyslexia, students can usually be identified as "at-risk" for reading failure when factors such as family history and early linguistic risk factors are considered. Ozernov-Palchik and Gaab (2016) described the "dyslexia paradox" where, unfortunately, dyslexia is typically not identified until a child is in second grade and has not learned to read as expected. The paradox is that early intervention is most effective when provided to children from Pre-K to Grade 1 prior to reading failure.

Ozernov-Palchik, O., & Gaab, N. (2016). Tackling the 'dyslexia paradox': Reading brain and behavior for early markers of developmental dyslexia. *WIREs Cognitive Science, 7*, 156–176. https://doi.org/10.1002/wcs.1383

What recommendations are suggested when assessing for dyslexia in middle- and high school students?

A comprehensive dyslexia assessment is important and can be completed using the TOD-C along with the TOD Rating Scales. These sources provide direct assessment of reading, spelling, and related skills/abilities from the TOD-C as well as current and historical perspectives of the examinee's reading/spelling performance from the examinee, parents, and teachers via the rating scales. Some students with dyslexia are not identified until middle or high school, especially students who are twice-exceptional, extremely hard-working, or who have had extensive explicit literacy instruction.

What warning signs could point to dyslexia in middle or high school students?

There are several warning signs to look for in middle or high school students with dyslexia. Examples include:

Has trouble keeping up with the volume of reading and written work.
Expresses frustration over the amount of time and energy it takes to read.
Reads slowly.
Needs to read material more than once because of limited fluency.
Has trouble using structural analysis to break apart unfamiliar words into syllables.
Has poor spelling and may spell the same word different ways.
Avoids reading and writing assignments.
Doesn't complete homework.
Has trouble learning a foreign language.

What are the best practices for assessing adults who may have dyslexia?

First, select an assessment that is normed for adults and includes content that is of an appropriate difficulty level. The TOD-C, which includes the TOD-S, is an assessment that is appropriate for adults. Second, collect relevant background information about the adult's education, work history, and family history. Have the adult complete a self-report rating scale designed to gather dyslexia-related information. The TOD-C Self-Rating Scale is designed for this purpose. The evaluator should also have experience in evaluating adults with dyslexia.

Many adults with dyslexia still exhibit slow reading rates; have difficulties with spelling; and may also have issues with attention, anxiety, and self-esteem.

How can the effects of ADHD be separated from dyslexia in an evaluation?

Dyslexia and ADHD are often comorbid, meaning they co-occur more often than would be expected by chance. The diagnostic process is somewhat similar for the two conditions, but the primary indicators differ. The primary indicator for a dyslexia diagnosis requires evidence of poor basic reading and spelling skills. The primary indicator for a diagnosis of ADHD requires evidence of a persistent pattern of inattention and/or hyperactivity-impulsivity that interferes with functioning or development.

Both types of evaluations require a thorough review of the individual's medical, family, and academic history as well as observation, permanent products from the classroom, and direct assessment. Much of this information can be provided through interviews and then supplemented from self, parent, and teacher rating scales, followed by direct assessment. The focus of this information is to determine the extent to which the examinee has the characteristics associated with either dyslexia (i.e., poor basic reading and spelling skills, difficulties in relevant linguistic processing skills) and/or ADHD (i.e., persistent patterns of inattention and/or hyperactivity-impulsivity that interfere with functioning or development).

Diagnostic indicators of ADHD are found in the Diagnostic and Statistical Manual-5-Text Revision (DSM-5-TR, 2022). Diagnosis of dyslexia may be guided by the DSM-5-TR or by state department of education criteria for special education eligibility. If an examiner identifies a sufficient number of indicators, such as inaccurate decoding, slow reading, and poor spelling, a diagnosis of dyslexia may be provided. Importantly, according to the DSM-5-TR, dyslexia is an alternative term used to refer to a pattern of reading-related learning difficulties and may be evidence of a Specific Learning Disorder. Similarly, if the examinee exhibits a sufficient number of specific indicators of (a): Inattention or (b) Hyperactivity/Impulsivity, or both, a diagnosis of ADHD may also be provided. An examiner uses the information from a psychoeducational assessment to determine if criteria for dyslexia and/*or* ADHD are present. For examinees who present with sufficient evidence of dyslexia *and* ADHD both diagnoses may be appropriate.

One other consideration is that some students with ADHD can pay attention in a one-to-one situation, such as during an assessment, but have difficulty sustaining attention in a classroom setting. Evaluations often provide short, focused tasks that change frequently, enhancing interest. A student's problems with attention and/or impulsive behavior may be more apparent during classroom observations than in a quiet, distraction-free, one-to-one setting.

American Psychiatric Association. (2022). *Diagnostic and statistical manual of mental disorders* (5th ed., Text Revision). https://doi.org/10.1176/appi.books.9780890425756

How can other learning disorders such as dysgraphia and dyscalculia complicate a dyslexia diagnosis?

Dyscalculia is a specific and persistent difficulty in understanding numbers, which can lead to a diverse range of difficulties with mathematics (British Dyslexia Association Handbook, 2022). Like dyslexia, dyscalculia is also a developmental learning disorder that affects the acquisition of mathematics. The primary linguistic risk factors found to be related to math disability include limitations in oral language, verbal working memory, processing speed, and rapid automatized naming. It is not uncommon for children who have difficulty automatizing letter names and sounds and words to also have difficulty automatizing math facts. In addition, lack of reading fluency or comprehension skills can negatively impact math problem solving. Dyscalculia is often comorbid with dyslexia (Pennington et al., 2019). For students who struggle with reading and mathematics, a comprehensive assessment of mathematical skills is recommended along with a comprehensive battery assessing reading, spelling, and related skills (e.g., Tests of Dyslexia).

Dysgraphia is a disorder of writing ability at any stage, including problems with letter formation/legibility, letter spacing, spelling, fine motor coordination, rate of writing, grammar, and composition (Chung et al., 2020, p. S46). It is sometimes characterized by impaired handwriting and spelling. Difficulty with handwriting can interfere with learning to spell words in isolation and written text. Children with dysgraphia may have only impaired handwriting, only impaired spelling (without reading problems), or both impaired handwriting and impaired spelling (International Dyslexia Association, n.d.). Individuals with dyslexia often have difficulty with written expression and poor spelling that contributes to weaknesses in handwriting and written expression more generally (Hebert et al., 2018). Poor spelling is associated with inhibited volume and sophistication of written expression, and those who exhibit these characteristics find writing to be more effortful than do peers; consequently, they avoid writing when possible (Wood et al., 2020). Individuals who struggle with learning to write often struggle with reading for the same reasons, as reading and writing involve many of the same skills. For example, reading requires decoding words using phonological ability of blending, and spelling requires encoding words using the phonological ability of segmenting. Further, writing relies on obtaining relevant information from reading and on rereading one's writing for errors (Hebert et al., 2018). Dyslexia and dysgraphia are often comorbid. For students with significant handwriting, spelling, and writing difficulties, a comprehensive assessment of written expression is recommended, in addition to a comprehensive test of reading, spelling, and relevant linguistic risk factors, all of which are included on the Tests of Dyslexia (TOD).

British Dyslexia Association Handbook. (2022). *Dyscalculia*. Retrieved from https://www.bdadyslexia.org.uk/dyscalculia

Chung, P. J., Patel, D. R., & Nizami, I. (2020). Disorder of written expression and dysgraphia: Definition, diagnosis, and management. *Translational Pediatrics, 9*(Suppl 1), S46–S54. https://doi.org/10.21037/tp.2019.11.01

Hebert, M., Kearns, D. M., Hayes, J. B., Bazis, P., & Cooper, S. (2018). Why children with dyslexia struggle with writing and how to help them. *Language, Speech, and Hearing Services in Schools, 49*, 843–863. https://doi.org/10.1044/2018_LSHSS-DYSLC-18-0024

International Dyslexia Association (n.d.). *Understanding dysgraphia*. Retrieved from https://dyslexiaida.org/understanding-dysgraphia/

Pennington, B. F., McGrath, L. M., & Peterson, R. L. (2019). *Diagnosing learning disorders: From science to practice* (3rd ed.). Guilford.

Wood, C., Schatschneider, C., & Wanzek, J. (2020). Matthew effects in writing productivity during second grade. *Reading and Writing, 33*, 1377–1398. https://doi.org/10.1007/s11145-019-10001-8.

How might an examiner clarify the overlap between developmental language disorders and dyslexia?

Dyslexia is often characterized as a localized weakness (e.g., the phonological component or module) within the larger language system. According to S. Shaywitz and Shaywitz (2020), the phonological module within the brain is where the sounds of the language are combined to form words and where the elements within these words are/or can be isolated as building blocks comprising these same basic sounds. This ability is sometimes referred to as phonological coding and has been described as the ability to use knowledge of letter-sound correspondences to read words. A second fundamental ability also contributes to printed word recognition—orthographic coding—which is the ability to recognize letter and word patterns to aid in pronunciation. Those with dyslexia may have deficits in both (Mather & Wendling, 2024), and both have been linked to specific and localized anomalies in the structure of the neural systems for reading (Seidenberg, 2017). Although dyslexia and developmental language disorders are comorbid, some problems within the language system are characterized as dyslexia, but others are not. Even though all language elements are inextricably linked, assessment experts disaggregate them for practical reasons. For example, individuals with dyslexia have difficulty acquiring the phonological, morphological, and orthographic aspects of written language, resulting in limitations in basic reading and spelling skills. In contrast, they often have strong vocabularies and good ability to comprehend spoken language.

Mather, N., & Wendling, B. J. (2024). *Essentials of dyslexia: Assessment and intervention* (2nd ed.). Wiley.

Seidenberg, M. (2017). *Language at the speed of sight: How we read, why so many can't, and what can be done about it.* Basic Books.

Shaywitz, S., & Shaywitz, J. (2020). *Overcoming dyslexia* (2nd ed.). Knopf.

How can sensory and executive function issues impact dyslexia and dyslexia assessment?

In some cases, sensory problems may underlie academic skill deficits. For example, individuals with significant hearing loss or auditory discrimination difficulties may be unable to discern the phonological aspects of the language, particularly the subtle differences in some speech sounds. Consequently, they will have problems mastering the phoneme-grapheme relationships necessary to develop proficiency in basic reading and spelling skills. Similarly, some vision problems may limit development of the orthographic processing skills necessary to master sight words and spelling patterns. When basic reading problems occur, visual and auditory acuity and related biological bases that potentially limit skill acquisition should be ruled out first. Similarly, poor executive functioning abilities may negatively impact the development of basic reading skills. In some situations, a neuropsychological assessment referral may be recommended if there are informal indicators of poor executive functioning (e.g., limited ability to set goals, plan and execute successful problem-solving strategies, monitor performance, and modify unsuccessful strategies as needed). Limitations in executive functioning can affect the acquisition of academic skills in general and may impact the ability to master early reading skills (e.g., impaired ability to set reading goals, having trouble learning strategies, or having difficulty persisting when tasks are challenging).

How can a dyslexia assessment be adapted for English learners?

According to Everatt et al. (2010), individuals who are learning to read in a language different from their native language will exhibit poor reading skills, at least temporarily. In addition, in bilingual settings, young learners have to cope with the demands of two languages simultaneously, and they may struggle with basic phonemic awareness because they have limited English vocabulary. Mather and Wendling (2024) noted that assessing an English learner for dyslexia is challenging and clinical judgment is important; they provide a summary of common evaluation practices from the literature though each has limitations as noted (e.g., Ortiz, 2011): (a) use of modified or adapted tests that might require eliminating or changing items, though such changes are not consistent with standardized administration procedures and may bias results, rendering the scores invalid; (b) use of an interpreter or translator, though examinees may not understand directions because of limited native language or lack of test content knowledge; (c) use of nonverbal tests, though these tests typically assess only cognitive abilities, which are less relevant for identifying dyslexia than the direct assessment of reading and spelling; (d) use of translated native-language tests, though these are typically standardized only on monolingual individuals in the native language; and (e) use of English language tests, though these may be biased, containing vocabulary words and directions unfamiliar to English learners. Mather and Wendling (2024) suggest some additional best practice strategies, such as beginning with early reading intervention and periodic measures of progress in reading and oral language over time. If reading development continues to lag behind oral language development, the examiner should then conduct standardized academic testing (in both languages if possible). Also, it is important to conduct interviews with parents and teachers and obtain rating scale data. The Tests of Dyslexia (TOD) includes parent rating scales in English and Spanish for both the TOD-Early and the TOD-Comprehensive. Ideally, the evaluation team would include an individual in the decision-making process who is fluent in the native language and/or is an expert in evaluating individuals from diverse backgrounds.

Everatt, J., Ovampo, D., Veii, K., Nenopolou, S., Smyth, I., al Mannai, H., & Elbeheri, G.(2010). Dyslexia in biscriptal readers. In N. Brunswick, S. McDougal, & P. de Mornay Davies (Eds.), *Reading and dyslexia in different orthographies* (pp. 221–246). Psychology Press.

Mather, N., & Wendling, B. J. (2024). *Essentials of dyslexia: Assessment and intervention* (2nd ed.). Wiley.

Ortiz, S. O. (2011). Separating cultural and linguistic differences (CLD) from specific learning disability (SLD) in the evaluation of diverse students: Differences or disorder? In D. P. Flanagan & V. C. Alfonso (Eds.), *Essentials of specific learning disability identification* (pp. 299–325). Wiley.

How can dyslexia be diagnosed when there aren't phonological weaknesses but reading difficulties exist?

First, it is critical to know the characteristic linguistic risk factors associated with dyslexia. Phonological weaknesses are limitations within oral language and have been the focus of research and instruction for years. For these reasons, individuals may have improved their phonological abilities through targeted instruction and may not currently exhibit a weakness in these skills. Phonological weaknesses, however, are not the only potential risk factors. Other linguistic risk factors (e.g., working memory, rapid automatized naming, orthographic processing) can contribute to reading difficulties. Second, it is important to identify the exact nature of the reading difficulties. Are the difficulties related to poor accuracy, poor fluency (e.g., slow reading of letters/words, poor understanding, lack of prosody), and/or poor spelling? Dyslexia may be identified not only by weaknesses in linguistic risk factors and reading and spelling, but also by the identification of cognitive and academic strengths as well. That is, many individuals with dyslexia have average or better overall general cognitive ability and typical academic functioning in non-affected areas (e.g., vocabulary, reasoning, math, science). Consequently, administration of a comprehensive test like the TOD may be needed to rule in/out dyslexia by assessing a wide range of abilities.

How do examiners know which tests to administer beyond those required to obtain the TOD-C Dyslexia Diagnostic Index?

Obtaining the DDI is an important step in an evaluation. The next step depends on the purpose for conducting the evaluation. If more information from the assessment is needed, look at the individual tests, composites, and indexes. The TOD Manual provides a roadmap for selecting additional tests via the Test Selection charts. The TOD-S and TOD-C Test Selection Chart is on page 11 of the TOD Manual and in Chapter 4 of this book. The TOD-S and TOD-E Test Selection Chart is on page 12 of the TOD Manual and in Chapter 3 of this book.

Further, a good understanding of the constructs measured is foundational to choosing specific tests. Several places in the TOD Manual provide help in developing an understanding of the constructs being measured. First, the Test Blueprint on page 4 presents the abilities measured by the TOD-S, TOD-C, and TOD-E. Pages 5 and 6 present descriptions of each test with more complete descriptions starting on page 66. Also, consult the following sections in the TOD Manual to help determine which additional tests to give: TOD Composites (p. 85), Comparing TOD Scores (p. 87), Further Diagnostic Considerations (p. 88), Identification of SLD (p. 91), and Qualitative Analyses with Instructional Implications (p. 99).

Some specific examples may help illustrate the process of determining which additional tests to give beyond Tests 1–9. If Tests 1–9 were administered, there would be a result for Irregular Word Spelling (5C). If the individual had difficulty with this test, an examiner would likely administer Regular Word Spelling (15C) to measure both types of spelling. Comparing the performance on these two types of spelling informs instruction. As another example, if the individual did poorly on Phonological Manipulation (4C), it might be helpful to administer the more basic phonological awareness tests, Blending (13C) and Segmenting (14C). If concerns exist about the individual's overall ability, administer Picture Analogies (10C). This test is combined with Picture Vocabulary (1S) to form the Vocabulary and Reasoning 2 composite score that gives an estimate of vocabulary and reasoning abilities. This composite can also be compared to the DDI, Linguistic Processing Index (LPI), and Reading and Spelling Index (RSI).

Other general things to consider when determining which additional tests to administer include:

Consider the referral question(s)/concerns and choose tests that assess skills/abilities of concern.
Consider areas of weakness as identified by the TOD Rating Scales or from other sources such as student work samples, observations, or referral questions.
Obtain composite scores for areas of weakness identified in Tests 1–9.

Obtain composite scores for major constructs of interest (e.g., phonological awareness, basic reading skills, reading fluency, orthographic processing, spelling, vocabulary and reasoning).

Obtain composite scores as needed to determine strengths and weaknesses and to satisfy diagnostic or special education eligibility guidelines.

What guidance is provided to help examiners decide what interventions are most appropriate to recommend?

The authors of the TOD had a goal to create comprehensive assessments and rating scales, but also to provide a resource that would address the issue of what to do after testing is completed. As a result, the TOD includes *Dyslexia Interventions and Recommendations, a Companion Guide to the TOD*. Each section of the guide covers a linguistic ability, a reading skill, or spelling skills that are assessed during a TOD administration. Relevant tests from the TOD are listed at beginning of each section. The ability or skill is introduced to enhance the reader's understanding of the construct. Guidance is then provided for selecting interventions, followed by specific recommendations and interventions. In addition, the guide provides a section on Accommodations, Self-advocacy/Strengths/and Transitions, a glossary of terms, and a reproducible Appendix on Teaching Students with Dyslexia. Once testing is completed, the examinee's identified weaknesses determine which sections of the guide to consult. The guide offers a developmental range of interventions and recommendations in each section. Choosing the most appropriate interventions or recommendations depends on the age or grade of the individual and the resources available.

Adapted from: WPS Frequently Asked Questions prepared by the TOD authors.

ANALYZING TOD SCORE REPORTS

The purpose of this Appendix is to provide additional practice in understanding and interpreting the Tests of Dyslexia (TOD) scores and score reports. For the first case, Derek, examples of information are presented that can be gleaned from administering and analyzing certain Tests of Dyslexia-Comprehensive (TOD-C) results, along with the TOD Rating Scales. Three additional cases are presented with test results and some questions to consider. The second case, Brock, presents results from the TOD-S. The third case, Elsa, presents results from the TOD-E. The final case, Amelia, presents results from the TOD-C. Answers to the questions are provided at the end of each case.

Case 1
Name: Derek Watson
Grade: 6

BACKGROUND

Derek is a sixth-grade student. He was first referred for an evaluation in the third grade and qualified as a student with a specific learning disability in the following areas: Basic Reading Skills, Reading Fluency, Reading Comprehension, and Written Expression. His sight word vocabulary was described as very limited and his writing as barely legible and full of spelling errors. The evaluator recommended that Derek receive specially designed instruction in basic reading, reading fluency, reading comprehension, and written expression. The evaluator also recommended that Derek be referred to the gifted program due to apparent strengths in verbal skills and general reasoning.

REASON FOR REFERRAL

Derek was referred this summer for an evaluation by his mother. She was concerned about his low reading and spelling skills as well as his negative attitude toward school. She wanted to know if Derek has dyslexia, and, if so, what the family should do to get him the help he needs. School personnel have also suggested that Derek should repeat the sixth grade.

TESTS ADMINISTERED

Derek was administered several tests from the TOD-C. Derek and his mother completed TOD-C Parent/Caregiver Rating Scales and Self-Rating Scales, respectively. Grade-based norms were used to determine Derek's scores on the TOD.

DDI, RSI, AND LPI

Derek's scores on the three TOD-C indexes are presented Figure B1.

Dyslexia Diagnostic Index (DDI), Reading and Spelling Index (RSI), and Linguistic Processing Index (LPI) Standard Scores					
TOD Index	**Sum of standard scores**	**Index standard score: Child age**	**Confidence interval: 90%**	**%ile rank**	**Descriptive range**
Dyslexia Diagnostic Index	580	59	55 - 63	0.3	Significantly Below Average
Reading and Spelling Index	254	60	53 - 67	0.4	Significantly Below Average
Linguistic Processing Index	326	73	67 - 79	4	Well Below Average

Descriptive ranges (based on standard scores): Significantly Below Average (69 and below); Well Below Average (70-79); Below Average (80-89); Average (90-109); Above Average (110-119); Well Above Average (120 and above).

Probability of dyslexia based on DDI standard score *	Extremely High Probability of Dyslexia

*Extremely Low (120 and above); Very Low (110-119); Low to Moderate (90-109); High (80-89); Very High (70-79); Extremely High (69 and below).

Figure B1   *Derek's DDI, RSI, and LPI Standard Scores*

The Dyslexia Diagnostic Index (DDI) is composed of the Reading and Spelling Index (RSI) and the Linguistic Processing Index (LPI). When interpreting the percentile rank, only 3 out of 1,000 grade- mates would have a DDI as low and only 4 out of 1,000 grade mates would have an RSI as low. (Note when the percentile rank includes a decimal, the comparison group is 1,000 individuals rather than 100). On the LPI, only 4 out of 100 grade mates would have a score as low. On the DDI, his index standard score is 59. For context, scores of 69 and below indicate an Extremely High Probability of Dyslexia. Figure B2 presents the Standard Score Profile.

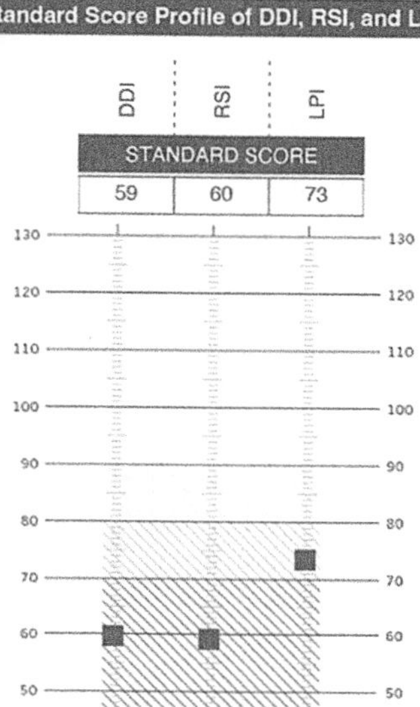

Figure B2   *Derek's Standard Score Profile of the DDI, RSI, and LPI*

DON'T FORGET

The TOD uses the following descriptors for the standard score ranges:

Description	Standard Score Range
Well Above Average	120 and above
Above Average	110–119
Average	90–109
Below Average	80–89
Well Below Average	70–79
Significantly Below Average	69 and below

TEST SCORES WITHIN THE DDI

The DDI includes eight tests. The standard score profile shows that Derek's Question Reading Fluency and Rapid Letter Naming scores are Extremely Low. In contrast, his Word Memory score fell within the Average range. When examining the scores on tests within the LPI (4C: Phonological Manipulation, 6C: Rapid Letter Naming, 8C: Word Pattern Choice, and 9C: Word Memory), his primary weakness was on the Rapid Letter Naming test, a measure of rapid automatized naming (RAN). When examining scores on tests within the RSI (2S: Letter and Word Choice, 3Sb: Question Reading Fluency, 5C Irregular Word Spelling, and 7C Pseudoword Reading), Derek's lowest score was on Question Reading Fluency. This score is consistent with his slow RAN, which is a strong predictor of reading rate. Figure B3 illustrates Derek's Standard Score Profile for the DDI.

Figure B4 illustrates a sample from the Standard Score Comparisons of Tests in the DDI showing how certain test scores compare to each other. Only 1–5% of the TOD standardization sample had significant differences of this size between the two tests.

> **CAUTION**
>
> The LPI is composed of four tests, each measuring a different linguistic processing ability that can affect reading and spelling development. In most cases, a student will not be low in all four areas, so it is important to review the scores on each of the four tests. The weakness may just be within one or two areas, such as slow RAN or a weakness in working memory.

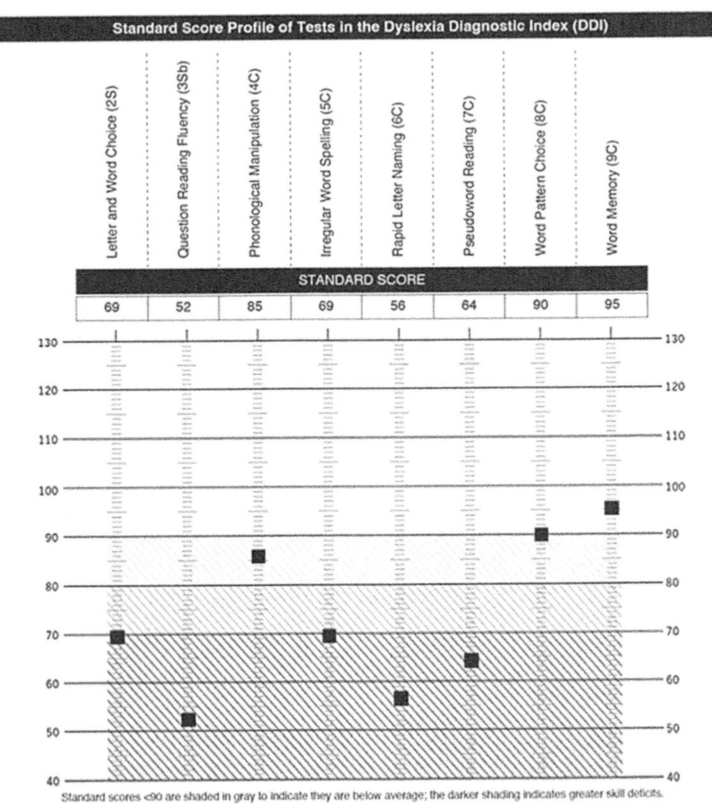

Figure B3 *Derek's Standard Score Profile of Tests in the DDI*

TOD-C COMPOSITE SCORES

The TOD-C composite scores indicate that both reading and spelling are significantly below average with linguistic processing weaknesses in both RAN and orthographic processing. In Derek's case, his vocabulary and reasoning scores are all Well Above Average. Dyslexia is often

Standard Score Comparisons of Tests in the DDI			
TOD test scores compared	Difference in standard scores	Significant difference	Percentage of sample with this difference
Question Reading Fluency vs. Word Memory	43	Yes	1%-5%
Question Reading Fluency vs. Word Pattern Choice	38	Yes	1%-5%
Rapid Letter Naming vs. Word Memory	39	Yes	1%-5%
Rapid Letter Naming vs. Word Pattern Choice	34	Yes	1%-5%

Comparisons significant at p<.05 are listed. Nonsignificant differences are not included in this table.

Figure B4   *Derek's Standard Scores Comparisons of Tests in the DDI*

Score Summary of TOD-C Composites					
TOD-C composite	Sum of standard scores	Composite standard score: Child age	Confidence interval: 90%	%ile rank	Descriptive range
Basic Reading Skills	124	63	57 - 69	1	Significantly Below Average
Spelling	139	68	62 - 74	2	Significantly Below Average
Rapid Automatized Naming	116	52	50 - 54	0.1	Significantly Below Average
Auditory Working Memory	181	89	81 - 97	23	Below Average
Orthographic Processing	159	73	63 - 83	4	Well Below Average
Vocabulary	234	119	110 - 128	90	Above Average
Reasoning	250	130	123 - 130	98	Well Above Average
Vocabulary and Reasoning 2	243	128	121 - 130	97	Well Above Average
Vocabulary and Reasoning 4	484	130	123 - 130	98	Well Above Average

Descriptive ranges (based on standard scores): Significantly Below Average (69 and below); Well Below Average (70-79); Below Average (80-89); Average (90-109); Above Average (110-119); Well Above Average (120 and above).

Figure B5   *Derek's Score Summary of TOD-C Composites*

Standard Score Comparisons of TOD-C Composites and Indexes			
TOD-C composite and Index scores compared	Difference in standard scores	Significant difference	Percentage of sample with this difference
Dyslexia Diagnostic Index vs. Vocabulary and Reasoning 4	71	Yes	<1%
Basic Reading Skills vs. Vocabulary and Reasoning 4	67	Yes	<1%

Figure B6   *Derek's Standard Score Comparisons of TOD-C Composites and Indexes*

described as "unexpected" reading failure because many other abilities are intact and inconsistent with difficulty learning to read. Figure B5 illustrates Derek's scores on the TOD composites.

Certain TOD-C composites can be compared to the indexes. When Derek's DDI is compared to the Vocabulary and Reasoning 4 (VR4) composite, less than 1% of the norm sample exhibits a difference of this magnitude. Similar results were obtained when Basic Reading Skills was compared to the VR4 composite. It is extremely unusual for Derek to be so far behind same-grade peers in reading given his advanced vocabulary and reasoning abilities. Figure B6 presents comparisons of the TOD-C composites and indexes.

SELECTING TESTS TO ADMINISTER

In some cases, evaluators will start the administration with the first nine tests of the TOD-C that create the DDI, RSI, and LPI. Although Test 1S: Picture Vocabulary does not contribute to these indexes, it can be reviewed to determine if the vocabulary score is higher than the reading scores. In contrast to the other tests, Derek's Picture Vocabulary test score was well above average. When comparing his Picture Vocabulary score to the DDI, less than 1% of same-grade individuals (based on the TOD standardization sample) would have a difference of that magnitude. Figure B7 illustrates standard score comparisons between the LPI and RSI and the DDI and Picture Vocabulary.

> **DON'T FORGET**
>
> Do not ask students to read quickly if they are not yet accurate.

After scoring the first nine tests, a decision should be made about additional tests to administer. In Derek's case, because his basic reading skills and reading fluency scores were so low, there was no point in administering any of the timed tests: 12C: Oral Reading Efficiency, 16C: Silent Reading Efficiency, 19C: Rapid Pseudoword Reading, or 20C: Rapid Irregular Word Reading.

Because Derek's score on 6C: Rapid Letter Naming was so low, the evaluator chose to administer the other RAN test, 17C: Rapid Number and Letter Naming, to obtain the RAN composite score and to confirm that RAN is a significant weakness. The evaluator also chose to administer 1S: Picture Vocabulary, 10C: Picture Analogies, 22C: Listening Vocabulary, and 23C: Geometric Analogies, to obtain the VR4 composite, to confirm Derek's strengths in these areas. The evaluator also administered 11C: Irregular Word Reading and 15C: Regular Word Spelling to learn more about Derek's ability to read and spell both phonically regular and irregular words. Because of time constraints, 13C: Blending and 14C: Segmenting were not administered during this first meeting. Given Derek's poor performance on 4C: Phonological Manipulation, these two tests should be administered in a follow-up evaluation because they measure more basic phonological skills.

ERROR ANALYSES

Instructional tips can be gained from analyzing the types of errors that a student makes when reading and spelling. As noted, Derek had a very low score on 3Sb: Question Reading Fluency.

Standard Score Comparisons of DDI, RSI, LPI, and PV-S			
Standard score	Difference in standard scores	Significant difference	Percentage of sample with this difference
Linguistic Processing Index vs. Reading and Spelling Index	13	Yes	20%-25%
Picture Vocabulary vs. Dyslexia Diagnostic Index	54	Yes	<1%

Figure B7 Derek's Standard Score Comparisons of the LPI vs. RSI and the DDI vs. Picture Vocabulary

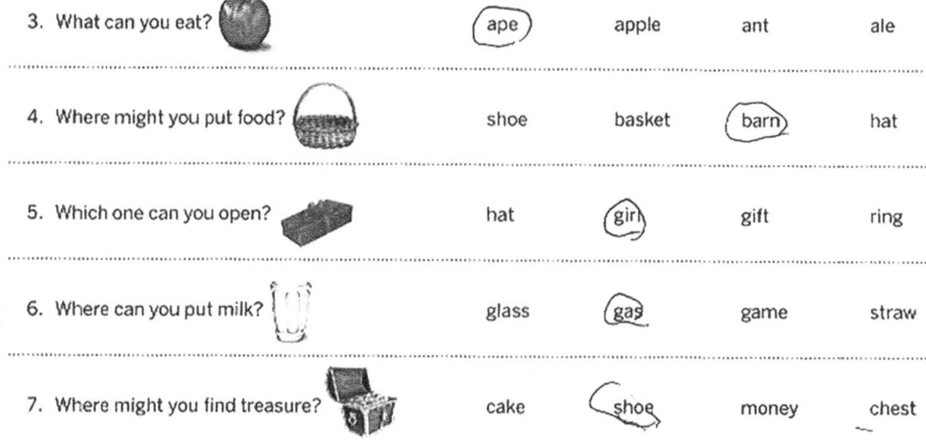

Figure B8   Derek's Responses on Question Reading Fluency

Figure B9   Derek's Responses on Irregular Word Spelling

Based on his errors, it is clear that he cannot read even relatively simple words. Figure B8 illustrates a few of his responses on Question Reading Fluency.

Based on the pattern of his responses on 5C: Irregular Word Spelling, it is apparent that he hears the sounds in words but does not know the correct spellings of those words. Figure B9 illustrates a few of his responses on Irregular Word Spelling.

On 7C: Pseudoword Reading, Derek confused the /b/ sound by producing a /d/ sound. Although he identified the first sound on several of the initial nonsense words, he only read one nonsense word correctly. On 11C: Irregular Word Reading, Derek was able to identify the individual letters but did not read any of the words correctly. He did, however, identify the word *off* as "of."

TOD-C RATING SCALES

Derek's mother completed the TOD-C Parent/Caregiver Rating Scale, and Derek completed the TOD-C Self-Rating Scale. Because this evaluation was conducted in the summer, a Teacher Rating Scale was not administered. On the Parent/Caregiver Rating Scale, his mother's ratings resulted in a T-score that indicated a Very High Risk for dyslexia. With the exceptions of General Reasoning and Verbal Comprehension, she noted that he had major difficulties in all areas. Figure B10 presents her Score Profile on the rating scale.

His mother also noted a family history of reading difficulties in another relative, but that relative was not specified. She noted a history of vision problems and that Derek had received both speech-language and reading support services in school. After reviewing this information, the evaluator may want to ask the mother additional questions about Derek's vision problems and family history, particularly whether his vision problems have been corrected. Figure B11 illustrates her responses to the background Information.

On the TOD-C Self-Rating Scale, similar to his mother's, Derek's ratings resulted in a T-score that indicated a Very High Risk for dyslexia. Both Derek and his mother agree that he has no weaknesses in General Reasoning and minor to some difficulty with Verbal Comprehension. Derek indicated he had some difficulty with phonological processing, memory, and reading comprehension with major difficulties in orthographic processing, basic reading skills, reading fluency, and spelling. Figure B12 illustrates Derek's Score Profile.

Derek was unaware of any family members with reading difficulties. He noted that he received extra help with reading from his in-class teacher who read to him when she had the time. He stated that he was not receiving any direct services. Figure B13 illustrates his responses on the background information.

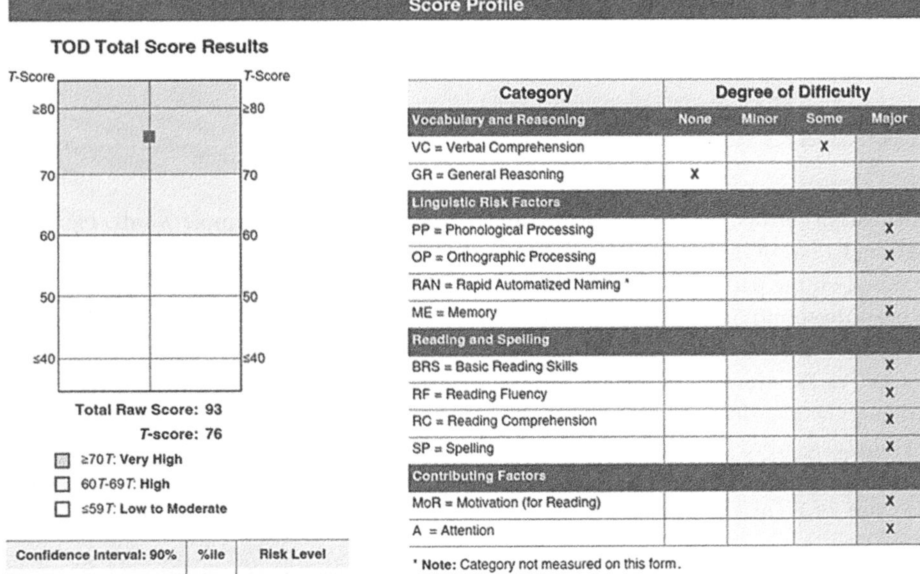

Category	Degree of Difficulty			
Vocabulary and Reasoning	None	Minor	Some	Major
VC = Verbal Comprehension			X	
GR = General Reasoning	X			
Linguistic Risk Factors				
PP = Phonological Processing				X
OP = Orthographic Processing				X
RAN = Rapid Automatized Naming *				
ME = Memory				X
Reading and Spelling				
BRS = Basic Reading Skills				X
RF = Reading Fluency				X
RC = Reading Comprehension				X
SP = Spelling				X
Contributing Factors				
MoR = Motivation (for Reading)				X
A = Attention				X

* **Note:** Category not measured on this form.

The Rating Scale *T*-score indicates a Very High Risk for dyslexia. Considerable difficulties in reading, spelling, and related skill areas are present. Item-level responses, as well as additional data from TOD tests, will be helpful in understanding the areas of difficulty.

Figure B10   *Derek's Score Profile of TOD-C Parent/Caregiver Rating Scale*

Background information	
The individual...	**Response**
1. Has a family history of reading difficulties.	Yes
If yes, please check all that apply:	Other Relative
If other relative, please specify:	No paternal history
2. Has/had an educational, medical, or behavioral diagnosis.	No
If yes, please specify:	
3. Has a history of vision problems.	Yes
4. Has a history of ear infections or tubes in ears.	No
5. Receives/received speech and/or language services.	Yes
6. Receives/received additional reading support services in school.	Yes
7. Receives/received extra outside tutoring for reading.	No
8. Has repeated (or is repeating) a grade.	No

Figure B11   *Derek's Mother's Responses on the Background Information*

Score Profile

TOD Total Score Results

Total Raw Score: 110

T-score: 70

- ≥70 T: **Very High**
- 60 T–69 T: **High**
- ≤59 T: **Low to Moderate**

Confidence Interval: 90%	%ile	Risk Level
66 - 74	98	Very High Risk

Category	Degree of Difficulty			
Vocabulary and Reasoning	None	Minor	Some	Major
VC = Verbal Comprehension		X		
GR = General Reasoning	X			
Linguistic Risk Factors				
PP = Phonological Processing			X	
OP = Orthographic Processing				X
RAN = Rapid Automatized Naming *				
ME = Memory			X	
Reading and Spelling				
BRS = Basic Reading Skills				X
RF = Reading Fluency				X
RC = Reading Comprehension			X	
SP = Spelling				X
Contributing Factors				
MoR = Motivation (for Reading)				X
A = Attention *				

* **Note:** Category not measured on this form.

The Rating Scale *T*-score indicates a Very High Risk for dyslexia. Considerable difficulties in reading, spelling, and related skill areas are present. Item-level responses, as well as additional data from TOD tests, will be helpful in understanding the areas of difficulty.

Figure B12   *Derek's Score Profile on the Self-Rating Scale*

Background information		Response
1.	One or more of my family members has/had difficulty with reading.	No
2.	One or more of my family members has/had difficulty with spelling.	No
3.	I have had ear infections or tubes in my ears.	No
4.	I receive/received extra help with reading.	Yes
	If yes, please specify:	In class teacher reads to me when she has time.

Figure B13   *Derek's Responses on the Background Information*

CONCLUSIONS

Results from this and past evaluations indicate that Derek is extremely intelligent but has severe dyslexia that has affected his reading and spelling development. His vocabulary and reasoning abilities are in the Well Above Average range in contrast to his extremely low reading and spelling scores. Despite years of being identified as a student with a specific learning disability, he has made very limited progress and essentially cannot read even first-grade text with accuracy. Derek requires systematic, intensive instruction in basic reading skills and spelling. He would benefit from enrollment in a school that specializes in instruction for students with dyslexia or, as an alternative, daily one-hour instruction five days a week from a reading specialist who is trained in structured literacy. Although he is receiving some accommodations in his current educational placement, he is not being taught how to read and spell words. Even though school personnel have discussed retention as an option, repeating a grade is not recommended as an appropriate solution to address Derek's needs.

Case 2
Name: Brock Bryant
Grade: 2

Midway through grade 1, Brock began participating in reading intervention at his school. He began after-school tutoring shortly after entering grade 2. Brock's teacher noted that he tends to mix up letters, numbers, and words. His grades in English/ Language Arts tend to be low, and his scores on the school's universal reading screeners are described as low. Thus, he was referred for a psychoeducational evaluation. As a first step in the assessment process, Brock was administered the TOD-S. His scores are shown in Figure B14.

1. **Do the TOD-S results indicate the need for further assessment? Why or why not?**
2. **Brock's Dyslexia Risk Index (DRI) standard score is equal to or higher than what percent of the norm group?**
3. **Is Brock's performance on the DRI unexpectedly low? Why or why not?**
4. **When Brock's Picture Vocabulary is compared to his DRI, what percentage of the sample would have a difference that size?**

Score Summary								
Test number	Test name	Raw score		Standard score	Confidence interval: 90%	%ile rank	Equivalent: Child age	Descriptive range
		Raw score	Ability score					
1S	Picture Vocabulary	19	121	105	94 - 116	63	9:0 to 9:5	Average
2S	Letter and Word Choice	13	102	85	75 - 95	16	6:4 to 6:7	Below Average
3Sb	Question Reading Fluency	23		93	88 - 98	32	7:4 to 7:7	Average

Dyslexia Risk Index (DRI)

Sum of standard scores for DRI (Letter and Word Choice + Reading Fluency)	DRI standard score: Child age	Confidence interval: 90%	%ile rank	Risk of dyslexia based on DRI*
178	87	79 - 95	19	At-Risk

* No to Low Risk (110 and above); Possible Risk (90-109); At-Risk (89 and below).

Standard Score Comparisons of TOD-S Tests and DRI

TOD-S scores compared	Difference in standard scores	Significant difference	Percentage of sample with this difference
Picture Vocabulary vs. Dyslexia Risk Index	18	Yes	20%
Picture Vocabulary vs. Letter and Word Choice	20	Yes	15%

Comparison between DDI and PV is included regardless of significance. For other comparisons, only those significant at p<.05 are listed.

Figure B14   *Brock's TOD-S Score Summary, DRI, and Standard Score Comparisons*

ANSWERS FOR CASE 2: BROCK

1. Yes, Brock's DRI is in the At-Risk range. In addition, his DRI is significantly lower than his Picture Vocabulary score.

2. His score is equal to or higher than 19% of the norm group. (Percentile rank of 19)

3. Yes, Brock's performance on the DRI is lower than would be expected when compared to his Picture Vocabulary score.

4. The difference between his Picture Vocabulary and DRI is significant and occurred in 20% or less of the norm group.

Case 3
Name: Elsa Harper
Grade: 1

Elsa will begin 2nd grade next month. Her parents opted for her to start kindergarten at age 6 due to her late summer birthdate and concerns about school readiness. She has a strong vocabulary, but she met developmental milestones a little late (e.g., delays in speech sound production, walking, and toilet training). Based on her performance on her school's universal reading screener, Elsa began receiving tiered instruction (Tier II) midway through kindergarten and has received more intensive instruction (Tier III) during the first grade. The extra instruction has

		Raw score						
Test number	Test name	Raw score	Ability score	Standard score	Confidence interval: 90%	%ile rank	Equivalent: Child grade	Descriptive range
1S	Picture Vocabulary	25	119	110	100 - 120	75	2 - Spring	Above Average
2S	Letter and Word Choice	16	94	86	78 - 94	18	K - Spring	Below Average
3Sa	Word Reading Fluency	13		81	75 - 87	10	K - Fall	Below Average

Score Summary

Dyslexia Risk Index (DRI)

Sum of standard scores for DRI (Letter and Word Choice + Reading Fluency)	DRI standard score: Child grade	Confidence interval: 90%	%ile rank	Risk of dyslexia based on DRI*
167	80	70 - 90	9	At-Risk

* No to Low Risk (110 and above); Possible Risk (90-109); At-Risk (89 and below).

Standard Score Comparisons of TOD-S Tests and DRI

TOD-S scores compared	Difference in standard scores	Significant difference	Percentage of sample with this difference
Picture Vocabulary vs. Dyslexia Risk Index	30	Yes	1%-5%
Picture Vocabulary vs. Letter and Word Choice	24	Yes	5%-10%
Picture Vocabulary vs. Word Reading Fluency	29	Yes	5%

Comparison between DDI and PV is included regardless of significance. For other comparisons, only those significant at p<.05 are listed.

Figure B15   *Elsa's TOD-S Score Summary, DRI, and Standard Score Comparisons*

focused primarily on phonological awareness and early phonics skills. She was referred for an assessment to determine the extent to which she exhibits characteristics of dyslexia. The TOD-S was administered digitally using a tablet, followed by the TOD-E a few days later. Grade-based norms were used to calculate her standard scores because she is a little older than the typical student who has just completed 1ˢᵗ grade. Figure B15 shows her scores on the TOD-S.

1. **Do the TOD-S results indicate the need for further assessment? Why or why not?**

2. **How uncommon is the difference between Elsa's Picture Vocabulary score and her DRI score? Letter and Word Choice score? Word Reading Fluency score?**

3. **Based on her performance on the TOD-S, Elsa was administered the TOD-E. Figure B16 presents her scores on the TOD-E. Which test scores are of most concern?**

4. **Some of Elsa's scores are in the average range for her grade placement. Given her history, why might Elsa's scores on Tests 4E Sounds and Pseudowords, 8E Early Segmenting, and 9E Letter and Sound Knowledge be in the average range?**

DON'T FORGET

Tests 2S through 9E make up the EDDI. Tests 5E, 6E, and 8E are the TOD-E linguistic processing tests that make up the ELPI. Tests 2S, 3E, 4E, 7E, and 9E make up the ERSI. Picture Vocabulary does not contribute to these scores but can be compared to other scores and can help determine unexpectedness or if there is a weakness in vocabulary.

Test number	Test name	Raw score		Standard score	Confidence interval: 90%	%ile rank	Equivalent: Child grade	Descriptive range
		Raw score	Ability score					
1S	Picture Vocabulary	25	119	110	100 - 120	75	2 - Spring	Above Average
2S	Letter and Word Choice	16	94	86	78 - 94	18	K - Spring	Below Average
3Sa	Word Reading Fluency	13		81	75 - 87	10	K - Fall	Below Average
4E	Sounds and Pseudowords	17		95	89 - 101	37	1 - Fall	Average
5E	Rhyming	8		77	71 - 83	6	K - Fall	Well Below Average
6E	Early Rapid Number and Letter Naming	34		76	67 - 85	5	< Start grade	Well Below Average
7E	Letter and Sight Word Recognition	25		92	88 - 96	30	1 - Fall	Average
8E	Early Segmenting	21		106	101 - 111	66	2 - Fall	Average
9E	Letter and Sound Knowledge	30		104	99 - 109	61	2 - Fall	Average

Descriptive ranges (based on standard scores): Significantly Below Average (69 and below); Well Below Average (70-79); Below Average (80-89); Average (90-109); Above Average (110-119); Well Above Average (120 and above)

Figure B16   *Elsa's TOD-E Score Summary*

5. On Early Rapid Number and Letter Naming, what does "<Start grade" mean?

Figure B17 presents Elsa's EDDI, ERSI, and ELPI scores

Early Dyslexia Diagnostic Index (EDDI), Early Reading and Spelling Index (ERSI), and Early Linguistic Processing Index (ELPI) Standard Scores

TOD Index	Sum of standard scores	Index standard score: Child grade	Confidence interval: 90%	%ile rank	Descriptive range
Early Dyslexia Diagnostic Index	734	87	84 - 90	19	Below Average
Early Reading and Spelling Index	457	88	83 - 93	21	Below Average
Early Linguistic Processing Index	277	90	86 - 94	25	Average

Descriptive ranges (based on standard scores): Significantly Below Average (69 and below); Well Below Average (70-79); Below Average (80-89); Average (90-109); Above Average (110-119); Well Above Average (120 and above).

Probability of dyslexia based on EDDI standard score *	High Probability of Dyslexia

*Extremely Low (120 and above), Very Low (110-119), Low to Moderate (90-109), High (80-89), Very High (70-79), Extremely High (69 and below)

Figure B17   *Elsa's EDDI, ERSI, ELPI Standard Scores*

6. Elsa's ELPI is in the average range. Why does the EDDI indicate High Probability of dyslexia?

7. The TOD-E provides a figure of statistically significant differences in scores between the EDDI and Picture Vocabulary and between the ELPI and the ERSI. Figure B18 shows Elsa's statistically significant differences. What relevance does the statistically significant difference between Elsa's Picture Vocabulary and her EDDI scores have for making a diagnosis of dyslexia?

Standard Score Comparisons of EDDI, ERSI, ELPI, and PV-S			
Standard score	Difference in standard scores	Significant difference	Percentage of sample with this difference
Early Dyslexia Diagnostic Index vs. Picture Vocabulary	26	Yes	1%-5%
Early Linguistic Processing Index vs. Early Reading and Spelling Index	7	No	

Figure B18   *Elsa's Standard Scores Comparisons of the EDDI vs. PV and ELPI vs. ERSI*

8. **Does the non-significant difference between Elsa's ELPI and her ERSI show the "expected" aspect of dyslexia? How does this relate to a diagnosis of dyslexia?**

   Figure B19 shows Elsa's scores on the TOD-E composites.

TOD-E composite	Sum of standard scores	Composite standard score: Child grade	Confidence interval: 90%	%ile rank	Descriptive range
Early Sight Word Acquisition	181	88	81 - 95	21	Below Average
Early Phonics Knowledge	176	86	80 - 92	18	Below Average
Early Basic Reading Skills	187	92	88 - 96	30	Average
Early Phonological Awareness	194	96	90 - 102	39	Average

Descriptive ranges (based on standard scores): Significantly Below Average (69 and below); Well Below Average (70-79); Below Average (80-89); Average (90-109); Above Average (110-119); Well Above Average (120 and above).

Figure B19   *Elsa's Scores on the TOD-E Composites*

9. **Do Elsa's TOD-E composite scores suggest she has dyslexia? Why or why not?**

10. **Considering Elsa's performance on the TOD-S and TOD-E individual tests and composites, and after referring to the *TOD's Dyslexia Interventions and Recommendations* guide, what instructional recommendations would you make for Elsa?**

ANSWERS TO CASE 3: ELSA

1. Yes, further assessment is indicated. Elsa's DRI is in the At-Risk range. Also, two of the three tests are below average – both of which are related to reading skills. Oral language/ vocabulary was Above Average.

2. All differences were significant. The difference between Elsa's Picture Vocabulary score and her DRI is very uncommon, occurring in only 1–5% of the norm sample; the difference between her Picture Vocabulary and her Letter and Word Choice occurred in only 5–10% of the norm sample and the difference between her Picture Vocabulary and Word Reading Fluency occurred in only 5% of the norm sample.

3. Elsa's scores on Tests 5E: Rhyming and 6E: Early Rapid Number and Letter Naming are of the most concern because they are in the Well Below Average range and because they are linguistic abilities that are often weak in individuals with dyslexia.

4. Elsa has participated in intensive intervention focused primarily on phonological awareness and early phonics skills, which are areas of performance assessed by Tests 4E, 8E, and 9E. These results show that the intervention likely was effective in building these early skills.

5. "<Start grade" means that her performance was lower than children entering Kindergarten, which is the start grade, or the lowest grade in the norm sample.

6. Elsa's performance on the ELPI is at the low end of average. The ELPI is comprised of two tests on which Elsa performed in the Well Below Average range (Test 5E: Rhyming and 6E: Early Rapid Number and Letter Naming), but she performed in the Average range on the third (Test 9E: Letter and Sound Knowledge). Elsa has received significant intervention in phonological skills, which has likely boosted her ability to identify first, last, and middle sounds and the letters that represent those sounds.

7. For most people, their level of proficiency in vocabulary is similar to their level of performance in reading and spelling. That is often not the case for individuals with dyslexia (like Elsa) whose reading and spelling performance is typically lower than vocabulary. Only 1–5% of the sample had a difference of that size between their Picture Vocabulary and EDDI scores. This is a pattern that represents the "unexpected" nature of dyslexia – good vocabulary ability, but poor reading skills.

8. Elsa's ELPI and ERSI are not significantly different, which exemplifies the "expected" relationship between linguistic processing and reading and spelling for individuals with dyslexia. If the underlying linguistic abilities are weak, then difficulties with reading and spelling are expected.

9. Elsa's scores on two of the TOD-E composites fell in the Below Average range despite intensive extra instruction. Yes, the scores are suggestive of dyslexia.

10. Elsa needs continued explicit, systematic, intensive intervention to build her reading and spelling skills. She appears to have benefitted from this in that some of her phonological and early phonics and word recognition skills are in the average range. Selected recommendations should focus on continued instruction in the ability to blend sounds fluently while reading words and to expand her sight word vocabulary. Her early encoding skills are weak, so she will benefit from learning to recognize and spell words simultaneously. Use of a phoneme-grapheme mapping program is recommended to build her orthographic knowledge, which will enhance her decoding and encoding skills. She needs practice reading both decodable texts and easy readers with basic sight words. Her vocabulary is a strength and can be used to help her remember words.

Case 4
Name: Amelia James
Grade: 2nd

REASON FOR REFERRAL

Amelia was referred by her second-grade teacher who was concerned about her slow reading and spelling development.

TOD-S

Amelia was administered the TOD-S. Figure B20 presents her scores.

1. **When analyzing the TOD-S results, what findings suggest a need for more testing?**

Score Summary								
Test number	Test name	Raw score		Standard score	Confidence interval: 90%	%ile rank	Equivalent: Child age	Descriptive range
		Raw score	Ability score					
1S	Picture Vocabulary	22	127	113	102 - 124	81	11:0 to 11:5	Above Average
2S	Letter and Word Choice	11	99	82	72 - 92	12	6:4 to 6:7	Below Average
3Sb	Question Reading Fluency	20		88	83 - 93	21	7:0 to 7:3	Below Average

Figure B20   *Amelia's TOD-S Score Summary*

Figure B21 shows Amelia's Dyslexia Risk Index (DRI) score.

2. **The DRI indicates that Amelia is at-risk for dyslexia. What does her percentile rank of 12 mean?**

Dyslexia Risk Index (DRI)				
Sum of standard scores for DRI (Letter and Word Choice + Reading Fluency)	DRI standard score: Child age	Confidence interval: 90%	%ile rank	Risk of dyslexia based on DRI*
170	82	74 - 90	12	At-Risk

* No to Low Risk (110 and above); Possible Risk (90-109); At-Risk (89 and below).

Figure B21   *Amelia's scores on the Dyslexia Risk Index*

Figure B22 compares Picture Vocabulary to the TOD-S tests and the DRI.

3. **What percentage of the sample would have a significant difference the same size as Amelia between Picture Vocabulary and the DRI?**

Standard Score Comparisons of TOD-S Tests and DRI			
TOD-S scores compared	Difference in standard scores	Significant difference	Percentage of sample with this difference
Picture Vocabulary vs. Dyslexia Risk Index	31	Yes	1%-5%
Picture Vocabulary vs. Letter and Word Choice	31	Yes	1%-5%
Picture Vocabulary vs. Question Reading Fluency	25	Yes	10%-15%

Comparison between DDI and PV is included regardless of significance. For other comparisons, only those significant at p<.05 are listed.

Figure B22   *Amelia's Standard Scores Comparisons of TOD-S Tests and DRI*

TOD-C RESULTS

Figure B23 presents Amelia's results on Picture Vocabulary and the eight tests of the DDI.

Test number	Test name	Raw score		Standard score	Confidence interval: 90%	%ile rank	Equivalent: Child age	Descriptive range
		Raw score	Ability score					
1S	Picture Vocabulary	22	127	113	102 - 124	81	11:0 to 11:5	Above Average
2S	Letter and Word Choice	11	99	82	72 - 92	12	6:4 to 6:7	Below Average
3Sb	Question Reading Fluency	20		88	83 - 93	21	7:0 to 7:3	Below Average
4C	Phonological Manipulation	22		87	81 - 93	19	6.0 - 6.3	Below Average
5C	Irregular Word Spelling	9		89	86 - 92	23	7.0 - 7.3	Below Average
6C	Rapid Letter Naming	29		75	65 - 85	5	< Start age	Well Below Average
7C	Pseudoword Reading	18		83	79 - 87	13	6.0 - 6.3	Below Average
8C	Word Pattern Choice	11		91	81 - 101	27	6.4 - 6.7	Average
9C	Word Memory	4		92	82 - 102	30	6.0 - 6.3	Average

Figure B23   *Amelia's scores on the Picture Vocabulary and the Tests that Compose the DDI*

4. What test score is of the most concern?

Figure B24 illustrates Amelia's results on the DDI, RSI, and LPI.

Dyslexia Diagnostic Index (DDI), Reading and Spelling Index (RSI), and Linguistic Processing Index (LPI) Standard Scores					
TOD Index	Sum of standard scores	Index standard score: Child age	Confidence interval: 90%	%ile rank	Descriptive range
Dyslexia Diagnostic Index	687	79	75 - 83	8	Well Below Average
Reading and Spelling Index	342	82	75 - 89	12	Below Average
Linguistic Processing Index	345	80	74 - 86	9	Below Average

Descriptive ranges (based on standard scores): Significantly Below Average (69 and below); Well Below Average (70-79); Below Average (80-89); Average (90-109); Above Average (110-119); Well Above Average (120 and above).

Probability of dyslexia based on DDI standard score *	Very High Probability of Dyslexia

*Extremely Low (120 and above); Very Low (110-119); Low to Moderate (90-109); High (80-89); Very High (70-79); Extremely High (69 and below).

Figure B24   *Amelia's DDI, RSI, and LPI Standard Scores*

5. Why does the DDI standard score indicate a Very High Probability of Dyslexia?

Figure B25 illustrates Amelia's results on the TOD-C Composites.

			Score Summary of TOD-C Composites		
TOD-C composite	Sum of standard scores	Composite standard score: Child age	Confidence interval: 90%	%ile rank	Descriptive range
Sight Word Acquisition	164	80	74 - 86	9	Below Average
Phonics Knowledge	166	82	78 - 86	12	Below Average
Basic Reading Skills	165	80	74 - 86	9	Below Average
Decoding Efficiency	165	81	78 - 84	10	Below Average
Spelling	174	86	80 - 92	18	Below Average
Reading Fluency	176	88	81 - 95	21	Below Average
Reading Comprehension Efficiency	168	82	77 - 87	12	Below Average
Phonological Awareness	265	85	79 - 91	16	Below Average
Rapid Automatized Naming	151	73	71 - 75	4	Well Below Average
Auditory Working Memory	176	85	77 - 93	16	Below Average
Orthographic Processing	173	83	73 - 93	13	Below Average
Vocabulary	229	116	107 - 125	86	Above Average
Reasoning	241	126	119 - 130	96	Well Above Average
Vocabulary and Reasoning 2	234	122	115 - 129	93	Well Above Average
Vocabulary and Reasoning 4	470	125	118 - 130	95	Well Above Average

Descriptive ranges (based on standard scores): Significantly Below Average (69 and below); Well Below Average (70-79); Below Average (80-89); Average (90-109); Above Average (110-119); Well Above Average (120 and above).

Figure B25   *Amelia's Score Summary of TOD-C Composites*

6. **All of her reading and spelling composite scores are Below Average. In contrast, her VR4 composite is Well Above Average. What does this suggest? What would it suggest if her VR4 composite was Well Below Average?**

PARENT/CAREGIVER RATING SCALE

Amelia's mother completed the Parent/Caregiver Rating Scale. Interestingly, she marked that Amelia had some difficulties in Verbal Comprehension and Minor difficulties in General Reasoning. With the exceptions of Phonological Processing and Attention (some difficulty), all other areas were of Major concern. Figure B26 presents the results of Amelia's mother's responses on the rating scale.

7. **What does the T-score of 73 on the rating scale mean? How would this score help support a diagnosis of dyslexia?**

8. **Figure B27 illustrates Amelia's mother's additional information in the Background section. After reviewing the Background Information provided by her mother, what else might be important to know?**

9. **What are some appropriate recommendations from Dyslexia Interventions and Recommendations, A Companion Guide to the Tests of Dyslexia (TOD™), given her pattern of scores?**

Score Profile

TOD Total Score Results

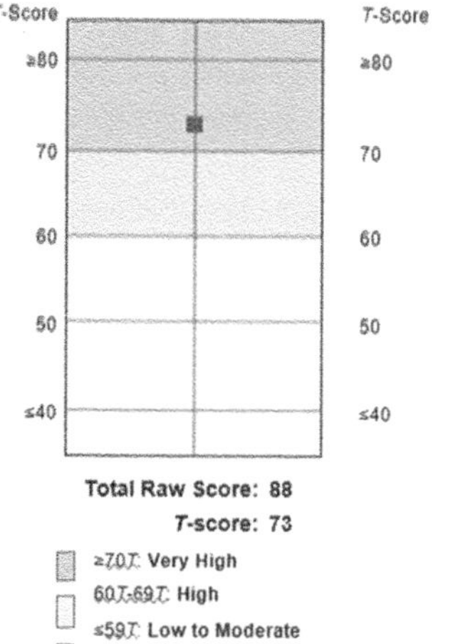

Total Raw Score: 88

T-score: 73

- ≥70*T*: Very High
- 60*T*–69*T*: High
- ≤59*T*: Low to Moderate

Confidence Interval: 90%	%ile	Risk Level
69 - 77	99	Very High Risk

Category	Degree of Difficulty			
	None	Minor	Some	Major
Vocabulary and Reasoning				
VC = Verbal Comprehension			X	
GR = General Reasoning		X		
Linguistic Risk Factors				
PP = Phonological Processing			X	
OP = Orthographic Processing				X
RAN = Rapid Automatized Naming *				
ME = Memory				X
Reading and Spelling				
BRS = Basic Reading Skills				X
RF = Reading Fluency				X
RC = Reading Comprehension				X
SP = Spelling				X
Contributing Factors				
MoR = Motivation (for Reading)				X
A = Attention			X	

* **Note:** Category not measured on this form.

The Rating Scale *T*-score indicates a Very High Risk for dyslexia. Considerable difficulties in reading, spelling, and related skill areas are present. Item-level responses, as well as additional data from TOD tests, will be helpful in understanding the areas of difficulty.

Figure B26   *Amelia's Score Profile on Parent/Caregiver Rating Scale*

Background information	
The individual...	Response
1. Has a family history of reading difficulties.	No
If yes, please check all that apply:	
If other relative, please specify:	
2. Has/had an educational, medical, or behavioral diagnosis.	Yes
If yes, please specify:	Add-inattentive
3. Has a history of vision problems.	No
4. Has a history of ear infections or tubes in ears.	No
5. Receives/received speech and/or language services.	Yes
6. Receives/received additional reading support services in school.	Yes
7. Receives/received extra outside tutoring for reading.	Yes
8. Has repeated (or is repeating) a grade.	No

Figure B27   *Amelia's Mother's Responses on Background Information*

ANSWERS TO CASE 4: AMELIA

1. The higher Picture Vocabulary score indicates that Amelia's low scores in reading are unexpected. In addition, Letter and Word Choice and Question Reading Fluency are both Below Average. More testing is needed to determine why Amelia's reading skills are below average when her vocabulary indicates above average ability.

2. The percentile rank of 12 indicates the percentage of scores in the distribution that were the same as or lower than Amelia's score. Amelia's percentile rank of 12 on the DRI indicates that her performance was the same as or better than only 12% of her age mates (or grade mates if grade norms were used).

3. 5% or less

4. Rapid Letter Naming. The result indicates the 5th percentile and <Start age which means that Amelia's score was lower than the score at the start age of 6–0. It is also of concern because RAN is a strong predictor of reading rate and may be related to Amelia's reading difficulties.

5. The DDI standard score was 79. That score falls in the standard score range of 70–79, which indicates a Very High Probability of Dyslexia.

6. Amelia's results are both unexpected and expected. The Well Above Average VR4 score that is well above her linguistic processing and reading and spelling abilities suggests that her reading and spelling difficulties are unexpected, which often occurs with students with dyslexia. Her difficulties, however, are somewhat expected as Phonological Manipulation and Rapid Letter Naming (which predict poor reading) and her reading and spelling abilities are low. In contrast, if the VR4 composite score was Well Below Average, then her low reading and spelling difficulties would be expected. With that pattern of scores the evaluator would likely consider the possibility of a coexisting disorder, such as a developmental language disorder.

7. The mother's ratings on the rating scale resulted in a T-score of 73. This score indicates a Very High Risk for Dyslexia. The higher the T-score, the greater the risk. Amelia's mother's qualitative observations help confirm Amelia's difficulties developing reading and spelling skills.

8. Prior to writing a report, it would be important to know when Amelia was diagnosed with ADHD-Inattentive Presentation. It would also be helpful to know when and for how long she received speech and language services, as well as the focus of those services. In addition, further information is needed regarding the nature and extent of reading interventions that Amelia has already received both in the home and school.

9. Specific recommendations should address Amelia's weaknesses in basic reading skills, reading rate, and spelling. A phoneme-grapheme mapping program would help develop Amelia's decoding and encoding skills.

TOD-E AND TOD-C DYSLEXIA PROFILES
(NOTE: FILLABLE FORMS ARE AVAILABLE ON THE WPS WEBSITE)

Dyslexia Profile

TOD-E®

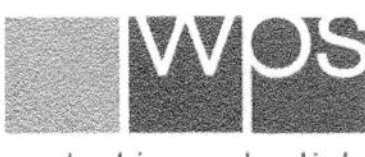

Nancy Mather, PhD   R. Steve McCallum, PhD   Sherry Mee Bell, PhD   Barbara J. Wendling, MA

Name		Date of birth	ID
School		Grade	Date

Enter the district, state, or country dyslexia definition:

International Dyslexia Association Definition (2025)

Dyslexia is a specific learning disability characterized by difficulties in word reading and/or spelling that involve accuracy, speed, or both and vary depending on the orthography. These difficulties occur along a continuum of severity and persist even with instruction that is effective for the individual's peers. The causes of dyslexia are complex and involve combinations of genetic, neurobiological, and environmental influences that interact throughout development. Underlying difficulties with phonological and morphological processing are common but not universal, and early oral language weaknesses often foreshadow literacy challenges. Secondary consequences include reading comprehension problems and reduced reading and writing experience that can impede growth in language, knowledge, written expression, and overall academic achievement. Psychological well-being and employment opportunities also may be affected. Although identification and targeted instruction are important at any age, language and literacy support before and during the early years of education is particularly effective.

Dyslexia affects reading at the single-word level; reading fluency and rate; and spelling. In turn, these difficulties affect reading comprehension and written expression.

SECTION 1: SUMMARY

A. EARLY READING AND SPELLING

Check areas of concern based on Below Average scores.[1]

- ☐ Letter–Sound Associations (Informal)
  - ☐ Letter Names
  - ☐ Letter Sounds
- ☐ Early Sight Word Acquisition
- ☐ Early Phonics Knowledge
- ☐ Early Basic Reading Skills
- ☐ Early Spelling Recognition (Letter and Word Choice)

B. EARLY LINGUISTIC PROCESSING

Check possible risk factors based on Below Average scores.

- ☐ Rhyming
- ☐ Early Segmenting
- ☐ Early Rapid Number and Letter Naming

SECTION 1: SUMMARY *(CONTINUED)*

C. VOCABULARY

Check if the Picture Vocabulary score is higher than the individual's scores in reading and spelling, based on Average or higher scores.

☐ Picture Vocabulary

D. ADDITIONAL RISK FACTORS

Check additional risk factors from history or TOD Rating Scales.

☐ Family history of reading or spelling difficulties

☐ Early speech–language difficulties

☐ Retained a grade

☐ Received extra reading help

E. RATING SCALE/BACKGROUND INFORMATION

Enter significant information from any completed TOD Rating Scales (Parent/Caregiver, Teacher) or background information.

TOD-E T-Score and Risk Level	Comments
TOD-E Parent/Caregiver:	
TOD-E Teacher:	

F. INFORMAL ASSESSMENT INFORMATION

Area Tested	Test Date			
Letter–Sound Knowledge		Number of Letters Known: Lowercase: _______ /26 Uppercase: _______ /26	List Letters Not Known:	☐ Poor ☐ Typical
		Number of Sounds Known: _______________ /44	List Sounds Not Known:	☐ Poor ☐ Typical

EXAMINER CONSIDERATIONS

☐ Data do not demonstrate characteristics of dyslexia.

☐ Data demonstrate characteristics of dyslexia.

☐ Data are consistent with district, state, or country guidelines for identification of dyslexia as a specific learning disability.

Comments

Evaluator(s)	Date

SECTION 2: SUMMARY OF SCORES

Indexes	Test Date	Probability of Dyslexia[2] (No Probability or Extremely Low to Extremely High Probability)	Below Average and Lower SS 40–89 PR 1–24	Average SS 90–109 PR 25–73	Above Average and Higher SS 110–130 PR 75–99
Early Dyslexia Diagnostic Index (EDDI)					
Early Reading and Spelling Index (ERSI)					
Early Linguistic Processing Index (ELPI)					

Area Tested		Test Date	Composite/Test	Below Average and Lower SS 40–89 PR 1–24	Average SS 90–109 PR 25–73	Above Average and Higher SS 110–130 PR 75–99
Reading and Spelling	Sight Word Acquisition		**Early Sight Word Acquisition Composite**			
			Letter and Word Choice Test			
			Letter and Sight Word Recognition Test			
	Phonics Knowledge		**Early Phonics Knowledge Composite**			
			Sounds and Pseudowords Test			
			Letter and Sound Knowledge Test			
	Basic Reading Skills		**Early Basic Reading Skills Composite**			
			Letter and Sight Word Recognition Test			
			Letter and Sound Knowledge Test			
	Reading Fluency/Rate		Word or Question Reading Fluency Test			
	Spelling Recognition		Letter and Word Choice Test			
Linguistic Processing	Phonological Awareness		**Early Phonological Awareness Composite**			
			Rhyming Test			
			Early Segmenting Test			
	Rapid Automatized Naming (RAN)		Early Rapid Number and Letter Naming Test			
Vocabulary	Vocabulary		Picture Vocabulary Test			

Comments

[1] High-ability students may have scores in the Average range and still have dyslexia.
[2] In some cases, only one or two of the linguistic processing scores making up the ELPI may be low, but they still may be indicative of dyslexia, especially when the ERSI is low and/or the student has already received strong instruction/intervention.

Dyslexia Profile

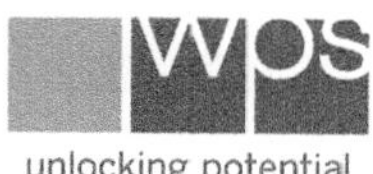

unlocking potential

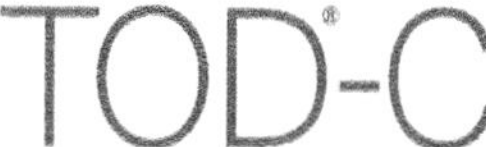

TOD®-C

Nancy Mather, PhD   R. Steve McCallum, PhD   Sherry Mee Bell, PhD   Barbara J. Wendling, MA

Name		Date of birth	ID
School		Grade	Date

Enter the district, state, or country dyslexia definition:

International Dyslexia Association Definition (2025)

Dyslexia is a specific learning disability characterized by difficulties in word reading and/or spelling that involve accuracy, speed, or both and vary depending on the orthography. These difficulties occur along a continuum of severity and persist even with instruction that is effective for the individual's peers. The causes of dyslexia are complex and involve combinations of genetic, neurobiological, and environmental influences that interact throughout development. Underlying difficulties with phonological and morphological processing are common but not universal, and early oral language weaknesses often foreshadow literacy challenges. Secondary consequences include reading comprehension problems and reduced reading and writing experience that can impede growth in language, knowledge, written expression, and overall academic achievement. Psychological well-being and employment opportunities also may be affected. Although identification and targeted instruction are important at any age, language and literacy support before and during the early years of education is particularly effective.

Dyslexia affects reading at the single-word level; reading fluency and rate; and spelling. In turn, these difficulties affect reading comprehension and written expression.

SECTION 1: SUMMARY

A. READING AND SPELLING

Check areas of concern based on Below Average scores.[1]

- ☐ Letter–Sound Associations (Informal)
  - ☐ Letter Names
  - ☐ Letter Sounds
- ☐ Sight Word Acquisition
- ☐ Phonics Knowledge
- ☐ Basic Reading Skills
- ☐ Decoding Efficiency
- ☐ Spelling
- ☐ Reading Fluency
- ☐ Reading Comprehension Efficiency

B. LINGUISTIC PROCESSING

Check possible risk factors based on Below Average scores.

- ☐ Phonological Awareness
- ☐ Rapid Automatized Naming (RAN)
- ☐ Auditory Working Memory
- ☐ Orthographic Processing
- ☐ Visual–Verbal Paired-Associate Learning (Symbol to Sound Learning)

The TOD-C Dyslexia Profile was created by Nancy Mather, Carla Proctor, and Sherry Mee Bell.

SECTION 1: SUMMARY *(CONTINUED)*

C. VOCABULARY AND REASONING

Check if the Vocabulary and/or Reasoning scores are higher than the individual's scores in reading and spelling, based on Average or higher scores.

- ☐ Vocabulary
- ☐ Reasoning
- ☐ Vocabulary and Reasoning 2
- ☐ Vocabulary and Reasoning 4

D. ADDITIONAL RISK FACTORS

Check additional risk factors from history or TOD Rating Scales.

- ☐ Family history of reading or spelling difficulties
- ☐ Early speech–language difficulties
- ☐ Retained a grade
- ☐ Received extra reading help

E. RATING SCALE/BACKGROUND INFORMATION

Enter significant information from any completed TOD Rating Scales (Self, Parent/Caregiver, Teacher) or background information.

TOD-C T-Score and Risk Level	Comments
TOD-C Self:	
TOD-C Parent/Caregiver:	
TOD-C Teacher:	

F. INFORMAL ASSESSMENT INFORMATION

Area Tested	Test Date			
Letter–Sound Knowledge		**Number of Letters Known:** Lowercase: _______ /26 Uppercase: _______ /26	List Letters Not Known:	☐ Poor ☐ Typical
		Number of Sounds Known: _______ /44	List Sounds Not Known:	☐ Poor ☐ Typical

EXAMINER CONSIDERATIONS

- ☐ Data do not demonstrate characteristics of dyslexia.
- ☐ Data demonstrate characteristics of dyslexia.
- ☐ Data are consistent with district, state, or country guidelines for identification of dyslexia as a specific learning disability.

Comments

Evaluator(s)	Date

SECTION 2: SUMMARY OF SCORES

Indexes	Test Date	Probability of Dyslexia[2] (No Probability or Extremely Low to Extremely High Probability)	Below Average and Lower SS 40–89 PR 1–24	Average SS 90–109 PR 25–73	Above Average and Higher SS 110–130 PR 75–99
Dyslexia Diagnostic Index (DDI)					
Reading and Spelling Index (RSI)					
Linguistic Processing Index (LPI)					

Area Tested		Test Date	Composite/Test	Below Average and Lower SS 40–89 PR 1–24	Average SS 90–109 PR 25–73	Above Average and Higher SS 110–130 PR 75–99
Reading and Spelling	Sight Word Acquisition		**Sight Word Acquisition Composite**			
			Irregular Word Reading Test			
			Rapid Irregular Word Reading Test			
	Phonics Knowledge		**Phonics Knowledge Composite**			
			Pseudoword Reading Test			
			Rapid Pseudoword Reading Test			
	Basic Reading Skills		**Basic Reading Skills Composite**			
			Pseudoword Reading Test			
			Irregular Word Reading Test			
	Decoding Efficiency		**Decoding Efficiency Composite**			
			Rapid Pseudoword Reading Test			
			Rapid Irregular Word Reading Test			
	Spelling		**Spelling Composite**			
			Irregular Word Spelling Test			
			Regular Word Spelling Test			
	Reading Fluency		**Reading Fluency Composite**			
			Word or Question Reading Fluency Test			
			Oral Reading Efficiency Test			
	Reading Comprehension Efficiency		**Reading Comprehension Efficiency Composite**			
			Word or Question Reading Fluency Test			
			Silent Reading Efficiency Test			

3

SECTION 2: SUMMARY OF SCORES *(CONTINUED)*

Area Tested	Test Date	Composite/Test	Below Average and Lower SS 40–89 PR 1–24	Average SS 90–109 PR 25–73	Above Average and Higher SS 110–130 PR 75–99
Linguistic Processing					
Phonological Awareness		**Phonological Awareness Composite**			
		Phonological Manipulation Test			
		Blending Test			
		Segmenting Test			
Rapid Automatized Naming (RAN)		**Rapid Automatized Naming (RAN) Composite**			
		Rapid Letter Naming Test			
		Rapid Number and Letter Naming Test			
Auditory Working Memory		**Auditory Working Memory Composite**			
		Word Memory Test			
		Letter Memory Test			
Orthographic Processing		**Orthographic Processing Composite**			
		Letter and Word Choice Test			
		Word Pattern Choice Test			
Visual–Verbal Paired-Associate Learning		Symbol to Sound Learning Test			
Vocabulary and Reasoning					
Vocabulary		**Vocabulary Composite**			
		Picture Vocabulary Test			
		Listening Vocabulary Test			
Reasoning		**Reasoning Composite**			
		Picture Analogies Test			
		Geometric Analogies Test			
Vocabulary and Reasoning		**Vocabulary and Reasoning 2 Composite**			
		Picture Vocabulary Test			
		Picture Analogies Test			
		Vocabulary and Reasoning 4 Composite			
		Picture Vocabulary Test			
		Picture Analogies Test			
		Listening Vocabulary Test			
		Geometric Analogies Test			

Comments

[1] High-ability students may have scores in the Average range and still have dyslexia.

[2] In some cases, only one or two of the linguistic processing scores making up the LPI may be low, but they still may be indicative of dyslexia, especially when the RSI is low and/or the student has already received strong instruction/intervention.

4

Chapter	Description	Source
One	Clinical Pattern of Dyslexia as Measured by the TOD (Table 1.1)	TOD Manual, p. 3/Western Psychological Services (WPS)
Two	Calculating the Chronological Age (Figure 2.1)	TOD-C Record Form, box on front cover/WPS
	Test Observation Worksheet (Figure 2.2)	TOD-C Record Form, box on front cover/WPS
Three	TOD-S and TOD-E Test Selection Chart (Figure 3.1)	TOD Manual, p. 12/WPS
Four	TOD-S and TOD-C Test Selection Chart (Figure 4.1)	TOD Manual, p. 11/WPS
Five	None	
Six	Melia's TOD-C Self-Rating Score Report Completed, Page 1 (Figure 6.1), Page 2 (Figure 6.2), Page 3 (Figure 6.3)	OES online scoring for Rating Scales/WPS
	William's Completed TOD-C Self-Rating Form Page 1 (Figure 6.4)	OES online scoring for Rating Scales/WPS
	William's Completed Background Information (Figure 6.5)	OES online scoring for Rating Scales/WPS
	Examples of William's Responses to Items (Figure 6.6)	OES online scoring for Rating Scales/WPS

(continued)

Chapter	Description	Source
	TOD-C Rater Comparison Report (Figure 6.7)	OES online scoring for Rating Scales/Western Psychological Services (WPS)
Seven	None	
Eight	Rules for Orthographic Mapping (Figure 8.2)	Adapted from Grace (2022)
Nine	TOD-S Score Report, part of page 1-Score Summary, DRI, SS to DRI for Aliza (Figure 9.1)	OES online scoring for TOD-S/WPS
	TOD-C Parent Rating Scale Report, part showing T Score Graph and Category with Degree of Difficulty Table (Figure 9.2)	OES online scoring for TOD-C Rating Scale/WPS
	TOD-C Teacher Rating Scale Report, Showing T Score Graph and Category with Degree of Difficulty Table (Figure 9.3)	OES online scoring for TOD-C Rating Scale/WPS
	TOD-S Score Report, part of page 1-Score Summary, DRI for Mr. Childs (Figure 9.5)	OES online scoring for TOD-S/WPS
	Dyslexia Risk Checklist (Figure 9.6)	TOD Manual, p. 79/WPS
	TOD-S Score Report, part of page 1-Score Summary, DRI for Tessa (Figure 9.7)	OES online scoring for TOD-S/WPS
	TOD-E Score Report, Index Scores Section for Tessa (Figure 9.8)	OES online scoring for TOD-E/WPS
	Descriptions of Indexes, Composites and Tests in Tessa's Case	Direct excerpts from the TOD-E narrative report generated by WPS OES
	TOD-E Score Report, Composite Scores Section for Tessa (Figure 9.9)	OES online scoring for TOD-E/WPS
	TOD-E Score Report, Individual Test Scores Section for Tessa (Figure 9.10)	OES online scoring for TOD-E/WPS
	Six Recommendations Taken Verbatim from Companion Guide	Dyslexia Interventions and Recommendations (WPS)
	TOD-E Parent/Caregiver Rating Scale Results (Figure 9.12)	OES online scoring for TOD-E Rating Scale/WPS

Chapter	Description	Source
Ten	Javier's TOD-S/TOD-C Score Report, Individual Test Scores Summary Section (Figure 10.1)	OES online scoring for TOD-C/WPS
	June's TOD-S Score Summary Report (Figure 10.2)	OES online scoring for TOD-C/WPS
	June's TOD-C Score Report for Individual Tests (Figure 10.3)	OES online scoring for TOD-C/WPS
	June's DDI Standard Score Profile (Figure 10.4)	OES online scoring for TOD-C/WPS
	June's TOD-C Composite Scores (Figure 10.5)	OES online scoring for TOD-C/WPS
	June's Parent Rating Scale Results (Figure 10.6)	OES online scoring for Parent Rating Scale/WPS
	June's Teacher Rating Scale Results (Figure 10.7)	OES online scoring for Parent Rating Scale/WPS
	Several Recommendations for June are taken from the TOD Companion Guide	Dyslexia Interventions and Recommendations (WPS)
	Gillian's TOD-S Score Summary Report (Figure 10.8)	OES online scoring for TOD-S/WPS
	Gillian's Index Scores (Figure 10.9)	OES online scoring for TOD-C/WPS
	Gillian's TOD-C Composite Scores (Figure 10.10)	OES online scoring for TOD-C/WPS
	Descriptions of Gillian's Composites and Tests are Verbatim from the TOD-C Report	OES online scoring for TOD-C/Western Psychological Services (WPS)
	Gillian's TOD-C Individual Test Scores (Figure 10.11)	OES online scoring for TOD-C/WPS
	Gillian's Spellings on Select Items in Test 5C (Figure 10.12)	Author created (but shows item content for 11–15 Test 5C IWS)
Appendix A	Commonly Asked Questions	Some are on WPS website; some new ones on the list that are author created.
Appendix B	Analyzing TOD Score Reports	
	Derek's Index Scores from TOD-C (Figure B.1)	OES online scoring for TOD-C/WPS
	Derek's SS Profile for DDI, RSI, and LPI (Figure B.2)	OES online scoring for TOD-C/WPS
	Derek's SS Profile of Tests in DDI (Figure B.3)	OES online scoring for TOD-C/WPS

(continued)

Chapter	Description	Source
	Derek's Standard Scores Comparisons of Tests in the DDI (Figure B.4)	OES online scoring for TOD-C/WPS
	Derek's TOD-C Composite Scores (Figure B.5)	OES online scoring for TOD-C/WPS
	Derek's Score Comparisons Composites/Indexes (Figure B.6)	OES online scoring for TOD-C/WPS
	Derek's Comparison of LPI vs. RSI and DDI vs. PV (Figure B.7)	OES online scoring for TOD-C/WPS
	Derek's Responses on Question Reading Fluency (Figure B.8)	Author created/QRF Items 3–7
	Derek's Responses on Irregular Word Spelling (Figure B.9)	Author created/IRW Items 10–11 and 17–20
	Parent Rating Scale Results-Derek's Mother (Figure B.10)	OES online scoring for Parent Rating Scale/WPS
	Derek's Mother's Responses to Background Information (Figure B.11)	OES online scoring for Parent Rating Scale/WPS
	Derek's Self-Rating Scale Results (Figure B.12)	OES for Self-Rating Scale/WPS
	Derek's Responses to Background Information (Figure B.13)	OES for Self-Rating Scale/WPS
	Brock's TOD-S Score Summery, DRI, and Standard Score Comparisons (Figure B.14)	OES online scoring for TOD-S/WPS
	Elsa's TOD-S Score Summary, DRI, and Standard Score Comparisons (Figure B.15)	OES online scoring for TOD-S/WPS
	Elsa's TOD-E Test Scores (Figure B.16)	OES online scoring for TOD-E/WPS
	Elsa's EDDI, ERSI, ELPI Standard Scores (Figure B.17)	OES online scoring for TOD-E/WPS
	Elsa's SS Comparisons EDDI vs. PV and ELPI vs. ERSI (Figure B.18)	OES online scoring for TOD-E/WPS
	Elsa's TOD-E Composite Scores (Figure B.19)	OES online scoring for TOD-E/WPS
	Amelia's TOD-S Test Scores (Figure B.20)	OES online scoring for TOD-S/WPS
	Amelia's TOD S DRI Results (Figure B.21)	OES online scoring for TOD-S/WPS
	Amelia's Standard Scores Comparisons of TOD-S Tests and DRI Figure B.22).	OES online scoring for TOD-S/WPS
	Amelia's Scores for Picture Vocabulary and the Tests That Compose the DDI (Figure B.23)	OES online scoring for TOD-C/WPS

Chapter	Description	Source
	Amelia's Scores on the Indexes: DDI, RSI, LPI (Figure B.24)	OES online scoring for TOD-C/WPS
	Amelia's Scores on TOD-C Composites (Figure B.25)	OES online scoring for TOD-C/WPS
	Amelia's Mother's Score Profile on Parent/Caregiver Rating Scale (Figure B.26)	OES online scoring for Parent Rating Scale/WPS
	Amelia's Mother's Responses on Background Information (Figure B.27)	OES online scoring for Parent Rating Scale/WPS
Appendix C	TOD-E and TOD-C Dyslexia Profiles	Author created/WPS reformatted

INDEX

Printed and bound by CPI Group (UK) Ltd, Croydon, CR0 4YY

23/06/2026